METASTATIC DISEASES

Novel Approaches in Diagnosis and Therapeutic Management

METASTATIC DISEASES

Novel Approaches in Diagnosis and
Therapeutic Management

Edited by
Sandeep Arora, PhD

Co-Edited by
Tapan Behl, PhD
Sukhbir Singh, PhD
Neelam Sharma, PhD
Saurabh Gupta, PhD

AAP APPLE
ACADEMIC
PRESS

First edition published 2022

Apple Academic Press Inc.
1265 Goldenrod Circle, NE,
Palm Bay, FL 32905 USA
4164 Lakeshore Road, Burlington,
ON, L7L 1A4 Canada

CRC Press
6000 Broken Sound Parkway NW,
Suite 300, Boca Raton, FL 33487-2742 USA
2 Park Square, Milton Park,
Abingdon, Oxon, OX14 4RN UK

© 2022 Apple Academic Press, Inc.

Apple Academic Press exclusively co-publishes with CRC Press, an imprint of Taylor & Francis Group, LLC

Library and Archives Canada Cataloguing in Publication

....

CIP data on file with Canada Library and Archives

....

Library of Congress Cataloging-in-Publication Data

Names: Arora, Sandeep, 1967- editor. | Behl, Tapan, editor. | Singh, Sukhbir, 1984- editor. | Sharma, Neelam, 1986- editor. | Gupta, Saurabh (Pharmacologist), editor.

Title: Metastatic diseases : novel approaches in diagnosis and therapeutic management / edited by Sandeep Arora ; co-edited by Tapan Behl, Sukhbir Singh, Neelam Sharma, Saurabh Gupta.

Description: 1st edition. | Palm Bay, FL : Apple Academic Press, 2021. | Includes bibliographical references and index. | Summary: "Metastatic Diseases: Novel Approaches in Diagnosis and Therapeutic Management opens new horizons for exploring modern therapeutic entities and emerging targets for combating the deadly disease of cancer. The authors provide a review of cancer along with descriptions of its molecular level mechanisms and emphasize the role of promising new therapies, including herbal therapies that can be utilized for the treatment of metastatic diseases. The chapters look at specific approaches that have been researched and developed and that have almost reached the standardization stage. One of the approaches focuses on intracellular mechanisms, particularly proteins, and the pathway involving or being regulated by the proteins that limit the metastatic cellular growths. In particular phosphoprotein enriched astrocytes are being extensively tried. Also discussed is transerythretin protein, which has been significantly studied for its involvement in formation and transportation of proteins in metastatic diseases. Other receptors and approaches examined include CXCR4, autophagy-inhibiting drugs, phosphoprotein-enriched astrocytes, spatiotemporal genetic analysis, tyrosine kinase inhibitors, and more. Also considered are advances in diagnostic systems like intra vital microscopy and molecular imaging, which further add to the arsenal in metastatic diseases, diagnosis, and management along with techniques like SAGA. These diagnostic methods and innovative methods of intervention by modification of epigenetic control of the immune system using immune checkpoint inhibitor s and phytopharmaceuticals provide newer and better dimensions to treatment of metastatic diseases. Key features: Discusses promising new therapies, including herbal therapies, for the treatment of metastatic diseases Explains the new areas that are widely explored by scientists, researchers, and scholars throughout the globe Explores new therapeutic molecules for cancer treatment The selection of appropriate treatment strategies presented in this volume provide deep insight into the adverse effects and contraindications that will be of immense benefit in the treatment and management of detrimental effects of this deadly disease. The volume will be beneficial for major laboratories working on cancer research and will also serve as a guide for researchers to explore new targets that can be beneficial for mankind"-- Provided by publisher.

Identifiers: LCCN 2020049549 (print) | LCCN 2020049550 (ebook) | ISBN 9781771889179 (hardcover) | 9781774638071 (softcover) | ISBN 9781003043249 (ebook)

Subjects: MESH: Neoplasm Metastasis--diagnosis | Neoplasm Metastasis--drug therapy

Classification: LCC RC263 (print) | LCC RC263 (ebook) | NLM QZ 203 | DDC 616.99/4--dc23

LC record available at https://lccn.loc.gov/2020049549

LC ebook record available at https://lccn.loc.gov/2020049550

ISBN: 978-1-77188-917-9 (hbk)
ISBN: 978-1-77463-807-1 (pbk)
ISBN: 978-1-00304-324-9 (ebk)

About the Editor

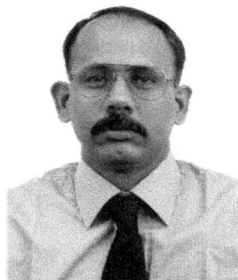

Sandeep Arora, PhD
Dean, Chitkara College of Pharmacy,
Chitkara University, Punjab, India; Professor,
Healthcare, Chitkara University, Rajpura,
Punjab, India

Sandeep Arora, PhD, MPharm, is Dean/Director of the Chitkara College of Pharmacy at Chitkara University, Punjab, India, as well Professor of Healthcare at Chitkara University, Rajpura, Punjab, India. He is also an industrial consultant. Dr. Arora is a seasoned pharma and academic professional with over 27 years of experience in pharma operations, quality management, academics, training, research, and consultancy planning and administration. An avid researcher and writer, he has published four books and 150 research publications (h index 17). He holds 18 patents and four trademarks, and has one registered company to his credit. He is an honorary editor of the journal *Advanced Drug Review*, editor of the *Journal of Pharmaceutical Technology, Research, and Management*, and honorary technical director and advisor to Natural Solutions, Mumbai, India. He and his team has received an IEDC (International Economic Development Council), Government of India, prototyping grant for his project related to the management of acute respiratory distress syndrome in COVID during Novate+ 2020, held at Chitkara University, Punjab, India. He and his team were shortlisted and eligible to apply for sustainability allowance from the Startup Himachal HACKATHON 2020, his project held at Chitkara University. He has delivered sessions as expert or keynote speaker and has chaired international conferences (University of Florida, Pfizer-IPA CPD Sessions, OMICS, and Conference Series Conferences at Thailand) on various topics relevant to pharmaceutical industry trends, technology, phytopharmaceuticals, regulatory affairs, etc. In addition to his pharmaceutical degrees, he also has certifications in business development, business strategy, EHS, and pharmacy technology.

About the Co-Editors

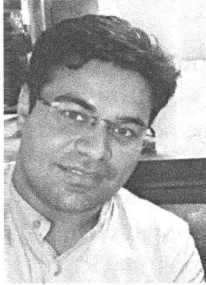

Tapan Behl, PhD
Associate Professor, Department of Pharmacology,
Chitkara College of Pharmacy, Chitkara University,
Rajpura, Punjab, India

Tapan Behl, PhD, MPharm, is currently working as an Associate Professor in the Department of Pharmacology, Chitkara College of Pharmacy, Chitkara University, Rajpura, Punjab, India. Dr. Behl carries a professional experience of over eight years in academics and research. His areas of interest include diabetes and associated complications, rheumatoid arthritis, preclinical ethical considerations, molecular pharmacology, pharmacotherapy for diabetic complications of the eye, drug transfusion across ocular barriers, and neuropathic pain and rheumatoid arthritis. Dr. Behl has more than 75 publications in various international and national journals of repute. He is also the author of two international books and has various book chapters to his credit. He has been invited as a guest speaker at various international and national conferences. Dr. Behl represents India as a voting delegate during the IUPHAR meeting and selection of IUPHAR 2026 in Kyoto, Japan. Dr. Behl has received many prestigious honors and awards for his work and academic excellence, including Academician of the Year Award–2018, Fellow of Society of Biomedical Laboratory Scientists, etc. He is also serving as a reviewer of many reputed journals in his field. Dr. Behl is also engaged in guiding students for their doctoral (PhD) work.

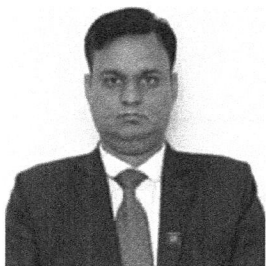

Sukhbir Singh, PhD
Associate Professor, Chitkara College of
Pharmacy, Chitkara University, Punjab, India;
Associate Head, Centre of Excellence,
Phytopharmaceutical, Chitkara College of
Pharmacy, Chitkara University, Punjab, India.

Sukhbir Singh, PhD in Pharmaceutical Science, is a pharmaceutical research professional with more than 12 years of experience in academics and research. Presently, he is Associate Professor and Associate Head, Centre of Excellence, Phytopharmaceutical, at the Chitkara College of Pharmacy, Chitkara University, Punjab, India. He is associated with industry-oriented courses held in collaboration with Chitkara University and established pharmaceutical industries, such as Dr. Reddy's Laboratories. He has 100 publications in various national and international journals (h-index 12 and I 10-index 13) and has published four books and 10 book chapters. He also has filed 12 patents to his credit. He has presented/published 40 review/research abstracts in various national/international conferences. He is also engaged with for consultancy projects on herbal/homeopathic formulations. He is an associate editor of *Open Access Journal of Pharmaceutical Research*. In 2017, he was been honored with a Research Excellence Award by the Honorable Chancellor of Chitkara University. He and his team has received an IEDC (International Economic Development Council), Government of India, prototyping grant for his project related to the management of acute respiratory distress syndrome in COVID during Novate+ 2020, held at Chitkara University, Punjab, India. He and his team were shortlisted and eligible to apply for sustainability allowance from the Startup Himachal HACKATHON 2020, his project held at Chitkara University. He has guided 16 MPharmacy students and 6 PhD students. His areas of interest in research are nanotechnology/liposome/niosomes/SEDDS based formulation development and solubility enhancement of BCS class II drugs. He has expertise in operation of various statistical analyses tools.

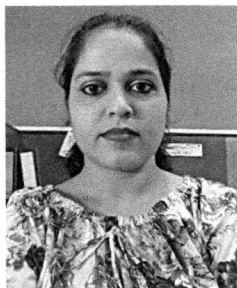

Neelam Sharma, PhD

Associate Professor, Chitkara College of Pharmacy, Chitkara University, Punjab, India; Associate Head, Centre of Excellence, Pharma Tech and Nanotechnology, Chitkara College of Pharmacy, Chitkara University, Punjab, India

Neelam Sharma, PhD in Pharmaceutical Science, is a pharmaceutical research professional with experience of more than 10 years in academics and research. Currently, she Associate Professor at the Chitkara College of Pharmacy, Chitkara University, Punjab, and Associate Head, Centre of Excellence, Pharma Tech and Nanotechnology, Chitkara College of Pharmacy, Chitkara University, Punjab, India. She has 90 publications in various national and international journals, three books, and 10 book chapters, and has filed 12 patents to her credit (h-index 9 and I-10-index 9. She has presented and published 40 review/research abstracts in various national/international conferences. She is engaged in four consultancy projects on herbal/homeopathic formulations. In 2016, she has been awarded a Certificate of Inventorship for her novel invention. She has supervised 10 M. Pharmacy students, and three students are pursuing PhDs under her guidance. She and her team (Dr. Sandeep Arora and Dr. Sukhbir Singh) have an IEDC (International Economic Development Council), Government of India, prototyping grant for the project related to the management of acute respiratory distress syndrome in COVID during Novate+ 2020, held at Chitkara University, Punjab, India, with an opportunity to pitch for university funding for research by Chitkara University Punjab. She and her team are shortlisted and eligible to apply for sustainability allowance from Startup Himachal HACKATHON 2020, for her project held at Chitkara University, Punjab. Her areas of interest in research are novel drug delivery systems such as nanoparticles, liposomes, phytosomes and solubility enhancement of BCS class II drugs. She also has expertise in operation of various statistical analyses tools.

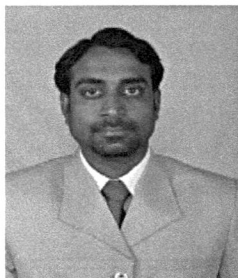

Saurabh Gupta, PhD
Associate Head, Department of Pharmacology,
Chitkara College of Pharmacy, Chitkara University,
Punjab, India

Saurabh Gupta, PhD, is an Associate Head of the Department of Pharmacology at Chitkara College of Pharmacy, Chitkara University, India. His research focuses on asthmatic pharmacology and cellular and molecular biology. He is serving as an editorial member of several reputed journals, including the *Austin Journal of Pharmacology and Therapeutics, World Journal of Pharmaceutical Research*, and *World Journal of Pharmacy and Pharmaceutical Sciences*. He is also an expert reviewer for the journals *International Immunopharmacology* and *Journal of Physiology and Pharmacology*. He has authored over 30 international and national research articles, two books, and a book chapter. Dr. Gupta is associated with many professional bodies and is a CPCSEA nominee and an elective member of the Indian Pharmaceutical Association, Madhya Pradesh State Branch, Indore, India.

Contents

Contributors

Sandeep Arora
Chitkara College of Pharmacy, Chitkara University, Punjab, India

Tapan Behl
Chitkara College of Pharmacy, Chitkara University, Punjab, India

Nidhi Garg
Chitkara College of Pharmacy, Chitkara University, Punjab, India

Ajmer Singh Grewal
Chitkara College of Pharmacy, Chitkara University, Punjab, India

Saurabh Gupta
Chitkara College of Pharmacy, Chitkara University, Punjab, India

Kiranjeet Kaur
Chitkara College of Pharmacy, Chitkara University, Punjab, India

Samir Mehndiratta
Taipei Medical University, Taipei, Taiwan

K. A. Shaima
Chitkara College of Pharmacy, Chitkara University, Punjab, India

Neelam Sharma
Chitkara College of Pharmacy, Chitkara University, Punjab, India

Pooja Sharma
Chitkara College of Pharmacy, Chitkara University, Punjab, India

Sukhbir Singh
Chitkara College of Pharmacy, Chitkara University, Punjab, India

Suman Baishnab
Chitkara College of Pharmacy, Chitkara University, Punjab, India

Abbreviations

67LR	67 kDa laminin receptor
A	adenine
AA	arachidonic acid
AAP	activatable aptamer probe
AB2	isostructural aluminum diboride
ADPh	antibody-dependent phagocytosis
Ag	silver
AIDS	acquired immune deficiency syndrome
AJCC	American Joint Committee on Cancer
ALL	acute lymphoid leukemia
AMBRA	activating molecule in Beclin1-regulated autophagy
AML	acute myeloidal leukemia
ANF	atrial natriuretic factor
AOM	azoxymethane
AP	alternate pathway
ApoG2	apogossypolone
ASOs	antisense oligonucleotides
ATG4	autophagy-related gene 4
Au	gold
AuNP	gold nanoparticles
BBB	blood-brain barrier
BCG	Bacillus Calmette-Guérin
Bcl-2	B-cell lymphoma 2
BCT	bruceantin
BH3	Bcl-2 homology 3
BIF 1	Bax-interacting factor 1
BIM SAHB	BIM stabilized α-helix of BCL-2
BM	basement membranes
BTK	Bruton's tyrosine kinase
C	cytosine
C1INH	C1 inhibitor
C4bp	C4b-binding protein

Ca²⁺	calcium ion

Ca^{2+} calcium ion
CAM chorioallantoic membrane
CaMKII calcium/calmodulin-dependent protein kinase II
cAMP cyclic adenosine monophosphate
CAR coxsackievirus-adenovirus receptor
CARD caspase activation and recruitment domain
CBC complete blood count
CFP cyan fluorescent protein
CHK1 check point kinase 1
CLL chronic lymphocytic leukemia
COX cyclooxygenase
CP classical pathway
CRC colorectal carcinoma
CsCl cesium chloride
CT computed tomography
CTAB cetyl trimethylammonium bromide
CTC circulating tumor cell
CTLA-4 cytotoxic T lymphocyte-associated antigen 4
CTLs cytotoxic T lymphocytes
Cy5 cyanine 5
CYP cytochrome P
DD death domain
DED death effector domain
DEP dielectrophoresis
DFCP double FYVE domain-containing protein
DHA dihyroxyartemisinin
DHFR dihydrofolate reductase
DNA deoxyribonucleic acids
DRAM damage-regulated autophagy modulator
ECOG Eastern Cooperative Oncology Group
EGFR epidermal growth factor receptor
EMT epithelial-to-mesenchymal transition
EpCAM epithelial cell adhesion molecule
EPR enhanced permeability and retention
ER endoplasmic reticulum
ERK1/2 extracellular signal-regulated kinases 1/2
ESCRT endosomal sorting complex required for transport
FACS fluorescence-activated cell sorters
FADD FAS associated death domain

FAP	familial amyloid polyneuropathy
FDA	Food and Drug Administration
Fe_3O_4	iron oxide
FH	factor H
FISH	fluorescent *in situ* hybridization
FOVs	fields of view
FPs	fluorescent proteins
G	guanine
GB	glioblastoma
GBM	glioblastoma multiforme
GDP	guanosine diphosphate
GFP	green fluorescent protein
GLUT4	glucose transporter 4
GPCRs	G-protein coupled receptors
GTP	guanosine triphosphate
HBV	hepatitis B virus
HCQ	hydroxychloroquine
HDAC	histone deacetylase
HDF	human diploid fibroblast
HER	human epidermal growth factor receptor
HIFU	high intensity focused ultrasound
HIV	human immunodeficiency virus
HSP70	heat shock protein 70
ICOS	inducible co-stimulator
ICP-MS	inductively combined plasma mass spectrometry
ICV	intracerebroventricular
IgG	immunoglobulins G
ILs	interleukins
IVM	intra-vital microscopy
JMD	juxta membrane domain
JNK	c-Jun N-terminal kinase
LAG3	lymphocyte activation gene 3
LMWHs	low-molecular-weight heparins
LNA	locked nucleic acid
LNPs	lipid nanoparticles
LP	lectin pathway
LPS	lipopolysaccharide
LT	liver transplantation
Mab	monoclonal antibody

mAbs	monoclonal antibodies
MAP	mitogen-activated protein
MCL	mantle cell lymphoma
MCTS	multicellular tumor spheroid
MEKi	mitogen-activated protein kinase inhibitor
MEN	multiple endocrine neoplasia
MMIA	multifunctional molecular imaging agents
MPM	multi-photon microscopy
MRI	magnetic resonance imaging
MSV	multistage vector
MTIC	monomethyl triazeno-imidazole-carboxamide
NaCl	sodium chloride
NES	nuclear exporting sequence
NPs	nanoparticles
NSCLC	non-small cell lung cancer
OFDI	optical frequency domain imaging
PCR	polymerase chain reaction
PD-1	programmed cell death protein 1
PDAC	pancreatic ductal adenocarcinoma
PD-L1	programmed death-ligand 1
PDMS	poly-dimethylsiloxane
PEA-15	phosphoprotein enriched astrocytes of 15 kDa
PEG	polyethylene glycol
PET	positron-emission tomography
PG	prostaglandin
PH	pleckstrin homology
PI	phosphoinositide
PI3K	phosphatidylinositol 3-kinase
PI3P	phosphatidyl inositol-3-phosphate
PKC	protein kinase C
PLD1/2	phospholipase D1 and D2
PML	promyelocytic leukemia
PNA	peptide nucleic acid
PNANs	polyvalent nucleic acid nanostructures
PSMA	prostate-specific membrane antigen
PTB	protein tyrosine binding
PTEN	phosphate and tensin homolog
Ptgs-1	prostaglandin-endoperoxide synthase 1
Ptgs-2	prostaglandin-endoperoxide synthase 2

PYD	pyrin domain
QD	quantum dot
RAR-alpha	retinoic acid receptor-alpha
RCC	renal cell carcinoma
RFP	red fluorescent protein
RGD	arginine-glycine-aspartic acid
RNA	ribonucleic acid
RNAi	RNA interference
ROS	reactive oxygen species
RSK2	ribosomal S6 kinase isozyme 2
RTKs	receptor tyrosine kinases
RT-PCR	reverse transcription polymerase chain reaction
SAXS	small-angle X-ray scattering
sc	simple cubic
SCA	senile cardiac amyloidosis
SCLC	small cell lung cancer
SDCM	spinning disk confocal microscopy
SDF1	stromal development factor 1
SGKs	SRC family kinases
SH2	SRC homology-2
SHG	second-harmonic
siRNA	small interfering RNA
SNA	spherical nucleic acid
SNARE	soluble N-ethylmaleimide-sensitive factor activating protein receptor
SPECT	single-photon emission computed tomography
SPIO	super paramagnetic iron oxide
SR	scavenger receptor
SSA	senile systemic amyloidosis
T	thymine
TCR	T-cell receptors
TEM	transmission electron microscopy
Th1	T lymphocyte and helper 1
TMD	transmembrane domain
TMIA	targeting molecular imaging agents
TNBC	triple negative breast cancer
TNF	tumor necrosis factor
TOR	target of rapamycin
TORC1	TOR complex 1

TP	terminal pathway
TRAIL	TNF-related apoptosis inducing ligand
TTR	transthyretin
ULK	UNC-51-like kinase
uPAR	urokinase plasminogen activator receptor
USP10	ubiquitin-specific peptidase 10
USPIO	ultra-small super paramagnetic iron oxide
UVRAG	ultraviolet radiation resistance-associated gene
VEGF-A	vascular endothelial growth factor A
VEGF-C	vascular endothelial growth factor C
Vps18	vacuolar protein sorting protein 18
VSM	vascular smooth muscle
WBCs	white blood cells
WHO	World Health Organization
WT	wild-type
YFP	yellow fluorescent protein

Preface

Metastatic diseases pose complicated issues in diagnosis and therapeutic management because of the limitations or hindrances observed in identifying the exact extent of nearby tissues' spread and involvement. The approaches in the management of metastatic diseases of various tissues are based on the efforts to localize and target the therapy on the cancerous cells and avoiding undue exposure of surroundings in the tissues, combining surgical, radiological, and chemotherapeutic interventions based on biopsy, and imaging for confirmation of metastatic stage.

Over the years, various oncolytic, anti-metabolite, and other agents have been developed and used in combination with radio-, chemo-, and surgical therapies, but with varying outcomes and post-treatment quality of life efficacy.

These outcomes have encouraged drug discovery development and clinical scientists to work on novel approaches for more efficacious and targeted treatment of metastatic diseases. Some of these approaches have been taken up for extensive development and have almost reached the standardization stage. One of the methods focuses on intracellular mechanisms, particularly proteins, and the pathway involving or being regulated by the proteins limiting the metastatic cellular growths. In particular, phosphoprotein-enriched astrocytes are being extensively tried. Also, transthyretin protein has been significantly studied for its involvement in the formation and transportation of proteins in metastatic diseases.

Specific receptors like CXCR4 are extensively investigated for their chemokine-related inflammatory activity and involvement in angiogenesis conditions and therapy managing the metastatic diseases.

Immune and inflammatory pathways, particularly the C3D complement systems and their activation, are being extensively investigated for their role in tumor-associated inflammation and possible ways to manage it. BH3 mimetics and other agents have been investigated, which play a role in apoptosis of normal and cancerous cells and help in designing therapies for cancerous cells. Various delivery platforms like spherical nucleic acid (SNA)-based drug delivery systems have been tried, making the therapies for metastatic diseases more targeted.

Advances in diagnostic systems like intravital microscopy and molecular imaging have further added to the arsenal in metastatic diseases, diagnosis, and management along with techniques like SAGA. These diagnostic methods and innovative methods of intervention by modification of epigenetic control of the immune system, using immune checkpoint inhibitors and use of phytopharmaceuticals have again given newer and better dimensions to the treatment of metastatic diseases.

The selection of appropriate treatment strategies with deep insight into the adverse effects and contraindications will prevent humanity from the detrimental effects of this deadly disease along with its complications.

—*Sandeep Arora, PhD*

CHAPTER 1

A Review on Cancer: From Clinical Perspective to Chemotherapy

SANDEEP ARORA and POOJA SHARMA

Chitkara College of Pharmacy, Chitkara University, Punjab, India

ABSTRACT

The primary trait of cancer is the unregulated growth and proliferation of abnormal cells. The normal physiological mechanism of the cells is not carried out with cancer cells, and they're not responsive to average cell growth, proliferation, and survival process sequences. The number of individuals diagnosed with cancer was around 1.4 million in 2007. Therefore, healthcare practitioners play an integral role in the diagnosis and treatment of cancer. To control drug-induced toxicities, this becomes necessary for a cancer patient to understand pharmacology and pharmacotherapy of chemotherapeutic agents. Perceptive and skilled physicians contribute to public treatment in the oncology unit. Carcinogenesis is a multistage mechanism that is genetically regulated. Owing to mutated cells that are developed with the association of carcinogens to normal cells, these mutated cells behave differently to their environment; excessive production of tumor tissues produces characteristics morphological and physiological changes in the initial phase of induction. This chapter describes cancer from the scientific point of view of suggested possible therapies.

1.1 INTRODUCTION

Unrestricted growth and spread of abnormal cells are the distinguishing features of cancer. Being unresponsive to normal cell growth, proliferation, and survival, cells' normal physiological function is not performed by the cancer cells. These cells can develop new tumors at a distant place by traveling through blood or lymph (metastasis); they also have a property to occupy adjacent normal tissue and separate from the primary tumor (metastasize). Their continuous growth and survival are promoted by their uncontrolled growth and their potential to prompt the formation of a blood vessel (Alldredge et al., 2012).

In 2007, the number of people diagnosed with cancer was about 1.4 million. It is essential to know anticancer drug pharmacology and pharmacotherapy in a cancer patient to manage drug-induced toxicities. In the oncology department, knowledgeable and trained health care professionals contribute extensively to patient care (DiPiro et al., 2017).

1.2   ETIOPATHOGENESIS

1.2.1   STEPS INVOLVED IN CARCINOGENESIS

Carcinogenesis is a genetically controlled multistage process. In the initial step of initiation, uncontrolled growth of neoplastic cells occurs due to the mutated cells which are formed with the interaction of carcinogens to normal cells, and these mutated cells respond differently to its environment. This is then followed by promotion, i.e., the second phase, in which cell alteration and mutated cell growth are observed over normal cells, induced further by carcinogens. The only difference between the two is that the promotion phase is reversible, whereas the initiation phase is irreversible. It may also be seen as the pointer to future chemoprevention strategies, including lifestyle and diet changes. Neoplastic growth marks the last stage of carcinogenesis, termed as progression; it is characterized by increased cell proliferation due to further genetic alteration. This phase includes tumor invasion into local tissues and metastases development (Calvo et al., 2005; Compagni and Christofori, 2000; Weston and Harris, 2003; Cotran et al., 1999).

1.2.2   CARCINOGENS

Chemical, physical, and biological agents constitute the three significant carcinogens (Weston and Harris, 2003). Chemical agents are discussed in Table 1.1 and are the associated cause of cancer. Also, ionization radiations and ultraviolet rays make up a part of the physical agents. These radiations cause the free radical formation known to damage the DNA (deoxyribonucleic acids) and result in mutations. Biological agents comprising of viruses may also become a cause for cancer; for example, the Burkitt's lymphoma is caused by the Epstein-Barr virus, and cervical cancer is caused due to the infection of human papillomavirus, age, gender, diet, growth factors, and chronic irritation from the other promoters of carcinogens (Weston and Harris, 2003).

TABLE 1.1   Cancer causing Drugs and Hormones in humans

Drug or Hormone	Cancer Caused
Alkylating agents (e.g., chlorambucil, mechlorethamine, melphalan, and nitrosoureas)	Leukemia
Anabolic steroids	Liver
Analgesics containing phenacetin	Renal, Urinary bladder
Anthracyclines (e.g., doxorubicin)	Leukemia
Antiestrogens (tamoxifen)	Endometrium
Coal tars (topical)	Skin
Estrogens:	
• Nonsteroidal (diethylstilbestrol)	Vagina/cervix, endometrium, breast
• Steroidal (estrogen replacement therapy, oral contraceptives)	Endometrium, breast, liver
• Immunosuppressive drugs (cyclosporine, azathioprine)	Lymphoma, skin

Source: Compagni and Christofori (2000).

1.2.3   GENES ENTAILED IN CARCINOGENESIS

Oncogenes and tumor suppressor genes are the genes associated with the process of carcinogenesis.

1.2.3.1   ONCOGENES

Oncogenes originate from proto-oncogenes or normal genes and play a significant role in carcinogenesis. All normal cells have proto-oncogenes, which monitor cellular function (cell cycle). Exposure to any carcinogenic agents causes an alteration in the genome of these proto-oncogenes via chromosomal rearrangement, point mutation, or gene amplification that, in turn, triggers the oncogenes. There is an increase in the probability of neoplastic transformation due to impaired cell growth, which results in a distinct growth advantage to the cell. This is all due to the oncogene's activation that produces an abundance of the abnormal gene product. HER (human epidermal growth factor receptor) is an example of oncogenes. Epidermal growth factor receptor or ErbB-1, HER-3, HER-2, and HER-4 are the four members present in this family having receptor tyrosine kinases (RTKs). In several cancers, proliferation, metastasis, angiogenesis, and cell survival happen once these receptors get activated, causing the acquiring of specialized features and rapid multiplication of cells through downstream signaling pathways and activation of receptor tyrosine kinase (Gross et al., 2004).

1.2.3.2   TUMOR SUPPRESSOR GENES

Tumor suppressor genes control cellular growth and proliferation (Calvo et al., 2005; Cotran et al., 1999; Weinberg, 1996). Failure to control cell growth occurs due to the mutations caused by carcinogens. Retinoblastoma and p53 genes are examples of tumor suppressor genes. In almost 50% of cancer cases, mutation of p53 is the major cause (Weinberg, 1996). Different type of malignancies including, breast cancer, cancer of the large intestine, lung, brain tumors, cervix, and anus; and osteogenic sarcoma occurs due to uncontrolled growth because of the mutation which stops the function of the normal p53 gene product from having control over the cell cycle. The following are examples of oncogenes and tumor suppressor genes (Table 1.2).

DNA repair gene (classified as tumor suppressor genes) is another important gene in carcinogenesis; this gene helps to repair the damaged DNA that may have developed during DNA replication (Cotran et al., 1999). Lack of this gene may result in the mutation of genes that further activate oncogenes via proto-oncogene. This condition can be seen in familial cancer of the colon and breast. Cell cycle regulation is under the stimulatory and inhibitory signals of oncogenes and tumor suppressor genes (Calvo et al., 2005; Weinberg, 1996). Such genes control the cell cycle clock.

TABLE 1.2 Summary of Tumor Suppressor Genes and Oncogenes

Oncogenes

Transcription Genes That Initiate Growth-Promoter Genes

Gene	c-MYC	N-MYC
Related Human Cancer	Leukemia and breast, colon, gastric, and lung carcinoma	Cancer found in adrenal glands, small cell lung carcinoma, and GBM

Growth Factor or Receptor Genes

Type	Erb-B1 or Epidermal Growth Factor Receptor	Erb-B2 or HER-2/neu	RET
Action/Activity	Codes expressing the epidermal growth factor (EGFR) receptor	Helps in the coding of a growth factor receptor	Helps in the coding of a growth factor receptor
Related Human Cancer	GBM, breast, head, and neck, and large intestine carcinoma	Breast, prostate, bladder, salivary gland, and ovarian carcinoma	Cancer of thyroid gland

Cytoplasmic Relays Genes for the Stimulatory Signaling Pathways

Gene	K-RAS	N-RAS
Action/Activity	Coding for guanine nucleotide-proteins with GTPase activity is conducted	
Related Human Cancer	Lung, ovarian, large intestine, and pancreatic cancers	Neuroblastoma, and acute leukemia

Genes for Other Molecules

Type	BCL-2	BCL-1 or PRAD1	MDM2
Action/Activity	Codes for a protein that obstructs apoptosis	Codes for cyclin D1, which is a cell-cycle clock stimulator	Protein antagonist of p53 tumor suppressor protein
Related Human Cancer	Indolent B-cell lymphomas	Breast, head, and neck cancers	Sarcomas

TABLE 1.2 *(Continued)*

Tumor Suppressor Genes

Gene	Protein Genes Whose Cellular Location is Unclear			
Type	BRCA1	BRCA2	VHL	MSH2, MLH1, PMS1, PMS2, MSH6
Action/ Activity	DNA repair, transcriptional regulation	DNA repair	Regulator of protein stability	DNA mismatch repair enzymes
Related Human Cancer	Breast and ovarian cancers	Breast cancer	Renal cell cancer	Hereditary nonpolyposis colorectal cancer

Gene	Protein Genes in Cytoplasm		
Type	APC	NF-1	NF-2
Action/Activity		Inhibition of the stimulatory RAS protein is coded by a signaling pathway step for a protein	Inhibition of the stimulatory RAS protein coded by a protein
Related Human Cancer	Colon and gastric cancer	Neurofibroma and leukemia	Meningioma, ependymoma, and schwannoma

Gene	Protein Genes in Nucleus	
Type	RB1	p53
Action/Activity	Codes for the pRB protein, a master brake of the cell cycle	Codes for the p53 protein, which can halt cell division and induce Apoptosis
Related Human Cancer	Retinoblastoma	Associated with a wide variety of cancers

Source: Cotran et al. (1999); Weinberg (1996).

1.2.4 TUMOR CLASSIFICATION

A tumor may surface from any of these four-primary tissues: connective tissue, epithelial tissue, lymphoid tissue, and nerve tissue. A benign tumor is named by adding the suffix -oma to the cell type, while for malignant sarcoma is added to the type of cell as a suffix (Table 1.3) exhibits the standard nomenclature of the tumor by the type of tissue (Cotran et al., 1999).

TABLE 1.3 Tumor Classification by the Type of Tissue

Tissue Origin	Connective Tissue			
	Fibrous tissue	**Bone**	**Smooth muscle**	**Striated muscle**
Benign	Fibroma	Osteoma	Leiomyoma	Rhabdomyoma
Malignant	Fibrosarcoma	Osteosarcoma	Leiomyosarcoma	Rhabdomyo-sarcoma
Tissue Origin	**Connective Tissue**	**Epithelial**		**Neural Tissue**
	Fat	Surface epithelium	Glandular tissue	Glial tissue
Benign	Lipoma	Papilloma	Adenoma	"Benign" gliomas
Malignant	Liposarcoma	Carcinoma (squamous, epidermoid)	Adenocarcinoma	Glioblastoma multiforme, astrocytoma
Tissue Origin	**Neural Tissue**		**Mixed Tumors**	
	Nerve sheath	Melanocytes	Gonadal tissue	
Benign	Neurofibroma	Pigmented nevus (mole)	Teratoma	
Malignant	Neurofibro-sarcoma	Malignant melanoma	Teratocarcinoma	

Source: DiPiro et al. (2017).

Tumors are mainly of two types: benign and malignant. Benign tumors are encapsulated, localized, and indolent non-cancerous growth. They are identical to their parent cell and once removed, they have very less chance of recurrence whereas malignant tumor occupies and destroys the surrounding tissue. These cells are genetically unstable and are unidentical of their cell of origin. Moreover, they do not act like normal cells, and this is known as anaplasia. It has a property to metastasize, and hence their recurrence chances are higher than a benign tumor.

1.2.5 PATHWAY OF METASTASIS

Hematogenous and lymphatic pathways are the two main pathways. Other rarely used modes of transmission include transabdominal spread and dissemination. Neoplastic cells are continuously shredded into the systemic or lymphatic circulations. This step occurs in the initial stage of the tumor but increases with time. Not every shed cell is a metastatic lesion (Stetler-Stevenson, 2005). The process of invasion and metastasis is a multistep process. After neoplastic alteration, both the malignant cells and host tissue are known to produce some substance that provokes new blood vessel formation in order to supply oxygen and nutrients to malignant cells; this process is termed as angiogenesis or neovascularization (Folkman and Kalluri, 2003). After that, tumor cells separate and spread into surrounding blood and lymph vessels, but not all cells survive the circulation; hence, these circulated cells should adhere to the vascular tissue and from that multiply inside the lumen vessel. This potentiates and serves as "fertilizer" for the proliferation of metastasis. Last, angiogenesis again stimulates continued growth and proliferation of cells. Figure 1.1 summarizes the functions acquired by a cell to survive as well as mechanisms by which the cancer cell achieves this function (Hanahan and Weinberg, 2000).

1.3 DIAGNOSING CANCER

The signs and symptoms vary and depend upon the type of cancer. The clinical aspect for adults and children is discussed in Table 1.4.

1.3.1 PHASES OF CANCER

American Joint Committee on Cancer's (AJCC's) TNM system is used all over the world to explain the type of cancer. General categorization is listed below:

1. **Tumor (T):** T (0–4) indicates the size and site of the tumor; i.e., the way most of the tumor grows into surrounding areas. The bigger and deeper the tumor, the more will be the aggregates.
2. **Node (N):** N (0–3) signifies the presence of cancer cells present inside the lymph nodes or not.

TABLE 1.4   Cancer Clinical Presentation

Forewarning Signs of Cancer in adults	• Discomfort in swallowing
	• Unhealing abrasion
	• Apparent difference in the size of mole
	• Wheeziness
	• Lump formation in mammary glands
	• Bowel movement becomes irregular.
	• Uncommon discharge or bleeding
Forewarning Signs of Cancer in Children	• Visible lack of color in the skin
	• Recurring fevers
	• Nausea and headaches
	• Continuous weight loss
	• Inflammation in neck or abdomen
	• Edema or constant soreness in bones
	• Pupil becomes white

Source: American Cancer Society (2007).

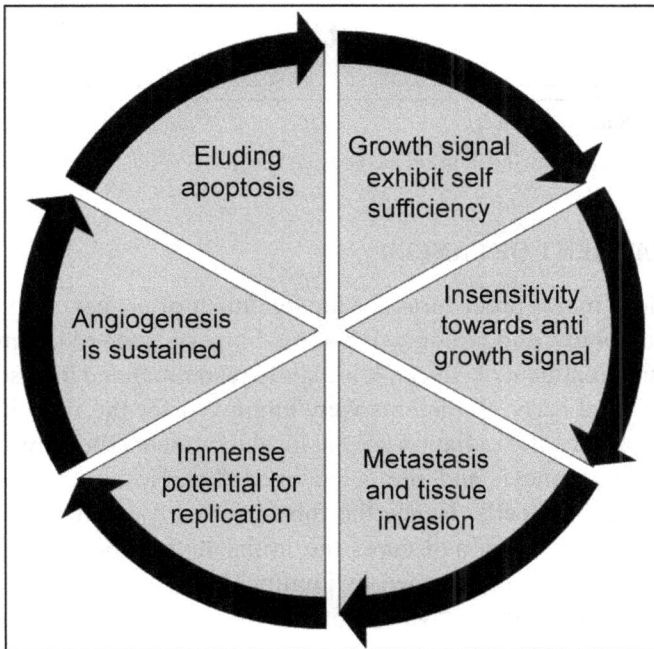

FIGURE 1.1   Mechanism of tumorigenesis (American Cancer Society, 2007).

3. **Metastasis (M):** M represents the stage in which cancer has spread
    to other parts of the body. M0 indicates that cancer has not spread,
    whereas M1 describes that it has spread.

1.3.1.1 STAGE GROUPING OF CANCER

Along with TNM, cancer stages have been categorized into four categories:
stages I, II, III, and IV (Figure 1.2). However, in some cases, stage 0 may
also be present.

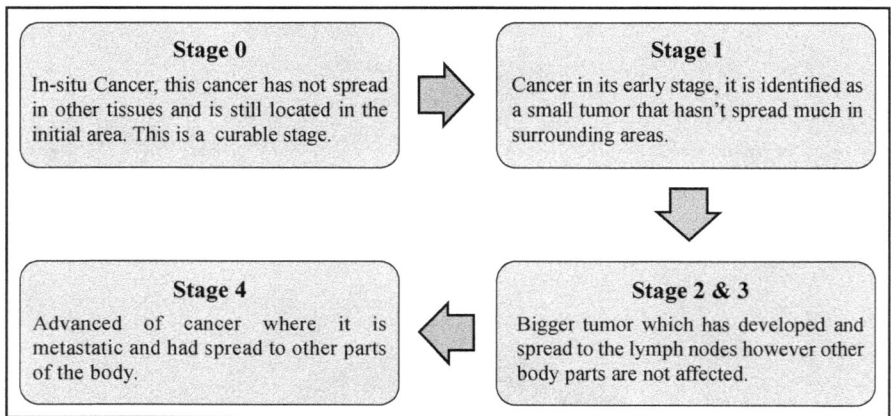

Stage 0
In-situ Cancer, this cancer has not spread in other tissues and is still located in the initial area. This is a curable stage.

Stage 1
Cancer in its early stage, it is identified as a small tumor that hasn't spread much in surrounding areas.

Stage 4
Advanced of cancer where it is metastatic and had spread to other parts of the body.

Stage 2 & 3
Bigger tumor which has developed and spread to the lymph nodes however other body parts are not affected.

FIGURE 1.2   Stages of cancer.
Source: American Society of Clinical Oncology (ASCO).

1.4 TREATMENT OF CANCER

There are four major procedures for the treatment of cancer: surgery, radiation, chemotherapy, and biological therapy. Surgery is the oldest method for
diagnosis and treatment of cancer. It is mainly recommended for a solid tumor
that is diagnosed early. Radiations were employed for the first time during
1800. Both surgery and radiation are the local treatment. Today most patients
have metastatic cancer, and these localized therapies cannot completely
eradicate the cancer cells. Hence the third treatment or the chemotherapy,
it reaches the circulation and cures the initial tumor and metastasis. Last
is biological therapy, also termed as immunotherapy or targeted therapies.
It basically involves the activation of the host's immune system to fight
cancer. It usually uses naturally occurring cytokines, which are produced
by recombinant DNA technology. Interferons and interleukins (ILs) serve

as examples. Targeted therapies include monoclonal antibodies (mAbs), tyrosine kinase inhibitors, and proteasome inhibitors (DiPiro et al., 2017).

Chances of recurrence of cancer after surgery or radiations are because some of the primary tumors may have metastasized before it was diagnosed. Moreover, these early metastases are too small and undetectable, so the name micrometastases. Hence, adjuvant therapy is being introduced to eradicate micrometastatic diseases following isolated treatments like radiation or surgery, or both. The prime purpose of using systemic medical care is to minimize the recurrences figures and extend survival. For example, additional methods are used in colorectal and breast cancers. Most of the cancer management uses combined modalities, for example, in the case of breast cancer (DiPiro et al., 2017).

1.4.1 CANCER MANAGEMENT PRINCIPLE: ONCOLOGY SURGERY

Patients with solid tumors are recommended surgery if the tumor is limited to the origin site. Treating an individual with surgery requires a specific ethical and psychological approach. Surgery as a means of cancer prevention is detailed in Table 1.5.

TABLE 1.5   Surgery as a Means of Cancer Prevention

Characteristic Situations	Colitis ulcerosa	Inherited colorectal cancer	Inherited breast carcinoma
Cancer	Cancer of colon	Cancer of colon	Cancer of mammary glands
Treatment	Colectomy	Colectomy	Mastectomy
Characteristic Situations	Undescended testicles	MEN1, MEN2 (Multiple endocrine neoplasia)	
Cancer	Cancer of testicles	Thyroid carcinoma	
Treatment	Orchidopexy	Thyroidectomy	

Source: DeVita et al. (1997).

Many surgical instruments have evolved, namely, fiberoptic endoscopy and laparoscopy that has changed into a prerequisite for intraperitoneal non-Hodgkin lymphoma's diagnosis, and when combined with ultrasonography, plays a very crucial part in cancer staging, like pancreatic and hepatic tumors (Berry and Maddern, 2000). Recently, nonoperative techniques have evolved that destroy the tumors caused by physical or chemical carcinogens such as arterial chemoembolization, cryotherapy, etc. (Luck and Maddern, 1999).

1.4.2   *PRINCIPLE OF CANCER MANAGEMENT: RADIATION THERAPY*

Ionizing radiation is used in this therapy for the treatment of malignant illness. Its high energy has 100 times more penetrating power than X-ray. Hence, the deep-seated tumors are treated by this therapy with very less radiations affecting the nearby areas (Partensky and Maddern, 1999; Price and Sikora, 2000). The penetrating power of radiotherapy is expressed as its energy and is calculated in terms of electron volts (eV). The simplest equipment used is a low energy orthovoltage machine, which can produce a beam of up to 250 KeV. The penetration of voltage is only 1–4 cm; hence, it is effective for treating skin cancers and bone metastases. But using millivoltage causes skin reactions. Another therapy called isotope-based radiotherapy uses sources that emit rays to produce higher energy beams. In the earlier times, radium was used for this purpose but later got replaced by cobalt as they produce higher energy and seem dependable.

Nowadays, linear accelerators are used as a standard. In this, charged subatomic particles or ions are accelerated to high speed by subjecting them to a series of oscillating electric potentials along a linear beamline. These machines can reliably produce beams of up to 20 MeV energy. It doesn't produce any skin reactions. Regarding the target, the dose is taken from clinical examination, X-rays, MRI, and CT scans. Radical radiotherapy is normally given in few regular doses in fractions 5 times a week. It enables the tumor cells to get administered with a lethal dose, during which surrounding cells get time to salvage and reconstruct the harm caused to the DNA due to radiation. The matter that has been always debated is the upper hand of cobalt machines as collated to the linear accelerators (Borras and Stovall, 1993).

"Short distance treatment" or the Brachytherapy is the technique in which radioactive substance is placed directly in contact with the tumor. It is effective for treating cervix cancer. In this procedure, cesium rods are put inside the uterus and in the vagina radioactive material is inserted. It reduces unwanted exposure of radiation in staff and relatives.

1.4.2.1   *SIDE EFFECTS OF RADIOTHERAPY*

Most people are tolerable to radiotherapy. Major adverse effects include mucous membranes becoming edematous and painful, and skin reaction may lead to severe cases of scarring and ulceration. Enteritis and diarrhea are caused by abdominal radiations.

1.4.3   CHEMOTHERAPY

1.4.3.1   CELL CYCLE

Normal and cancer cells reproduce in the same manner, through the cell cycle phenomenon. Figure 1.3 describes the cell cycle and the activity of phases for commonly used antineoplastic agents (Buick, 1994). The initial phase of the cell cycle termed as M phase is the Mitosis phase that lasts about 30–60 min and cell division occurs in that phase. After the first phase, the cell enters either to G0 or G1 phase. G0 is a dormant phase called the resting phase. In phase G1, the cell manufactures necessary enzymes for DNA synthesis. Next is the S phase, i.e., the synthesis phase, which lasts for 10–20 hrs. Flow cytometry is an instrument that measures the percentage of cells in the S phase, and it is the major signal for tumor cell proliferation. Then, after that, the G2 phase or premitotic phase occurs for 2–10 hr. In this phase, the cell prepares itself for cell division by manufacturing ribonucleic acid (RNA) and specialized proteins, as well as the mitotic spindle apparatus. After which, again, the M phase starts, and the cycle completes. The cell cycle is controlled by external mitogens, including cytokines, hormones, and growth factors and genes, namely proto-oncogenes and tumor suppressor genes. Numerous anticancer drugs affect the proliferation of cells (both normal and cancerous cells); these are called cell-cycle phase-specific agents. The S phase is mainly affected by antimetabolites, and alkylating agents have an effect on the multiphase of the cell cycle, for example, nitrogen mustard. Cell cycle consideration is important for scheduling chemotherapy; hence knowledge of the cell cycle is very crucial. At any given time, the tumor cell may be at any particular phase in the cycle. The phase-specific agents of the cell cycle are known as schedule dependent, while cell-cycle phase-nonspecific drugs activity depends on their dose, and hence these are called dose-dependent (Dang et al., 2003; Chabner et al., 2001) (Figure 1.3).

1.4.3.2   MECHANISM OF ACTION OF ANTINEOPLASTIC AGENTS

A summary of the mechanism of action of various antineoplastic agents is discussed in Table 1.6.

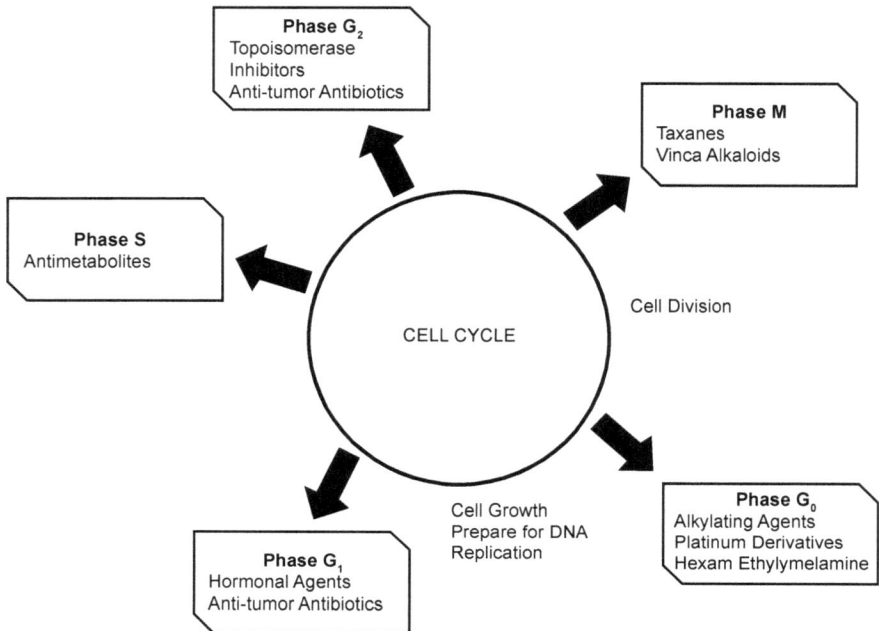

FIGURE 1.3   The cell cycle and the activity phases for commonly used antineoplastic agents (DiPiro et al., 2017).

1.4.4   ANTINEOPLASTIC AGENTS

1.4.4.1   ANTIMETABOLITES

1.4.4.1.1   Pyrimidine Analogs

1. **Fluorouracil (5-FU):** 5-FU is a fluorinated analog of the naturally occurring pyrimidine uracil. It is a prodrug and metabolizes to an active form called fluorodeoxyuridine monophosphate. In the presence of folates, fluorodeoxyuridine monophosphate tightly binds and interferes with the thymidylate synthase functions. This enzyme is essential for thymidine production, one of the amino acids in DNA, and other. Other metabolites of 5-FU, the triphosphate nucleotide, and causes hindrance in RNA function. Both mechanisms produce the cytotoxic 5-FU (Pizzorno et al., 2003).
2. **Cytarabine:** It forms an arabinose analog of cytosine. Its phosphorylation takes place in tumor cells to form active triphosphate

TABLE 1.6 Mechanism of actions of antineoplastic agents

Drugs	Mechanism of Action
(Phosphonacetyl)-L-aspartate	Inhibition of pyrimidine biosynthesis
Hydroxycarbamide	Inhibition ribonucleotide reductase
Capecitabine 5-Fluoracil	Inhibit dTMP synthesis
Cytarabine, Fludarabine, Cladribine and Gemcitabine	Inhibit DNA synthesis
Bleomycin	Damages DNA
Cisplatin, Carboplatin and Dacarbazine	Cross- linking of DNA
Vinea alkaloids and Taxanes	Inhibit function of microtubules
6-Mercaptopurine	Inhibition of biosynthesis of ring
6-Thioguanine	Inhibition of interconversions of nucleotide
Methotrexate	Inhibit purine ring biosynthesis
Teniposide, Irinotecan and Topotecan	Damages DNA and prevent reconstruction
Dactinomycin and Anthracyclinrs	Inhibition of synthesis of RNA

Source: DiPiro et al. (2017).

form. This active form inhibits DNA polymerase; it also inhibits the replication of DNA. A deaminase enzyme, mainly cytidine deaminase, opposes the activation of the active triphosphate form by converting it into an inactive form. Renal impairment and hepatic impairment cause the accumulation of a high level of active form that causes neurotoxic effect (Pizzorno et al., 2003; Johnson, 2000; Smith et al., 1997).

3. **Gemcitabine:** It is a fluorine alternative deoxycytidine parallel associated with cytarabine in composition. Its mode of action is the same as that of cytarabine. It inhibits DNA polymerase and also ribonucleotide reductase. This enzyme converts ribonucleotides into the deoxyribonucleotide forms. When compared to cytarabine, gemcitabine bioavailability is more and also having greater penetration to the cell membrane (Pizzorno et al., 2003; Johnson, 2000; Venook et al., 2000).

4. **Azacytidine and Decitabine:** Both antineoplastic agents were used for the patient of myelodysplastic syndrome, a disorder of hematopoietic cell maturation that can progress to acute myeloid leukemia. They both incorporate directly into DNA and inhibit the methyltransferase, which causes hypomethylation of DNA, resulting in cellular differentiation and apoptosis (Silverman et al., 2002; McKeage and Croom, 2006).

1.4.4.1.2 *Purines and Purine Antimetabolites*

1. **6-Mercaptopurine and 6-Thioguanine:** They are the synthetic analogs of the naturally occurring purines: guanine and adenine. Both drugs are converted to ribonucleotides that result in inhibition of biosynthesis of purine. It has been observed that co-administration of these agents with purine increases interconversion reactions and results in serious toxicity (Pizzorno et al., 2003).

2. **Fludarabine Monophosphate:** It is an analog of purine adenine. It inhibits DNA polymerase resulting in chain termination, and also inhibits transcription. Its toxicity is myelosuppression. It is basically an immunosuppressive; thus, there is a chance of opportunistic infection resulting in a decline of the CD4 counts (Pizzorno et al., 2003; Plosker and Figgitt, 2003).

3. **Pentostatin and Cladribine:** Both these agents are analogs of purine nucleoside. Cladribine is converted to its working form that incorporates into DNA and causes inhibition of synthesis of DNA along with chain termination. Pentostatin is an inhibitor of adenosine deaminase, this enzyme is important in the base metabolism of purine, and a high concentration is found in the lymph tissue. Moreover, it also causes immunosuppression; hence there is a chance of opportunistic infections (Pizzorno et al., 2003; Johnson, 2000).

1.4.4.1.3 *Antifolates*

Folate is essential for DNA synthesis. Dietary folates are being converted to tetrahydro forms, containing four hydrogens on the pteridine ring, this conversion is carried out by dihydrofolate reductase (DHFR) enzyme, and this tetrahydrofolate is essential for thymidylate and purine synthesis. Deficiency of either thymidine or purines prevents the synthesis of DNA. Methotrexate is an antifolate that inhibits the DHFR enzyme; lack of tetrahydrofolate forms results in a deficiency of thymidine or purines that alter the DNA synthesis. Resistance to antifolate caused by amplification of DHFR slows the rate of thymidylate synthesis, decreased affinity of DHFR for MTX, and lack of polyglutamation within tumor cells. Therapeutic monitoring is a very crucial parameter for methotrexate. Cytotoxic effect of methotrexate is observed as above 5×10^{-8} M. To recover from toxic effects of this agent, Leucovorin is recommended until levels fall below 5×10^{-8} M (Kamen et al., 2003).

1.4.4.2   DRUGS TARGETING MICROTUBULES

1.4.4.2.1   Vinca Alkaloids

Vinblastine, vinorelbine, and vincristine are natural alkaloids extract from the vinca plant. These are inhibitors of mitosis. Both vinorelbine and vinblastine cause myelosuppression with increasing dose, and vincristine shows neurotoxic effects. They act on the tubulin protein that polymerizes to form a microtubule. Vinca alkaloids cause an imbalance between polymerization and depolymerization of microtubules. This result in the accumulation of cell in mitosis and also induce apoptosis (Rowinsky, 2003).

1.4.4.2.2   Taxanes

Docetaxel and paclitaxel are natural plant alkaloid having antimitotic activity. Paclitaxel is produced semi synthetically from the European yew plant, whereas docetaxel is selected from 10-diacetyl baccatin III (Rowinsky, 2003). Taxanes cause microtubule disassembling and stimulate tubulin polymerization, which results in the formation of improper, non-functional toxicity. Moreover, taxanes also inhibit the process of angiogenesis. Toxicity of docetaxel and paclitaxel causes fluid retention and neurotoxicity, respectively (Krieger, 2002).

1.4.4.2.3   Topoisomerase Inhibitors

Topoisomerase is a key enzyme of DNA replication and transcription. It forms a strand break to reduce the torsional strain during the process of DNA unwinding. They form gaps through which DNA strands can pass, and then they reseal. There are two types of Topoisomerase: II and I. Topoisomerase I produces single-strand breaks, whereas topoisomerase II generate double-strand breaks (Rubin and Hait, 2003). Anticancer drugs that attack the topoisomerase enzyme are camptothecins, anthracyclines, and epipodophyllotoxins.

1.   **Camptothecin Derivatives:** It is a plant alkaloid isolated from *Camptotheca acuminata* and has the potential of inhibiting DNA topoisomerase I. This drug produces severe toxicity. Its analogs are irinotecan and topotecan and are synthesized in order to reduce toxicity and improve therapeutic effects. Both these analogs inhibit the activity of the topoisomerase I enzymes through the formation of SN-38 (Rubin and Hait, 2003; Ulukan and Swaan, 2002; Raymond et al., 2002).

2. **Etoposide and Teniposide:** These are podophyllotoxin derivates that are isolated from the mayapple or mandrake plant. It has two mechanisms; first, it interferes with microtubule formation by binding to tubulin, and second, it inhibits topoisomerase II, causing the breaking of DNA strands (Rubin and Hait, 2003). Clinically it was found that both are cross-resistant. It also affects the cell cycle, i.e., they arrest the cells in S or early G2 phase. Hence, its effect is shown much better in divided doses rather than a single dose.

3. **Anthracene Derivatives:** The members of anthracene derivatives are daunorubicin, epirubicin, idarubicin mitoxantrone, and doxorubicin, and out of them mostly used is doxorubicin. Also, they are topoisomerase inhibitors. Intercalating agents are those compounds that incorporate between DNA's base pair. The planar group of anthracene ring complex is responsible for intercalating with DNA. Those results in changes in their structures that interfere with the synthesis of DNA and RNA and also inhibit the topoisomerase II. Moreover, anthracyclines also undergo electron reduction as a result of which free radicals are formed. The final step needs iron. Iron binds to anthracyclines, and their iron-anthracycline complexes bind with the DNA and react quickly with hydrogen peroxide to produce the hydroxyl radicals that actually responsible for cleaving the DNA. Mitoxantrone has a similar mechanism as other derivatives, but their potency for free radical formation is much less (Rubin and Hait, 2003; Danesi et al., 2002).

1.4.4.3   ALKYLATING AGENTS

This is the oldest and useful antineoplastic agent. All alkylating agents act by forming a covalent bond of the alkyl group with the nucleophilic groups of nucleic acids and proteins. The binding site of the alkyl group is a seven-nitrogen group of guanines, this interaction causes cross-linking in the two strands of DNA or between the two bases inside the same DNA strand that causes the death of the cell and inhibits replication of DNA (Colvin, 2003).

1.4.4.3.1   Cyclophosphamide and Ifosfamide

These are nitrogen mustard derivatives. Both activated by mixed hepatic oxidase enzymes, including the cytochrome P450 (CYP) 2B6 and CYP3A4/5 isoenzymes. The active metabolic product of cyclophosphamide is phosphoramide mustard, and another metabolite is 4-hydroxycyclophosphamide; it is cytotoxic. Moreover, ifosfamide is hepatically activated to ifosfamide mustard (Colvin, 2003).

1.4.4.3.2   Non-Classic Alkylating Agents

These are antineoplastic agents that act like alkylators, but their structure does not resemble with classic alkylating agents. It includes dacarbazine, procarbazine, temozolomide, the heavy metal compounds, and some antitumor antibiotics (Colvin, 2003).

1. **Dacarbazine, Procarbazine, and Temozolomide:** Both dacarbazine and procarbazine undergo demethylation to the same active intermediate (monomethyl triazine-imidazole-carboxamide [MTIC]) that interrupt in the replication of DNA by causing guanine methylation and also inhibit DNA, RNA, and protein synthesis. Temozolomide can easily cross the blood-brain barrier (BBB), hence can be therapeutically used for brain tumor tissue (Colvin, 2003; Stupp et al., 2001).
2. **Heavy Metal Compounds:** Heavy metals include platinum derivatives, namely cisplatin, carboplatin, and oxaliplatin. They are used in colorectal cancer. Their mechanisms involve the formation of intra-strand cross-links or adduct between neighboring guanines, this major illicit bending of DNA, and also cause damage to the cells by damaging the normal conformation of DNA and prevent the pairing of base-pair with each other. Toxicity includes nephrotoxicity, ototoxicity, peripheral neuropathy, emesis, and anemia (Colvin, 2003). While carboplatin causes hematologic toxicity (Colvin, 2003; Guminski et al., 2002).

1.4.4.4   MISCELLANEOUS AGENTS

1.4.4.4.1   Bleomycin

It is an antitumor antibiotic; basically, it is a mixture of fungal Streptomyces species, and its strength is expressed in units of drug activity. One unit is approximately equal to 1 mg of polypeptide protein. Its mechanism involves the binding of iron bleomycin complex to DNA. This complex reduces to form free radicals that cause the breaking of strands of DNA. It affects the G2 phase of the cell cycle and also in mitosis (Lazo, 1999).

1.4.4.4.2   Hydroxyurea

It is a ribonucleotide reductase inhibitor; it targets the S phase of the cell cycle, resulting in the formation of abnormal DNA strands (Pizzorno et al., 2003).

1.4.4.4.3   L-Asparaginase

It is an enzyme produced by *Escherichia coli* and other bacteria. L-asparagine is degraded by the enzyme L-asparaginase, which depletes existing supplies and inhibits protein synthesis (Kurtzberg et al., 2003).

1.4.4.4.4   Arsenic Trioxide

It is effective for the treatment of acute promyelocytic leukemia (PML). Also, it induces programmed cell death or apoptosis (Soignet et al., 2001).

1.4.5   PRINCIPLES OF PATIENT MANAGEMENT DURING CHEMOTHERAPY

1.4.5.1   ASSESSMENT OF PATIENT FOR CHEMOTHERAPY

The four aspects of patient assessment are discussed in the following subsections.

1.4.5.1.1   Patient's Clinical Status and Performance

The Eastern Cooperative Oncology Group (ECOG) scale is used to grade this (Oken et al., 1982).

Phase 0
• Fully active, able to carry on all pre-disease performance without restriction.

Phase 1
• Restricted in strenuous physical activity but able to carry out work of a light sedentary nature.

Phase 2
• Restricted in strenuous physical activity but able to carry out work of a light sedentary nature.

Phase 3
• Capable of only limited self-care, confined to bed or chair more than 50% of waking hours.

Phase 4
• Completely disabled, cannot carry on any self-care, totally confined to bed or chair.

Usually, patients with ECOG grade more than two are not considered suitable for chemotherapy. The chemotherapy-sensitive cancers such as lymphoma and small cell lung cancers (SCLCs) are the only exceptions.

1.4.5.1.2   Kind and Seriousness of Side Effects From Previous Chemotherapy Cycles

Life-threatening side effects should be examined by the physicians. Firstly, the type and severity of side effects should be ruled out. For example, it is expected that peripheral neuropathy is common if a patient with breast cancer undergoes taxane chemotherapy, but there is a need for dose reduction of the subsequent cycle if the patient has a neutropenic fever in mid-cycle. The precedent that is given by the NCI that contains the common terminologies for the adverse events is applied for the grading of toxicity (Oken et al., 1982).

1.4.5.1.3   Blood (Hematological) Parameters

The count of platelets that is greater than $100 \times 10^9/L$ is required in the safer management of chemotherapy. In the case of cisplatin and carboplatin, renal function is important, and for docetaxel, liver function is important.

1.4.5.1.4   Non-Hematological Toxicity

The following are the common examples of non-hematological toxicity and antineoplastic agents that need to be taken into consideration:

Diarrhea	5-FU-based, Irinotecan, Oxaliplatin, Taxotere
Neuropathy	Cisplatin, Oxaliplatin, Taxanes, and Vinca alkaloids
Autotoxicity	Cisplatin.
Renal Impairment	Cisplatin.
Pulmonary Toxicity	camptothecin and gemcitabine

The examination of the physical conditions to be followed, intravenous infection sites, and side effects.

1.4.5.2   TERMINATION OF CHEMOTHERAPY

1. Cessation of treatment is necessary when there are any life-threatening or severe dose-limiting toxicity.
2. Treatment may have to be stopped if the cancer is not curable and other toxic side effects are caused.
3. Termination of therapy is required in case of deteriorating performance status and organ function.
4. In order to improve symptom management, comfort and care unit referral are done in the case of patients with metastatic disorders even when they are currently undergoing treatment.

1.4.5.3   COMMON REACTIONS OR SIDE EFFECTS OF THE CHEMO DRUGS

Some of the common adverse effects of the antineoplastic agents are discussed in Table 1.7.

TABLE 1.7   Common Adverse or Side Effects of the Antineoplastic Agents

Drugs Used in Chemo Treatment	Reactions/Side Effects
Cisplatinum/Platinol	Functions of the kidney, levels of magnesium, peripheral neuropathy
Gemcitabine	Pneumonitis, peripheral edema
Taxol/Paclitaxel	Peripheral neuritis, flu-like symptoms

TABLE 1.7 *(Continued)*

Drugs Used in Chemo Treatment	Reactions/Side Effects
Cytophosphane or CP/IFO (Ifex)	Functions of the kidney, brain dysfunction resulting in confusion.
Capecitabine	Inflammation of mucous membrane, palmoplantar erythrodysesthesia, and angina pectoris
Erbitux	Acneiform rash
Avastin	Hypertension and proteinuria

1.4.5.4   EMESIS IN CHEMOTHERAPY

Reasons for nausea in chemotherapy undergoing patients are:

1. related to chemotherapy; and
2. medications are comparable to opioids and other causes like gastro-esophageal reflux disease.

1.4.5.4.1   Chemotherapy Agent's Emetogenic Potential (Hesketh, 2008)

1. High (>90%):
   - Cisplatin > 50 mg/ml;
   - Dacarbazine;
   - Cyclophosphamide > 1.5 g/ml.

2. Minimal:
   - Bleomycin;
   - Herceptin;
   - Cetuximab;
   - Vincristine;
   - Vinorelbine.

1.4.5.4.2   Antiemetics

1. **Substance P Antagonist:** Emend.
2. **Serotonin 5-HT3 Receptor Antagonists:** Zofran.
3. **Dopamine Antagonists: Benzamides:** Metoclopramide.
4. **Histamine H1 receptor antagonist/Antihistamines:** Promethazine.

1.4.5.5   SUMMARY OF MANAGEMENT OF COMMON CANCERS

Various types of regimens for cancer chemotherapy are presented in Table 1.8.

TABLE 1.8   Summary of Various Types of Regimens for Cancer Chemotherapy

Type of Cancer	Regimen and specific drugs
Breast Cancer	
Taxotere, adriamycin, and cyclophosphamide	Docetaxel
FEC	5-Fluorouracil
AC or DD	Adriamycin
Taxotere and cyclophosphamide	Cytophosphane
Bowel and Colon Cancer	
FOLFOX	Eloxatin, Continuous infusion Fluorouracil (5-FU)/ Adrucil and Folinic acid
XELOX	Eloxatin, Xeloda
FOLFIRI	Camptosar, Continuous infusion Fluorouracil (5-FU)/ Adrucil and Folinic acid
XELIRI	Camptosar, Xeloda
	Eloxatin, Xeloda
	Camptosar, Continuous infusion Fluorouracil (5-FU)/ Adrucil and Folinic acid
	Camptosar, Xeloda
Cancer Affecting the Gastric/Lower Esophageal Parts	
ECX	Epirubicin, Cisplatin, Capecitabine
ECF	Epirubicin, Cisplatin, 5-Fluorouracil
EOX	Epirubicin, Oxaliplatin, Capecitabine
Head and Neck Cancer	
TPF	5-Fluorouracil, Cisplatin
Cancer of Testicles	
BEP	Bleomycin, Cisplatin, Etoposide (VP-16)

1.4.5.6   BREAST CANCER

Tamoxifen may be considered as the only option. Tamoxifen is administered daily for over 5 years, especially in those patients who are in more danger.

In women who are postmenopausal-unless contraindicated, aromatase inhibitors are the preferred therapy for endocrine. Tamoxifen is used in patients who cannot accept or bear AI. In terms of disease control in post-menopausal patients, AIs are considered superior to Tamoxifen. Regular calcium and vitamin D supplement are recommended in patients who are on AIs as they are reported with osteopenia in most cases.

1.4.5.6.1   Regimens for the Chemotherapy

- In case of either decreased/less or average risk: TC administered in 4 cycles, or 6 cycles of FEC.
- Increased/more risk: 6 cycles of TAC or 3 cycles of FEC. Aprepitant (Emend) is required for anthracycline or carboplatin containing regimes and 5HT3 antagonist is needed for all breast cancer adjuvant regimes.

1.4.5.6.2   Medicines Administered Before Surgery in Breast Cancer

Chemotherapy regimens given to the patients have a treatment that is similar to adjuvant regimens. In HER's-2 positive diseases or triple-negative, it is found to be more effective. In some instances, breast conservation may be possible to achieve.

1.4.5.6.3   Radiotherapy After Surgery

Following the removal of a distinct portion of the breast, radiotherapy decreases the rate of repetition.

The invasion of cancer into the blood vessels and/or lymph nodes is a lymphovascular invasion (LVI or lymphovascular space invasion).

1.4.5.7   GASTRO-INTESTINAL CANCER

1.4.5.7.1   Malignant/Cancerous Cells in the Tissue of Anus

Concurrent radiations are given to the majority of the patients.

Regimen: Along with radiation for 5–6 weeks, administration of Mito-mycin C on Day 1 and on Days 1 to 4 and 29 to 32 5-fluorouracil administrations should take place. Cisplatin can be altered with Mitomycin C as part of the combination of chemotherapy.

1.4.5.7.2   Gastroesophageal Cancer

- **Regimen:** 5-Fluorouracil and cisplatin are given to the patient. If cisplatin is contraindicated, FOLFOX 6 can be sustained.
- **Medications Provided before Surgery:** Along with radiation, 5-fluorouracil and cisplatin has to be administered. Neo-adjuvant and adjuvant are also conducted in patients.

1.4.5.7.3   Cancer of the Gastroesophageal Junction or Stomach That Is Advanced or Metastatic

- **For Positive Adenocarcinoma of HER 2 Disease:** Along with trastuzumab, cisplatin, 5-fluorouracil is provided.
- **For Negative Cancers of HER-2:** The regimes used may either be a single agent (Paclitaxel or docetaxel) or a combination (EOX and ECF).

1.4.5.8   HEAD AND NECK CANCERS

1. **Resectable Disease:** Surgical adjuvant radiotherapy, along with chemotherapy, significantly improves the overall survival of the high-risk disease.
2. **Preservation of Organ or Unresectable Disease:** Chemo-radio-therapy, after which induction chemotherapy is held.
3. Abnormal renal function or cardiac issues, if not fit for weekly cisplatin.
4. **Head and Neck Metastatic Cancer:** Clinical trials on (Cisplatin or Carboplatin) and 5FU.

1.4.5.9   CANCER CAUSED IN THE LUNGS

1.4.5.9.1   Cancers in the Non-Small Cell

In stages I, II, and III, surgical resection provides a good chance of cure:

1. **For 1b, II, or III Resected Stage:** Additional treatment to enhance the effectiveness of cisplatin is given to improve the survival of the elderly.
2. **Stage III:** Chemo-radiation can improve survival for patients who are unresectable.

3. Cisplatin with Etoposide is the preferred regimen that is concurrent with radiation. In patients who are unfit for Cisplatin, other alternatives are used.
4. **Stage IV (Stage that is Not Curable IIIb):** Testing for mutations that have the potential to cause cancer, such as epidermal growth factor receptor (EGFR), is conducted.

If the response of the patient is good, then the enlistment in the clinical trial of immunotherapy with chemotherapy is contemplated.

For those patients who are unfit for the clinical trials, platinum doublet chemotherapy is considered as first-line therapy. For select elderly patients, single-agent docetaxel is reasonable.

As for second-line treatment, therapy with an anti-PDL-1 antibody is contemplated if the first-line treatment fails. For patients with poor (ECOG>2), palliative supportive care is reasonable.

1.4.5.9.2   Lung Cancer of Small Cell

1. Along with radiation, cisplatin, and etoposide × 4 cycles is given.
2. Carboplatin and etoposide are administered for a cycle of 6 in extensive-stage.

In selected patients, it is useful to treat them with mesothelioma surgical decortication, while in other phases, every three weeks, cisplatin and alimta 500 mg/ml is given.

1.4.5.10   GYNECOLOGICAL CANCERS

1.4.5.10.1   Cancer in the Ovary

1. **1st Stage:** Surgical interventions.
2. **2nd Stage:** Consists of debulking surgery, BSO/TAH (This can be useful in selected stage 4). First, neoadjuvant chemotherapy is followed by the patient undergoing surgery as well as chemotherapy. This is mainly provided to patients who are unfit for surgery. Without compromising outcomes, the surgical morbidity of debulking procedures may be reduced by this approach.

3. **Relapsed Disease:** The interval since the last exposure to platinum may be the criteria on which the choice of the agent may depend (i.e., platinum-sensitive versus resistant). Carboplatin/calyx, carboplatin/ gemcitabine, and topotecan are the protocols included.

1.4.5.10.2   Cancer in the Cervix

- For the early treatment of disease, surgery and chemoradiotherapy along with cisplatin are given weekly.
- For the metastatic treatment, Gemcitabine, Platinum/Taxol are the treatment provided to the patients.

1.4.5.11   CANCERS THAT AFFECT THE GENITO-URINARY SYSTEM OF THE BODY

1.4.5.11.1   Cancer Affecting the Prostate

The stages of the disease and sensitivity of the hormone are the condition on which the treatment depends:

1. **Early Stage Disease:** The treatment conditions which the patient has to undergo consist of surgery, radiotherapy, or just observation. The treatment procedure or method depends on several factors like age, serum PSA levels, etc. For the disease that is inoperable, it is seen that essential or primary radiotherapy will have possibilities of cure. Androgen deprivation therapy is sometimes administered in selected high-risk patients (after/before radiotherapy). The aim is to extend survival and improve the condition of living in the case of incurable metastatic disease.

2. **Hormone Sensitive Disease:** For the patients who suffer from hormone-sensitive tumors, GnRH agonist is used for their treatment. It is controversial whether anti-androgens are continued beyond. In some cases, the withdrawal of the trial of anti-androgens conducted on the patients may aid them when the combining of anti-androgen and GnRH agonist takes place. When six doses of Docetaxel each of 75 mg/ml is utilized, accompanied by chemotherapy is found to be a good option to use as the survival in the patients with metastatic disease is improved.

3. **Hormone Refractory Disease:** When cases where the disease has grown even when the treatment of hormonal change is undergoing, those patients are the ones that come under the category of hormone-refractory disease. In order to treat bone metastases, intravenous bisphosphonates are used. Chemotherapy is usually delayed for asymptomatic disease. Prednisone 5 mg BD and docetaxel (75 mg/ml) and. may be used for the treatment of symptomatic metastases. Another option is palliative care. External beam radiotherapy is well used for the responding of localized bone pain.

1.4.5.11.2   Renal Cell Carcinoma (RCC)

Tyrosine kinase inhibitors (Sunitinib or Pazopanib) are used in the treatment of metastatic renal cell carcinoma (RCC). After these methods of therapy fail, the treatment can be done with the help of sorafenib. Other second-line options available are everolimus and axitinib.

1.4.5.11.3   Urinary Bladder Cancer

Adjuvant intravesical therapies, as well as surgery, are used to treat non-muscle invasive disease. Surgery is used to treat muscle-invasive disease. Survival is improved with the help of pre-op Cisplatin-based chemotherapy.

Management of inoperable diseases can be with radiotherapy with or without chemotherapy along with cisplatin is given weekly. Only the treatment of chemotherapy or the care provided by any unit for terminally ill patients can be provided. Chemotherapy or palliative care alone is required for the management of metastatic disease.

KEYWORDS

- **cytochrome P**
- **dihydrofolate reductase**
- **epidermal growth factor receptor**
- **human epidermal growth factor receptor**

- interleukins
- monomethyl triazine-imidazole-carboxamide
- multiple endocrine neoplasia
- ribonucleic acid

REFERENCES

Alldredge, B. K., Corelli, R. L., Ernst, M. E., Guglielmo, B. J., Jacobson, P. A., Kradjan, W. A., & Williams, B. R., (2012). *Koda-Kimble and Young's Applied Therapeutics: The Clinical Use of Drugs*. Lippincott Williams and Wilkins: New York.

American Cancer Society, (2007). *Warning Signs of Cancer*. American Cancer Society: Atlanta.

Berry, D. P., & Maddern, G. J., (2000). Other in situ ablative techniques for unresectable liver tumors. *Asian J. Surg., 23,* 22–31.

Borras, C., & Stovall, J., (1993). *Design Requirements for Megavoltage Radiotherapy X-Ray Machines for Cancer Treatment in Developing Countries*. Los Alamos Laboratories: New Mexico.

Buick, R. N., (1994). Cellular basis of chemotherapy. In: Dorr, R. T., & Von, H. D. D., (eds.), *Cancer Chemotherapy Handbook* (2nd edn., pp. 3–14). Elsevier: New York.

Calvo, K. R., Petricoin, E. F., & Liotta, L. A., (2005). Genomics and proteomics. In: De Vita, V. T., Hellman, S., & Rosenberg, S. A., (eds.), *Cancer: Principles and Practice of Oncology* (7th edn., pp. 51–72). Philadelphia: Lippincott Williams and Wilkins.

Chabner, B. A., Ryan, D. P., Paz-Ares, L., Carbonero, R., & Calabresi, P., (2001). Antineoplastic agents. In: Hardman, J. G., Limbird, L. E., & Gilman, A. G., (eds.), *Goodman and Gilman's the Pharmacologic Basis of Therapeutics* (10th edn., p. 1381). McGraw-Hill: New York.

Colvin, M., (2003). Alkylating agents. In: Kufe, D. W., Pollock, R. E., Weichselbaum, R. R., Bast, R. C., Gansler, T. S., & Holland, J. F., (eds.), *Holland-Frei Cancer Medicine* (6th edn.). BC Decker: Hamilton.

Compagni, A., & Christofori, G., (2000). Recent advances in research on multistage tumorigenesis. *Br. J. Cancer, 83,* 1–5.

Cotran, R. S., Kumar, V., & Collins, T., (1999). Neoplasia. In: Cotran, R. S., Kumar, V., & Collins, T., (eds.), *Robbins' Pathologic Basis of Disease* (pp. 260–328). Philadelphia: WB Saunders.

Danesi, R., Fogli, S., Gennari, A., Conte, P., & Del Tacca, M., (2002). Pharmacokinetic-pharmacodynamic relationships of the anthracycline anticancer drugs. *Clin. Pharmacokinet., 41,* 431–444.

Dang, C., Gilweski, T. A., Sarbone, A., & Norton, L., (2003). Chemotherapy: Cytokinetics. In: Kufe, D. W., Pollock, R. E., & Weichselbaum, R. R., (eds.), *Cancer Medicine* (6th edn., pp. 645–668). BC Decker: Hamilton, Ont.

DeVita, V. T., Rosenberg, S. A., & Lawrence, T. S., (1997). *DeVita, Hellman, and Rosenberg's Cancer: Principles and Practice of Oncology*. Lippincott, Williams & Wilkins: Philadelphia.

DiPiro, J. T., Talbert, R. L., Yee, G. C., Wells, B. G., & Posey, L. M., (2017). *Pharmacotherapy: A Pathophysiologic Approach*. McGraw Hill Professional: New York.

Folkman, J., & Kalluri, R., (2003). Tumor angiogenesis. In: Kufe, D. W., Pollock, R. E., & Weichselbaum, R. R., (eds.), *Cancer Medicine* (6th edn., pp. 161–194). Hamilton, Ont: BC Decker.

Gross, M. E., Shazer, R. L., & Agus, D. B., (2004). Targeting the HER-kinase axis in cancer. *Semin. Oncol., 31*(3), 9–20.

Guminski, A. D., Harnett, P. R., & DeFazio, A., (2002). Scientists and clinicians test their metal—Back to the future with platinum compounds. *Lancet Oncol., 3*, 312–318.

Hanahan, D., & Weinberg, R. A., (2000). The hallmarks of cancer. *Cell, 100*, 57–70.

Hesketh, P. J., (2008). Chemotherapy-induced nausea and vomiting. *N. Eng. J. Med., 358*(23), 2482–2494.

Johnson, S. A., (2000). Clinical pharmacokinetics of nucleoside analogs: Focus on hematological malignancies. *Clin. Pharmacokinet., 39*, 5–26.

Johnstone, R. W., Ruefli, A. A., & Lowe, S. W., (2002). Apoptosis: A link between cancer genetics and chemotherapy. *Cell, 108*, 153–164.

Joshi, A., Sabesan, S., Varma, S., & Otty, Z., (2016). *Medical Oncology Handbook for Junior Medical Officers* (4th edn.). James Cook University: Townsville, Australia.

Kamen, B. A., Cole, P. D., & Bertino, J. R., (2003). Folate antagonists. In: Kufe, D. W., Pollock, R. E., & Weichselbaum, R. R., (eds.), *Cancer Medicine* (6th edn., pp. 727–738). BC Decker: Hamilton, Ont.

Krieger, J. A., Stanford, B. L., Ballard, E. E., & Rabinowitz, I., (2002). Implementation and results of a test dose program with taxanes. *Cancer J., 8*, 337–341.

Kurtzberg, J., Yousem, D., & Beauchamp, Jr. N., (2003). Asparaginase. In: Kufe, D. W., Pollock, R. E., & Weichselbaum, R. R., (eds.), *Cancer Medicine* (6th edn., pp. 823–830). DC Becker: Hamilton, Ont.

Lazo, J. S., (1999). Bleomycin. *Cancer Chemother. Biol. Response Modif., 18*, 39–45.

Luck, A. J., & Maddern, G. J., (1999). Intraoperative abdominal ultrasonography. *Br. J. Surg., 86*, 5–16.

McKeage, K., & Croom, K. F., (2006). Decitabine: In myelodysplastic syndromes. *Drugs, 66*, 951–958.

Oken, M., Creech, R. H., Tormey, D. C., Horton, J., Davis, T. E., McFadden, E. T., & Carbone, P. P., (1982). Toxicity and response criteria of the eastern cooperative oncology group. *Am. J. Clin. Oncol., 5*, 649–655.

Partensky, C., & Maddern, G. J., (1999). Pancreatectomy after neoadjuvant chemo radiation for potentially resectable exocrine adenocarcinoma of the pancreas. In: Mornex, F., Mazeron, J. J., Droz, J. P., & Marty, M., (eds.), *Concomitant Chemoradiation: Current Status and Future*. Elsevier: Paris.

Pizzorno, G., Diasio, R. B., & Cheng, Y. C., (2003). Pyrimidines and purine antimetabolites. In: Kufe, D. W., Pollock, R. E., & Weichselbaum, R. R., (eds.), *Cancer Medicine* (6th edn., pp. 739–757). BC Decker: Hamilton, Ont.

Plosker, G. L., & Figgitt, D. P., (2003). Oral fludarabine. *Drugs, 63*, 2317–2323.

Price, P., & Sikora, K., (2000). *Treatment of Cancer* (4th edn.). Chapman and Hall: London.

Raymond, E., Boige, V., Faivre, S., Sanderink, G. J., Rixe, O., Vernillet, L., Jacques, C., et al., (2002). Dosage adjustment and pharmacokinetic profile of irinotecan in cancer patients with hepatic dysfunction. *J. Clin. Oncol., 20*, 4303–4312.

Rowinsky, E., (2003). Microtubule-targeting natural products. In: Kufe, D. W., Pollock, R. E., & Weichselbaum, R. R., (eds.), *Cancer Medicine* (6th edn., pp. 791–810). BC Decker: Hamilton, Ont.

Rubin, E. H., & Hait, W. N., (2003). Anthracylines and DNA intercalators/epipodophyllotoxins/camptothecins/DNA topoisomerases. In: Kufe, D. W., Pollock, R. E., & Weichselbaum, R. R., (eds.), *Cancer Medicine* (6th edn., pp. 781–790). BC Decker: Hamilton, Ont.

Silverman, L. R., Demakos, E. P., Peterson, B. L., Kornblith, A. B., Holland, J. C., Odchimar-Reissig, R., Stone, R. M., et al., (2002). Randomized controlled trial of azacitidine in patients with the myelodysplastic syndrome: A study of the cancer and leukemia group B. *J. Clin. Oncol., 20*, 2429–2440.

Slamon, D., Eiermann, W., Robert, N., Pienkowski, T., Martin, M., Press, M., Mackey, J., et al., (2011). Breast Cancer International Research Group. Adjuvant trastuzumab in HER2-positive breast cancer. *N. Eng. J. Med., 365*(14), 1273–1283.

Smith, G. A., Damon, L. E., Rugo, H. S., Ries, C. A., & Linker, C. A., (1997). High-dose cytarabine dose modification reduces the incidence of neurotoxicity in patients with renal insufficiency. *J. Clin. Oncol., 15*, 833–839.

Soignet, S. L., Frankel, S. R., Douer, D., Tallman, M. S., Kantarjian, H., Calleja, E., Stone, R. M., et al., (2001). United States multicenter study of arsenic trioxide in relapsed acute promyelocytic leukemia. *J. Clin. Oncol., 19*, 3852–3860.

Stetler-Stevenson, W. G., (2005). Invasion and metastases. In: DeVita, V. T., Hellman, S., & Rosenberg, S. A., (eds.), *Cancer: Principles and Practice of Oncology* (7th edn., pp. 113–127). Philadelphia: Lippincott Williams & Wilkins.

Stupp, R., Gander, M., Leyvraz, S., & Newlands, E., (2001). Current and future developments in the use of temozolomide for the treatment of brain tumors. *Lancet Oncol., 2*, 552–560.

Ulukan, H., & Swaan, P. W., (2002). Camptothecins: A review of their chemotherapeutic potential. *Drugs, 62*, 2039–2057.

Venook, A. P., Egorin, M. J., Rosner, G. L., Hollis, D., Mani, S., Hawkins, M., Byrd, J., et al., (2000). Phase I and pharmacokinetic trial of gemcitabine in patients with hepatic or renal dysfunction: Cancer and leukemia group B 9565. *J. Clin. Oncol., 18*, 2780–2787.

Weinberg, R. A., (1996). How cancer arises. *Sci. Am., 275*, 62–71.

Weston, A., & Harris, C. C., (2003). Chemical carcinogenesis. In: Kufe, D. W., Pollock, R. E., & Weichselbaum, R. R., (eds.), *Cancer Medicine* (6th edn., pp. 267–278). Hamilton, Ont: BC Decker.

CHAPTER 2

Phosphoprotein-Enriched Astrocytes as Potential Anticancer Agents

SANDEEP ARORA and NIDHI GARG

Chitkara College of Pharmacy, Chitkara University, Punjab, India

ABSTRACT

Phosphoprotein enriched astrocytes of 15 kDa (PEA-15) is a small protein that was first found in brain astrocytes around two decades back. It was found that PEA-15 was ubiquitously expressed in other human tissues. It is an endogenous substrate of protein kinase C (PKC) and highly enriched in astrocytes. Later, it was found to be expressed more widely among various tissues and species having two phosphorylation sites: Ser104 and Ser116. Various studies evidently suggested the indulgence of PEA-15 in regulating signaling pathways of various intracellular proteins enrolling its use as a therapy in multiple disorders like diabetes mellitus, cardiovascular diseases, neurological disorders, and cancer. Thus, it has been represented to be a novel target in the therapy of cancer and metastasis.

2.1 INTRODUCTION

Phosphoprotein enriched astrocytes of 15 kDa (PEA-15) is a small protein first identified in brain astrocytes about two decades ago (Araujo et al., 1993) and found to be ubiquitously expressed in other human tissues (Danziger et al., 1995; Estelles et al., 1996). This protein contains a site for protein kinase C (PKC) and is recognized as an endogenous substrate for PKC (Araujo et al., 1993). The first 80 amino acids of PEA-15 contain the death effector domain (DED) sequence found in proteins that regulate apoptotic-signaling pathways. The DED of PEA-15 can bind to both the Fas-associated death domain (FADD) and caspase 8 (Condorelli et al., 1999; Kitsberg et al., 1999). The other 51 amino acids having two phosphorylation sites: Ser104 and Ser116 (Estelles et al., 1996). Ser104 is the target for PKC (Araujo et al., 1993), whereas Ser116 is the target for calcium/calmodulin-dependent protein kinase II (CaMKII) (Kubes et al., 1998) and protein kinase B/Akt (Trencia et al., 2003).

In previous studies, it has been demonstrated that PEA15 regulated intracellular signaling and plays an important role in various processes, including cancer, diabetes mellitus, metabolic disorders, and nervous system diseases, and cardiovascular diseases (Mohammed et al., 2016; Wei et al., 2015). In type 2 diabetes, PEA 15 was found to be expressed in fibroblasts, skeletal muscle, and adipose tissues (Condorelli et al., 1998). This protein also inhibits membrane association of insulin-sensitive glucose transporter 4 (GLUT4) with phospholipase D1 and D2 (PLD1/2), which further activates PKC-α and -β, and blocks insulin-induction PKC-ζ activity (Condorelli et al., 1999; Renault et al., 2003) whereas the overexpression of PEA-15 in type 2 diabetic patients is considered as a common defect which is responsible for decreased insulin sensitivity in type 2 diabetic patients (Kitsberg et al., 1999).

PEA 15 serves as a multiprotein binding molecule, thereby modulating the function of a number of key cellular processes, including proliferation, apoptosis, and glucose metabolism (Greig and Nixon, 2014). These processes are regulated because of its distinctive interaction with different signaling proteins, e.g., Binding of PEA-15 with the protein named Fas-associated death domain (FADD) and inhibit apoptosis induced by Fas/TNF (tumor necrosis factor)-α and blocks the recruitment and activation of caspase-8 (Ramos et al., 2000). It was also reported that PEA-15 also activates extracellular signal-regulated kinases 1 and 2 (ERK1/2) in the mitogen-activated protein (MAP) kinase pathway (Haling et al., 2010). Interaction of PEA-15 to p90 ribosomal S6 kinase isozyme 2 (RSK2), making it clinically appropriate as a biomarker for use in cancer therapies and diabetes (Danziger et al., 1995; Renault et al., 2006), despite all the protein was not that significant to gain importance among the research community of major diseases, such as cancers and type 2 diabetes, necessitating the need of exploration of the potential role of PEA-15 in cancer.

2.2   STRUCTURE OF PEA-15

PEA-15 protein has been identified in phosphate-labeled astrocytes in the cells. It has been found in three different phosphorylated forms, such as monophosphorylated, bisphosphorylated, and unphosphorylated. PEA-15 is having an NH2-terminal DED and a COOH-terminal tail with irregular structure (Kubes et al., 1998). PEA-15 gene present on human chromosome 1q21–22, which is mainly found in mammals, and all overexpressed in human tissues (Kubes et al., 1998). Two different serine phosphorylation sites were identified in the protein. One is Ser104, which represents a PKC substrate (Park et al., 2007). The second is Ser116, which is represented by phosphorylated by Ca2/calmodulin kinase II (CaMKII) (24) and by PKB (Wei et al., 2014). PEA-15 consists of DED proteins that are involved in the cascade of apoptosis. This provides the first evidence of a cellular role for PEA-15 (Ramos et al., 1998). DED, along with death domain (DD), pyrin domain (PYD), and caspase activation and recruitment domain (CARD), constitutes the superfamily of death structural domain, which is composed of canonical six-helix bundle fold (Twomey et al., 2012; Formstecher et al., 2001). The nuclear export of ERK and cytosolic accumulation is promoted by the N-terminal of the DED having a leucine-rich nuclear exporting sequence (NES) (Ramos et al., 1998). All functions of PEA-15 are exerted through protein-protein interactions because it has no catalytic activities (Valmiki et al., 2009). To interact with its binding partners, PEA-15 has different surfaces, such as PEA-15 interacts with FADD-DED using a surface patch adjacent to helix α2 (Twomey et al., 2012). It utilizes both DED residues on helices α1, α5, and α6 and C-terminal tail residues to bind with ERK2 (Twomey et al., 2013). Therefore, PEA 15 behaves like a multiprotein binding molecule and regulates multiple numbers of cellular functions such as proliferation, apoptosis, and glucose metabolism (Valmiki et al., 2009).

2.3   CELLULAR FUNCTION OF PEA-15

One of the most important cellular functions of PEA-15 is binding with extracellular signal-regulated kinases 1/2 (ERK1/2) protein (Formstecher et al., 2001). ERK1 and ERK2 are members of the MAP kinase family and regulates various aspects of cell signaling, which activate MAP kinase and MEK1/2 and phosphorylates ERK1/2 on both serine and threonine residues (Ramos et al., 2008). This phosphorylated ERK1/2 is further responsible for various signaling outcomes such as cytoplasm interaction, and this includes interaction with the ETS transcription factor, Elk-1, which further induces proliferation. Recent evidence demonstrated that PEA-15 behaves like an "anchor" of cytoplasm for ERK1/2 (Formstecher et al., 2001). PEA-15 binds with ERK1/2 in different types of cells, such as astrocytes in the brain, fibroblasts, T-lymphocytes, testicular Sertoli cells, and vascular smooth muscle (VSM) cells (Formstecher et al., 2001; Buonomo et al., 2012). Overexpression of PEA-15 in cells decreases the nuclear translocation of ERK1/2, which further reduces the activation of nuclear substrates such as phosphorylation of the ETS transcription factor (Formstecher et al., 2001). At the same time, altered levels of PEA-15 does not affect the activation of cytoplasmic substrates induced by ERK1/2 (non-nuclear).

ERK1/2 interacts with its substrates through two docking domains; one is D-domain, and the other is a docking site for ERK, FXFP (DEF) motif. Recent studies have shown that within this complex regulatory signal, PEA-15 plays a unique role as a downstream regulator for ERK1/2 via its ERK1/2 binding properties. PEA-15 is located centrally and regulates the proliferation and apoptosis of ERK1/2. Therefore, the role of PEA-15 is emerging in various diseases. It has been found that in diabetes mellitus, the up-regulation of PEA-15 controls the uptake of glucose and insulin sensitivity, and whereas in the brain, distinctive expression of PEA-15 is associated with various neurological disorders. PEA-15 is also involved in the treatment of atherosclerosis because it regulates the proliferation of VSM cells in cardiovascular diseases. Therefore, the involvement of PEA-15 in different disease states raises its potential of being an effective therapeutic target for the treatment of the same.

2.4   PARADOXICAL ROLE OF PEA-15 IN CANCER

Cancer is the abnormal growth of cells and the formation of malignant tumors that attack and metastasize the nearby healthy tissues and other parts of the body. In the normal situations, inactive cells transform into active proliferative cancerous cells with different acquired capabilities such as the autogrowth patterns and the stimuli causing endless replications posing resistance to anti-growth signals apoptosis and destruction by the immune system, angiogenetic properties, reprogramming of energy metabolism and the ability to invade adjoining tissue resulting in the formation of tumor and metastasis (Kondoh et al., 2005). PEA-15, due to its intracellular function, has been found to be involved in the dysregulation of these pathological diseases. Furthermore, PEA 15 has been reported to have both tumor suppressor as well as promoter properties because various studies demonstrated that it inhibits the invasion and proliferation of some cancerous cells (Gawecka et al., 2012; Stassi et al., 2005; Garofalo et al., 2007) while upregulating the resistance to TRAIL-mediated apoptosis in different cancer types (Hanahan et al., 2000). This again divulges the role of PEA-15, either a prognostic marker or a therapeutic target in specific cancer subsets (Hanahan et al., 2011). Furthermore, various factors like smoking and dietary habits also contribute to the pathogenesis of mutations caused by either producing oncogenes or tumor suppressor genes with a recessive loss of function (Kondoh et al., 2005). Conclusively, it can be averred that for over more than two hundred different types of cancer, which influences the global population, there is an imminent necessity to develop a deeper understanding of disease progression, which would ultimately carve out a path for developing better therapeutics.

2.5   ROLE OF PEA-15 IN TUMOR SUPPRESSION

The central role of the MAP kinase signaling pathway in regulating cell proliferation, cell differentiation, apoptosis, and the localization of ERK1/2 majorly defines the fate of the tumorous cells (Bartholomeusz et al., 2010). PEA-15 prevents the invasion and proliferation of tumor cells via increasing cytoplasmic localization of activated ERK1/2 cells (Bartholomeusz et al., 2008). Furthermore, it also inhibits tumor progression in triple-negative breast cancer (Buonomo et al., 2012), and human ovarian cancer (Bock et al., 2010). Similarly, PEA-15 inhibits fibroblast motility and wound closure through this ERK1/2-dependent pathway (Bartholomeusz et al., 2006). PEA-15 promotes autophagy of glioma cells by modifying the signals of c-Jun N-terminal Kinase (JNK) (Botta et al., 2010). The antitumor activity of E1A in ovarian cancer has been found to be associated with PEA-15 translocalization of ERK from the nucleus to the cytoplasm (Watanabe et al., 2010). Furthermore, it is also used as a marker in glioblastoma (GB) as it modulates coxsackievirus-adenovirus Receptor (CAR) and adenoviral infectivity via ERK-mediated signals in glioma cells(Funke et al., 2013). The high expression level of PEA-15 was found to be inversely correlated with the malignancy grade of astrocytic tumors and positively correlated to longer overall survival (Nagarajan et al., 2014). Moreover, in colorectal carcinoma (CRC), PEA-15 expression was also suggested to be negatively correlated with the malignancy stage in the case of CRC. Furthermore, increased expression of PEA-15 inhibits the invasion and proliferation of CRC cells. It also significantly protects CRC cells from apoptosis via cytotoxic drugs (Shieh et al., 1997).

Association of PEA-15 was found with cell cycle arrest and checkpoints in malignant cells. PEA-15 plays an important role in promoting damage-induced G2/M checkpoints. PEA-15 and tumor suppressor proteins like p53 are stabilized by the mechanism of DNA damage induced overexpression that involves suppression of proteasome-mediated degradation and polyubiquitin. PEA-15 protein levels are higher in the G2/M phase of the cell cycle and thus defect in this phase by ERK1/2 due to increased activation of CDC25C results in elevation of CDK1/cyclin B. PEA-15 inhibits ERK-dependent, c-JUN-mediated transcriptional activation of CDK6 and hence controls the progression of the cell cycle. It is also found to suppress CDK6 activity alternatively by regulating the RAS mediated neoplastic transformation. In a recent study, it has been shown that by promoting DNA hypermethylation, PEA-15 was epigenetically silenced in lung, breast, and colorectal and breast cancer tissues (Lee et al., 2015). In another study, it has been shown that PEA-15 also activates the proliferation in human diploid fibroblast (HDF) senescent cells and reduced progression of G1 arrested cells significantly to S-phase (Kuramitsu et al., 2009). Hence, the above findings suggest the potential role of PEA-15 in regulating genomic integrity by promoting and regulating cell cycle checkpoints. Downregulation of PEA-15 results in various genomic DNA mutations with the acceleration in the cell cycle.

2.6   ROLE OF PEA-15 IN CANCER PROMOTER

The tumorigenic potential of PEA-15 has been suggested in various types of cancer. It is recognized to be upregulated in various types of cancers, which includes malignant pleural mesothelioma cells (Formisano et al., 2005), enduring cancer cells (e.g., MCF-7 and HeLa cells) (Eramo et al., 2005), non-small cell lung cancer (NSCLC) cells (Hanahan et al., 2000), breast cancer cells (Heikaus et al., 2008), renal cell carcinomas (RCCs) (Sulzmaier et al., 2012) and GB (Zanca et al., 2010). Overexpressing PEA-15 showed four times elevation in papilloma cells as compared to wild type littermates that suggest their potential role in tumor formation and progression of cancer (Menard et al., 1998).

In NSCLC, Rac1 gets activated by interacting with PEA-15, which results in the modification of invasion and migration (Menard et al., 1998). PEA-15 was found in well-differentiated tumor areas, and it also regulates the entry of cells in the colorectal region (Formisano et al., 2012). 67 kDa laminin receptor (67LR) is recommended to be for the metastasis marker. It has been found that

PEA-15 interacts with 67LR and results in a significant increase in its migration and proliferation (Sulzmaier et al., 2012; Bartholomeusz et al., 2012). PEA-15 transforms kidney epithelial cells and further potentiates ERK1/2 signaling during H-Ras (a proto-oncogene) activation (Debatin et al., 2004). Also, in patients with triple-negative breast cancer (TNBC), PEA-15 is found to be correlated with high ERK1/2 levels, which are further associated with their short survival rates (Kim et al., 2000). These highlights have shown the contribution of PEA-15 in the progression of the tumor via various processes of cells.

Apart from TRAIL resistance, PEA-15 has been shown to be associated with cell death through other mechanisms. The interleukin (IL)-4 and -10, cytokines upregulate PEA-15, which induces resistance to Fas activation or CD95 in the case of thyroid cancer (Eckert et al., 2008). The overexpression of PEA-15 and various other anti-apoptotic proteins induced by IL-4 in cancers like colon, breast, colon, and lung tumors results in resistance to apoptosis (Mourtata et al., 2009). Similarly, its overexpression affects GB cells by increasing resistance to apoptosis, which is associated with glucose deprivation. Moreover, perinecrotic areas also get affected by PEA-15, which results in the elevation of phosphorylation at its Ser116 region (Seigelin et al., 2008). However, dephosphorylation of PEA-15 is important in preventing lymphoma and leukemia through protein phosphatase 4-induced apoptosis of T cells (Festuccia et al., 2008).

Therapeutically to suppress tumor formation, reduction in resistance to apoptotic signaling in cancerous cells could be a potential target. So in GB cells, treatment with epigallocatechin-3-gallate (a flavonoid) through Akt (PKB)-dependent mechanism along with TRAIL down-regulates expression of PEA-15 that could be beneficial in inducing apoptosis in tumor cells (Diageler et al., 2008). Moreover, a chemotherapeutic drug decitabine sensitizes cells that are resistant to TRAIL-mediated apoptosis by reducing PEA-15 and other anti-apoptotic proteins in prostate cancer (Greig et al., 2014). Doxorubicin (a potent chemotherapeutic agent) regulates numerous pro-apoptotic proteins and some anti-apoptotic proteins such as PEA-15 when microarray analysis of liposarcoma cultures was analyzed (Bartholomeusz et al., 2008).

2.7 THERAPEUTIC TARGET OF PEA-15 IN CANCER

Several therapeutic interventions have been developed for diseases such as cancer, diabetes type-2, neurological disorders, and cardiovascular diseases by targeting PEA-15 (Lee et al., 2012). It is an endogenous protein that has been clinically found to elucidate salubrious effects for patients suffering from different kinds of cancers (Stassi et al., 2012; Xei et al., 2013). At two different sites of phosphorylation, mutation of serine residues of PEA-15 occurs by transforming it either into an alanine (A), which then represents the non-phosphorylated state, or into aspartic acid (D) to imitate the phosphorylated state. Previous studies have reported that the concentration of phosphorylated PEA-15 has been found to be higher in the tissues with ovarian cancer than normal tissues in the vicinity. Also, the study has added that the non-phosphory-latable PEA-15 S104A/S116A mutant (PEA-15-AA) form causes more potent inhibition of tumor cell migration and in vivo angiogenesis as compared to phosphomimetic S104D/S116D mutant (PEA-15-DD) (Shin, M et al., 2015). Furthermore, it has been reported that resistance to paclitaxel may develop following the downregulation of PEA-15 in ovarian cancer cells (Xei et al., 2012). PEA-15 may also play an important role in promoting the ER-anchored protein tyrosine phosphatase, which has been reported to dephosphorylate EGFR and thus involved in the downregulation of EGFR signaling in TNBC cells (Xei et al., 2015). Therefore, PEA-15 may possibly act through inhibiting protein kinase activities or via enhancing tumor phosphatase activities and potentially may develop as a novel therapeutic strategy for the treatment of various neurodegenerative diseases and tumorous cells (Twomey et al., 2013; Zanca et al., 2008; Sulzmaier et al., 2012).

2.8   CONCLUSION

PEA-15, a small endogenous protein, has been found to regulate the cellular pathways, which subsequently determine the fate of the cancerous cells. PEA-15 also possesses potential therapeutic value and is free from life-threatening side effects or higher cellular toxicity. All these positive traits may prove PEA-15 to be an effective agent for the treatment of a different form of cancer.

KEYWORDS

- **astrocytes**
- **coxsackievirus-adenovirus receptor**
- **death effector domain**

- **extracellular signal-regulated kinases**
- **phosphoprotein enriched astrocytes**
- **protein kinase C**

REFERENCES

Araujo, H., Danziger, N., Cordier, J., Glowinski, J., & Chneiweiss, H., (1993). Characterization of pea-15, a major substrate for protein kinase c in astrocytes. *J. Biol. Chem., 268*, 5911–5920.

Bartholomeusz, C., Gonzalez-Angulo, A. M., Liu, P., Hayashi, N., Lluch, A., Ferrer-Lozano, J., et al., (2012). High ERK protein expression levels correlate with shorter survival in triple-negative breast cancer patients. *Oncologist, 17*, 766–774.

Bartholomeusz, C., Itamochi, H., Nitta, M., Saya, H., Ginsberg, M. H., & Ueno, N. T., (2006). Antitumor effect of E1A in ovarian cancer by cytoplasmic sequestration of activated ERK by PEA15. *Oncogene, 25*, 79–90.

Bartholomeusz, C., Rosen, D., Wei, C., Kazansky, A., Yamasaki, F., Takahashi, T., Itamochi, H., et al., (2008). PEA-15 induces autophagy in human ovarian cancer cells and is associated with prolonged overall survival. *Cancer Res., 68*, 9302–9310.

Böck, B. C., Tagscherer, K. E., Fassl, A., Krämer, A., Oehme, I., Zentgraf, H. W., Keith, M., & Roth, W., (2010). The PEA-15 protein regulates autophagy via activation of JNK. *J. Biol. Chem., 285*, 21644–21654.

Botta, G., Perruolo, G., Libertini, S., Cassese, A., Abagnale, A., Beguinot, F., Formisano, P., & Portella, G., (2010). PED/PEA-15 modulates coxsackievirus-adenovirus receptor expression and adenoviral infectivity via ERK-mediated signals in glioma cells. *Hum. Gene Ther., 21*, 1067–1076.

Buonomo, R., Giacco, F., Vasaturo, A., Caserta, S., Guido, S., Pagliara, V., Garbi, C., Mansueto, G., Cassese, A., Perruolo, G., et al., (2012). PED/PEA-15 controls fibroblast motility and wound closure by ERK1/2-dependent mechanisms. *J. Cell. Physiol., 227*, 2106–2116.

Condorelli, G., Vigliotta, G., Cafieri, A., Trencia, A., Andalo, P., Oriente, F., Miele, C., et al., (1999). PED/PEA-15: An anti-apoptotic molecule that regulates Fas/TNFR1-induced apoptosis. *Oncogene, 18*, 4409–4415.

Condorelli, G., Vigliotta, G., Iavarone, C., Caruso, M., Tocchetti, C. G., Andreozzi, F., Cafieri, A., Tecce, M. F., Formisano, P., Beguinot, L., et al., (1998). PED/PEA-15 gene controls glucose transport and is overexpressed in type 2 diabetes mellitus. *EMBO J., 17*, 3858–3866.

Daigeler, A., Klein-Hitpass, L., Chromik, M. A., Muller, O., Hauser, J., Homann, H. H., et al., (2008). Heterogeneous *in vitro* effects of doxorubicin on gene expression in primary human liposarcoma cultures. *BMC Cancer, 8*, 313.

Danziger, N., Yokoyama, M., Jay, T., Cordier, J., Glowinski, J., & Chneiweiss, H., (1995). Cellular expression, developmental regulation, and phylogenic conservation of pea-15, the astrocytic major phosphoprotein and protein kinase c substrate. *J. Neurochem., 64*, 1016–1025.

Debatin, K. M., & Krammer, P. H., (2004). Death receptors in chemotherapy and cancer. *Oncogene 23*, 2950–2966.

Eckert, A., Bock, B. C., Tagscherer, K. E., Haas, T. L., Grund, K., Sykora, J., et al., (2008). The PEA-15/PED protein protects glioblastoma cells from glucose deprivation-induced apoptosis via the ERK/MAP kinase pathway. *Oncogene, 27*, 1155–1166.

Eramo, A., Pallini, R., Lotti, F., Sette, G., Patti, M., Bartucci, M., et al., (2005). Inhibition of DNA methylation sensitizes glioblastoma for tumor necrosis factor-related apoptosis-inducing ligand-mediated destruction. *Cancer Res., 65*, 11469–11477.

Estellés, A., Yokoyama, M., Nothias, F., Vincent, J. D., Glowinski, J., Vernier, P., & Chneiweiss, H., (1996). The major astrocytic phosphoprotein pea-15 is encoded by two MRNAs conserved on their full length in mouse and human. *J. Biol. Chem., 271*, 14800–14806.

Farina, B., Doti, N., Pirone, L., Malgieri, G., Pedone, E. M., Ruvo, M., & Fattorusso, R., (2013). Molecular basis of the PED/PEA15 interaction with the c-terminal fragment of phospholipase d1 revealed by NMR spectroscopy. *Biochim. Biophys. Acta, 1834*, 1572–1580.

Festuccia, C., Gravina, G. L., D'Alessandro, A. M., Millimaggi, D., Di Rocco, C., Dolo, V., et al., (2008). Down modulation of dimethyl transferase activity enhances tumor necrosis factor-related apoptosis-inducing ligand-induced apoptosis in prostate cancer cells. *Int. J. Oncol., 33*, 381–388.

Formisano, P., Perruolo, G., Libertini, S., Santopietro, S., Troncone, G., Raciti, G. A., et al., (2005). Raised expression of the anti-apoptotic protein ped/pea-15 increases susceptibility to chemically induced skin tumor development. *Oncogene, 24*, 7012–7021.

Formisano, P., Ragno, P., Pesapane, A., Alfano, D., Alberobello, A. T., Rea, V. E., et al., (2012). PED/PEA-15 interacts with the 67 kD laminin receptor and regulates cell adhesion, migration, proliferation, and apoptosis. *J. Cell Mol. Med., 16*, 1435–1446.

Formstecher, E., Ramos, J. W., Fauquet, M., Calderwood, D. A., Hsieh, J. C., Canton, B., Nguyen, X. T., Barnier, J. V., Camonis, J., Ginsberg, M. H., et al., (2001). PEA-15 mediates cytoplasmic sequestration of ERK MAP kinase. *Dev. Cell, 1*, 239–250.

Funke, V., Lehmann-Koch, J., Bickeboller, M., Benner, A., Tagscherer, K. E., Grund, K., et al., (2013). The PEA-15/PED protein regulates cellular survival and invasiveness in colorectal carcinomas. *Cancer Lett., 335*, 431–440.

Garofalo, M., Romano, G., Quintavalle, C., Romano, M. F., Chiurazzi, F., Zanca, C., et al., (2007). Selective inhibition of PED protein expression sensitizes B-cell chronic lymphocytic leukemia cells to TRAIL-induced apoptosis. *Int. J. Cancer, 120*, 1215–1222.

Glading, A., Koziol, J. A., Krueger, J., & Ginsberg, M. H., (2007). PEA-15 inhibits tumor cell invasion by binding to extracellular signal-regulated kinase 1/2. *Cancer Res., 67*, 1536–1544.

Greig, F. H., & Nixon, G. F., (2014). Phosphoprotein enriched in astrocytes (PEA)-15: A potential therapeutic target in multiple disease states. *Pharmacol. Therap., 143*, 265–274.

Haling, J. R., Wang, F., & Ginsberg, M. H., (2010). Phosphoprotein enriched in astrocytes 15 kDa (PEA-15) reprograms growth factor signaling by inhibiting threonine phosphorylation of fibroblast receptor substrate 2α. *Mol. Biol. Cell, 21*, 664–673.

Hanahan, D., & Weinberg, R. A., (2000). The hallmarks of cancer. *Cell, 100*, 57–70.

Hanahan, D., & Weinberg, R. A., (2011). Hallmarks of cancer: The next generation. *Cell, 144*, 646–674.

Heikaus, S., Kempf, T., Mahotka, C., Gabbert, H. E., & Ramp, U., (2008). Caspase-8 and its inhibitors in RCCs *in vivo*: The prominent role of ARC. *Apoptosis, 13*, 938–949.

Kim, K., Fisher, M. J., Xu, S. Q., & El-Deiry, W. S., (2000). Molecular determinants of response to TRAIL in killing of normal and cancer cells. *Clin. Cancer Res., 6*, 335–346.

Kitsberg, D., Formstecher, E., Fauquet, M., Kubes, M., Cordier, J., Canton, B., Pan, G., et al., (1999). Knock-out of the neural death effector domain protein PEA-15 demonstrates that its expression protects astrocytes from tnfα-induced apoptosis. *J. Neurosci., 19*, 8244–8251.

Kondoh, K., Torii, S., & Nishida, E., (2005). Control of map kinase signaling to the nucleus. *Chromosoma, 114*, 86–91.

Kubes, M., Cordier, J., Glowinski, J., Girault, J. A., & Chneiweiss, H., (1998). Endothelin induces a calcium-dependent phosphorylation of pea-15 in intact astrocytes: Identification of ser104 and ser116 phosphorylated, respectively, by protein kinase c and calcium/calmodulin kinase ii *in vitro. J. Neurochem., 71*, 1307–1314.

Kuramitsu, Y., Miyamoto, H., Tanaka, T., Zhang, X., Fujimoto, M., Ueda, K., et al., (2009). Proteomic differential display analysis identified up regulated astrocytic phosphoproteinPEA-15 in human malignant pleural mesothelioma cell lines. *Proteomics, 9*, 5078–5089.

Lee, J., Bartholomeusz, C., Krishnamurthy, S., Liu, P., Saso, H., Lafortune, T. A., Hortobagyi, G. N., & Ueno, N. T., (2012). PEA-15 unphosphorylated at both serine 104 and serine 116 inhibits ovarian cancer cell tumorigenicity and progression through blocking beta-catenin. *Oncogenesis, 1*, e22.

Lee, Y. Y., Kim, H. S., & Lim, I. K., (2015). Down regulation of PEA-15 reverses g1 arrest, and nuclear and chromatin changes of senescence phenotype via perk1/2 translocation to nuclei. *Cell Signal, 27*, 1102–1109.

Menard, S., Tagliabue, E., & Colnaghi, M. I., (1998). The 67 kDa laminin receptor as a prognostic factor in human cancer. *Breast Cancer Res. Treat, 52*, 137–145.

Mohammed, H. N., Pickard, M. R., & Mourtada-Maarabouni, M., (2016). The protein phosphatase 4-PEA15 axis regulates the survival of breast cancer cells. *Cell Signal, 28*, 1389–1400.

Mourtada-Maarabouni, M., & Williams, G. T., (2009). Protein phosphatase 4 regulates apoptosis in leukemic and primary human T-cells. *Leuk Res., 33*, 1539–1551.

Nagarajan, A., Dogra, S. K., Liu, A. Y., Green, M. R., & Wajapeyee, N., (2014). PEA15 regulates the DNA damage-induced cell cycle checkpoint and oncogene-directed transformation. *Mol. Cell. Biol., 34*, 2264–2282.

Park, H. H., Lo, Y. C., Lin, S. C., Wang, L., Yang, J. K., & Wu, H., (2007). The death domain superfamily in intracellular signaling of apoptosis and inflammation. *Ann. Rev. Immunol., 25*, 561–586.

Ramos, J. W., Hughes, P. E., Renshaw, M. W., Schwartz, M. A., Formstecher, E., Chneiweiss, H., & Ginsberg, M. H., (2000). Death effect or domain protein PEA-15 potentiates Ras activation of extracellular signal receptor-activated kinase by an adhesion-independent mechanism. *Mol. Biol. Cell, 11*, 2863–2872.

Ramos, J. W., Kojima, T. K., Hughes, P. E., Fenczik, C. A., & Ginsberg, M. H., (1998). The death effector domain of PEA-15 is involved in its regulation of integrin activation. *J. Biol. Chem., 273*, 33897–33900.

Renault, F., Formstecher, E., Callebaut, I., Junier, M. P., & Chneiweiss, H., (2003). The multifunctional protein PEA-15 is involved in the control of apoptosis and cell cycle in astrocytes. *Biochem. Pharmacol., 66*, 1581–1588.

Renault-Mihara, F., Beuvon, F., Iturrioz, X., Canton, B., De Bouard, S., Leonard, N., Mouhamad, S., et al., (2006). Phosphoprotein enriched in astrocytes-15 kDa expression inhibits astrocyte migration by a protein kinase C delta-dependent mechanism. *Mol. Biol. Cell, 17*, 5141–5152.

Shieh, S. Y., Ikeda, M., Taya, Y., & Prives, C., (1997). DNA damage-induced phosphorylation of p53 alleviates inhibition by mdm2. *Cell, 91*, 325–334.

Shin, M., Lee, K. E., Yang, E. G., Jeon, H., & Song, H. K., (2015). PEA-15 facilitates EGFR dephosphorylation via ERK sequestration at increased ER-PM contacts in TNBC cells. *FEBS Lett., 589*, 1033–1039.

Siegelin, M. D., Habel, A., & Gaiser, T., (2008). Epigallocatechin-3-gallate (EGCG) down regulates PEA15 and thereby augments TRAIL-mediated apoptosis in malignant glioma. *Neurosci. Lett., 448*, 161–165.

Stassi, G., Garofalo, M., Zerilli, M., Ricci-Vitiani, L., Zanca, C., Todaro, M., et al., (2005). PED mediates AKT-dependent chemo resistance in human breast cancer cells. *Cancer Res., 65*, 6668–6675.

Sulzmaier, F. J., Valmiki, M. K., Nelson, D. A., Caliva, M. J., Geerts, D., Matter, M. L., et al., (2012). PEA-15 potentiates H-Ras-mediated epithelial cell transformation through phospholipase D. *Oncogene, 31*, 3547–3560.

Sulzmaier, F., Opoku-Ansah, J., & Ramos, J. W., (2012). Phosphorylation is the switch that turns PEA-15 from tumor suppressor to tumor promoter. *Small GTPases, 3*, 173–177.

Trencia, A., Perfetti, A., Cassese, A., Vigliotta, G., Miele, C., Oriente, F., Santopietro, S., Giacco, F., Condorelli, G., Formisano, P., et al., (2003). Protein kinase b/akt binds and phosphorylates PED/PEA-15, stabilizing its anti-apoptotic action. *Mol. Cell. Biol., 23*, 4511–4521.

Twomey, E. C., & Wei, Y., (2012). High-definition NMR structure of PED/PEA-15 death effector domain reveals details of key polar side chain interactions. *Biochem. Biophys. Res. Commun., 424*, 141–146.

Twomey, E. C., Cordasco, D. F., & Wei, Y., (2012). Profound conformational changes of PED/PEA-15 in ERK2 complex revealed by NMR backbone dynamics. *Biochim. Biophys. Acta, 1824*, 1382–1393.

Twomey, E. C., Cordasco, D. F., Kozuch, S. D., & Wei, Y., (2013). Substantial conformational change mediated by charge-triad residues of the death effector domain in protein-protein interactions. *PLoS One, 8*, e83421.

Vaidyanathan, H., & Ramos, J. W., (2003). RSK2 activity is regulated by its interaction with PEA-15. *J. Biol. Chem., 278*, 32367–32372.

Valmiki, M., & Ramos, J., (2009). Death effector domain-containing proteins. *Cell. Mol. Life Sci., 66*, 814–830.

Viparelli, F., Cassese, A., Doti, N., Paturzo, F., Marasco, D., Dathan, N. A., Monti, S. M., Basile, G., Ungaro, P., Sabatella, M., et al., (2008). Targeting of PED/PEA-15 molecular interaction with phospholipase d1 enhances insulin sensitivity in skeletal muscle cells. *J. Biol. Chem., 283*, 21769–21778.

Watanabe, Y., Yamasaki, F., Kajiwara, Y., Saito, T., Nishimoto, T., Bartholomeusz, C., Ueno, N., et al., (2010). Expression of phosphoprotein enriched in astrocytes 15 kDa (PEA-15) in astrocytic tumors: A novel approach of correlating malignancy grade and prognosis. *J. Neurooncol., 100*, 449–457.

Wei, Y., & Twomey, E. C., (2014). NMR spectroscopic characterization of death domain super family proteins: Structures, dynamics, and interactions. In: Rao, D. K., (ed.), *Nuclear Magnetic Resonance (NMR): Theory, Applications, and Technology* (pp. 83–110). Nova Science Publishers, Inc.: Hauppauge, NY, USA.

Wei, Y., (2015). On the quest of cellular functions of PEA-15 and the therapeutic opportunities. *Pharmaceuticals (Basel), 8*, 455–473.

Xie, X., Bartholomeusz, C., Ahmed, A. A., Kazansky, A., Diao, L., Baggerly, K. A., Hortobagyi, G. N., & Ueno, N. T., (2013). Bisphosphorylated PEA-15 sensitizes ovarian cancer cells to paclitaxel by impairing the microtubule-destabilizing effect of SCLIP. *Mol. Cancer Ther., 12*, 1099–1111.

Xie, X., Tang, H., Liu, P., Kong, Y., Wu, M., Xiao, X., Yang, L., Gao, J., Wei, W., Lee, J., et al., (2015). Development of PEA-15 using a potent non-viral vector for therapeutic application in breast cancer. *Cancer Lett., 356*, 374–381.

Zanca, C., Cozzolino, F., Quintavalle, C., Di Costanzo, S., Ricci-Vitiani, L., Santoriello, M., et al., (2010). PED interacts with Rac1 and regulates cell migration/invasion processes in human non-small cell lung cancer cells. *J. Cell Physiol., 225*, 63–72.

Zanca, C., Garofalo, M., Quintavalle, C., Romano, G., Acunzo, M., Ragno, P., et al., (2008). PED is over expressed and mediates TRAIL resistance in human non-small cell lung cancer. *J. Cell Mol. Med., 12*, 2416–2426.

CHAPTER 3

Autophagy-Modulating Drugs as Complements to Cancer Chemotherapy

SANDEEP ARORA and SUKHBIR SINGH

Chitkara College of Pharmacy, Chitkara University, Punjab, India

ABSTRACT

Autophagy is a progressive conserved process that comprises cellular self-ingestion. It consists of Greek words 'auto' imply self and 'phagia' denote eating. It is cellular decomposition procedure wherein prolonged living proteins, and mutilation organelles are confiscated and contained by intra-cytoplasmic binary walled autophagosomes that mingle with lysosomes where lipids and proteins are hydrolyzed into amino and fatty acids that can contribute energy in the nutrient-deprived environment. Cancer is a complex process, and autophagy exerts its effect in numerous ways. Therefore, autophagy inhibiting drugs act as complements to cancer chemotherapy. This chapter briefly summarizes fundamental components of the autophagy process and types of autophagy mechanisms, i.e., microautophagy, chaperone-mediated autophagy, and macroautophagy. ATG5/7-independent and ATG5/7-dependent signaling pathways and numerous factors, i.e., insulin/IGF-1, mTOR, DRAM & p53, and FOXO & ROS, which regulate autophagy have also been discussed. This chapter also recapitulates autophagy inducers and several novel autophagy inhibitors for modulation for cancer therapy.

3.1 INTRODUCTION

The aptitude of malignant cells to elude apoptotic cell killing is an eminent basis for their endurance and assertiveness. Autophagy is an invariant, evolutionary mechanism that involves cellular self-ingestion. It is made up of Greek phrases 'auto' implying self and 'phagia' implying feeding. It is a process of cell decay in which intracytoplasmic binary walled autophagosomes incorporate prolonged living proteins as well as mutilation organelles that integrate with lysosomes whereby lipids and proteins are hydrolyzed into amino, and fatty acids which can provide energy to the nutrition-deprived environment are confiscated. Throughout autophagic progression, flat membrane organelles termed "phagophores" develop in the cytosol and augments to confiscate cytoplasmic substance into double-membrane things coined "autophagosomes." Upon the union of autophagosomes with lysosomes, the requisition load is ruined and reused in the form of innovative structure blocks for cell or organism to utilize (Figure 3.1) (Darby, 2017).

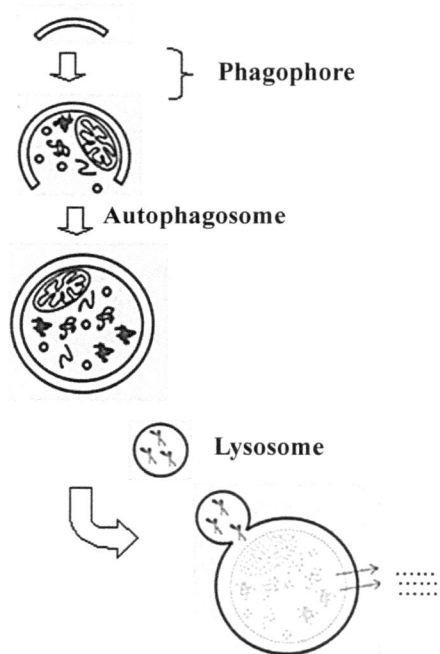

FIGURE 3.1 A simple outline of the autophagic process.

Cancer is a complex phenomenon, and in many aspects, autophagy confers its impact. The fact that autophagy has tumor-suppressive as well as stimulating roles, renders it an appealing theme in research related to cancer. The tumor suppressor role of autophagy is interceded through scavenging of injured oxidative organelles, consequently avoiding accretion of contaminated oxygen radicals, which could trigger the genome. Unexpectedly, nevertheless, during several instances, autophagy may additionally endorse the continued existence of cancer cells on cancerous growth. Autophagy participates in cytoprotective endurance pathway under cancerous circumstances through autophagy obstructing long-lasting destruction of tissue and cell death that could guide to cancer instigation and development to facilitate improved aptness to endure with distorted metabolism and in antagonistic tumor micro-environment. Paradoxically, nevertheless, in several circumstances, autophagy might support the continued existence of malignancy cells when tumors have growth. This is accredited to the capability of autophagy to support cell persistence under circumstances of deprived nutrient perfusion, regularly countenanced by metastasizing cancer cells and solid tumors. Three distinguished autophagic mechanisms corresponding to the method of cargo delivery to lysosome have been depicted in Figure 3.2 (Hoyer-Hansen and Jaattela, 2008; Mizushima et al., 2008; Maiuri et al., 2009).

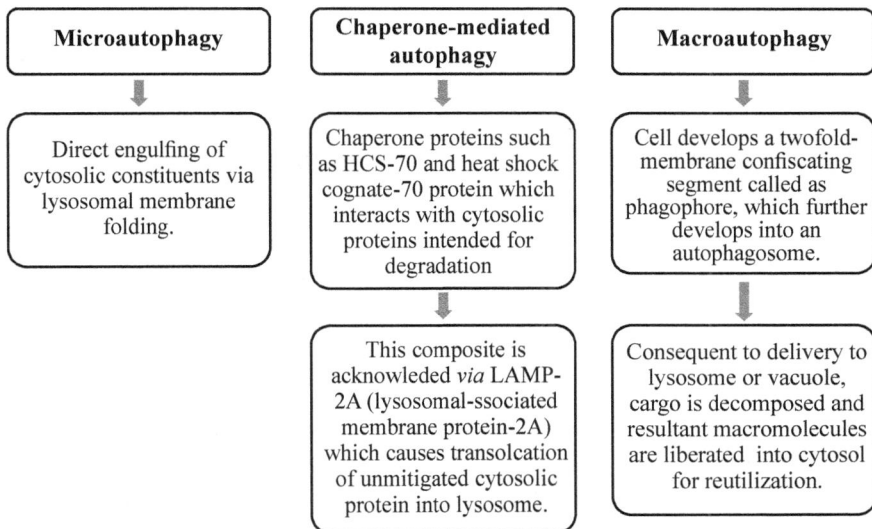

FIGURE 3.2   Types of autophagy mechanisms.

3.2   FUNDAMENTAL COMPONENTS OF AUTOPHAGY PROCESS

The fundamental components of the autophagic process include phagophore development, elongation, and phagosomes multimerization, cargo selection, and fusion of lysosomes (Figure 3.3).

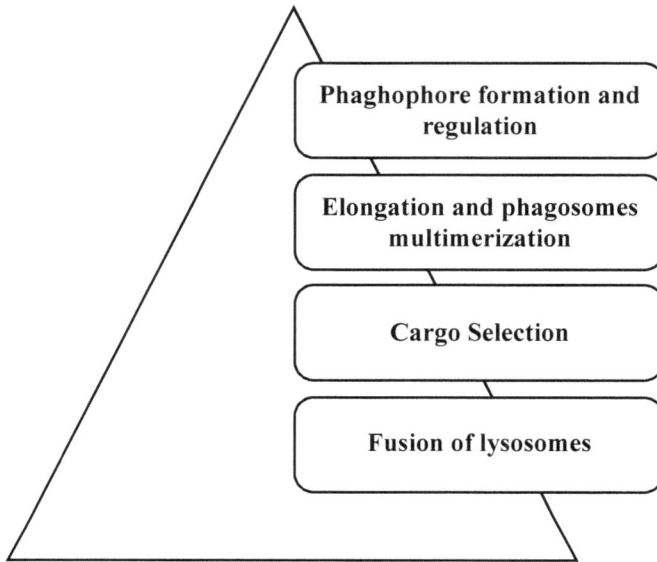

FIGURE 3.3   Fundamental components of the autophagy process.

3.2.1   *PHAGOPHORE DEVELOPMENT AND REGULATION*

The preliminary stage of phagophore membrane development in mammals involves the target of rapamycin (TOR) kinase as a molecular sensor to distinctive stress responses (i.e., hypoxia, insulin signaling, and nutrient depletion), which plays a fundamental role in autophagy control (Klionsky, 2007; Yorimitsu and Klionsky, 2005; Kamada et al., 2010). Preliminary nutrient starvation inactivates TOR kinase, which leads to hypophosphory-lated Atg13 that demonstrates an augmented affinity for Atg1 kinase and develops a complex with scaffold-like protein Atg17. Therefore, starvation management enhances the affinity among Atg13, Atg1, and Atg17. Atg13 and Atg17 are mutually essential for appropriate supervision of the kinase activity of Atg1. Successively, Atg1 standardizes the transmembrane protein Atg9. The kinase action of Atg1 is superfluous; yet, it restrains the dynamics of Atg9 recruitment to phagophore in an Atg17-dependent pathway. Atg9 is concerned in lipid import from distinctive sources like endoplasmic reticulum (ER), mitochondria, endosomes, Golgi bodies, nuclear envelope and furthermore augments the assembly of integral phagophore membrane (Axe et al., 2008; Simonsen and Tooze, 2009; Sekito et al., 2009).

3.2.2 ELONGATION AND MULTIMERIZATION OF PHAGOSOMES

Developed phagophore gets elongated on binding to Vps34 (vesicular protein sorting), which is a class III PI3 kinases. Elongated phagophore further binds to Beclin1, which augments its catalytic action to produce phosphatidyl inositol-3-phosphate (PI3P), which is a noteworthy localization signal in assisting the fusion during autophagosome formation (Axe et al., 2008; Simonsen and Tooze, 2009). Vps34-Beclin1 interaction is up-regulated through proteins, for instance, UVRAG (ultraviolet radiation resistance-associated gene), AMBRA (the activating molecule in Beclin1-regulated autophagy protein 1), and BIF 1 (Bax-interacting factor 1). On the contrary, this interaction is down-regulated via Bcl-XL, Bcl-2, and Rubicon (Funderbur et al., 2010). Ubiquitin, like conjugation systems, which are important constituent for vesicle elongation progression, has been represented in Figure 3.4.

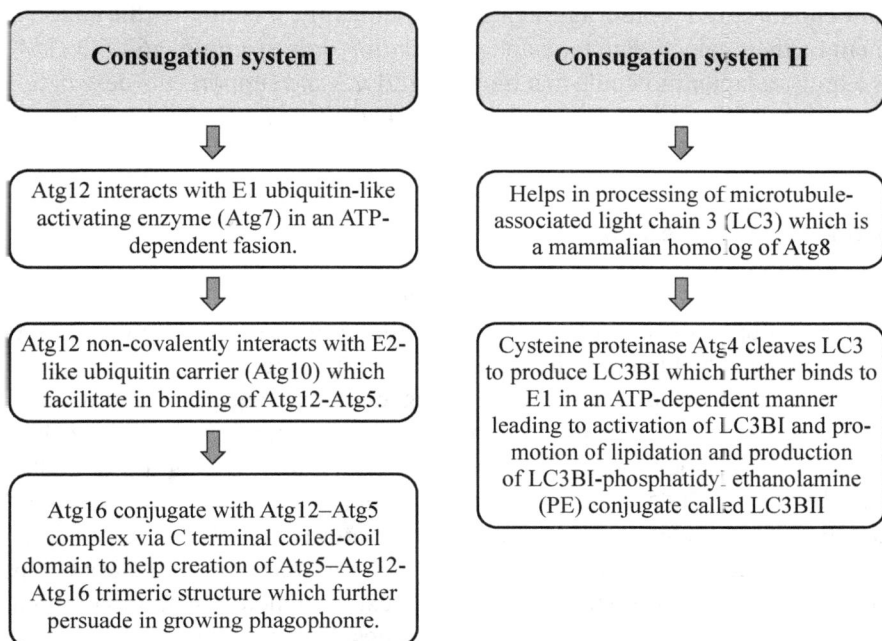

Consugation system I	Consugation system II
⬇	⬇
Atg12 interacts with E1 ubiquitin-like activating enzyme (Atg7) in an ATP-dependent fasion.	Helps in processing of microtubule-associated light chain 3 (LC3) which is a mammalian homolog of Atg8
⬇	⬇
Atg12 non-covalently interacts with E2-like ubiquitin carrier (Atg10) which facilitate in binding of Atg12-Atg5.	Cysteine proteinase Atg4 cleaves LC3 to produce LC3BI which further binds to E1 in an ATP-dependent manner leading to activation of LC3BI and promotion of lipidation and production of LC3BI-phosphatidyl ethanolamine (PE) conjugate called LC3BII
⬇	
Atg16 conjugate with Atg12–Atg5 complex via C terminal coiled-coil domain to help creation of Atg5–Atg12-Atg16 trimeric structure which further persuade in growing phagophonre.	

FIGURE 3.4 Ubiquitin-like conjugation system for vesicle elongation progression (Geng and Klionsky, 2008).

Sequentially, the multimerization of phagosomes instigates on activation of an Ulk1/2 ("UNC-51-like kinase ½") parallely complex. Activated Ulk1/2 allies with starting membrane of phagophore and Vps34 complex is conscripted to phagophore and phosphorylates phosphoinositides (PIs) which leads to the synthesis of PI3P and DFCP1 (double FYVE domain-containing protein) and WIPI1/WIPI2 (WD repeat protein-interacting with PIs) which contributes to elongating membrane (Kabeya et al., 2000; Hanada et al., 2007; Geng and Klionsky, 2008; Fujita et al., 2008; Kamada et al., 2010).

3.2.3 CARGO SELECTION

Autophagy is an indiscriminate method as it seems to engulf the cytoplasm arbitrarily. Electron micrographs illustrate that autophagosomes accumulate mitochondria, ER, and Golgi membranes within them. However, developing a phagophore membrane can selectively interact with organelles and protein aggregates. LC3B-II imparts the function of "receptor" at phagophore and interrelates with "adaptor" molecules on the target comprising damaged mitochondria and protein aggregates. Consequently, it facilitates the endorsement of their selective uptake and degradation. For example, p62/SQSTM1 is a multi-adapter molecule that binds Atg8/LC3 and supports the destruction of polyubiquitinated protein aggregates (Okamoto et al., 2009; Ichimura and Komatsu, 2010; Weidberg et al., 2011).

3.2.4 LYSOSOMAL FUSION

Autophagosomes are fused with lysosomes to produce "auto-lysosomes," where acidic lysosomal elements digest the entire cargos. Minor GTPases such as Rab7, "soluble N-ethylmaleimide-sensitive factor activating protein receptor" (SNARE), "endosomal sorting complex required for transport" (ESCRT), and class C Vps proteins contribute strategic roles in synchronized vesicular docking and fusion with target modules (Kimura et al., 2008; Atlashkin et al., 2003; Jager et al., 2004; Martens et al., 2008). Both UVRAG and Rubicon modulates autophagosomal maturity. UVRAG has an independent function in absolute maturation step through engaging class C Vps proteins, consequently stimulating Rab7 fusion, which assists in combination with lysosomes and later with endosomes. Rubicon continues to be part of a complex containing diverse proteins, for instance, UVRAG, hVps15, and hVps34, and thereby restrain autophagosomal maturation (Matsunaga et al., 2010; Zhong et al., 2009).

3.3   SIGNALING PATHWAYS REGULATING AUTOPHAGY

There are two foremost autophagy regulating pathways that were revealed subsequently:

- ATG5/7-independent; and
- ATG5/7-dependent.

ATG5/7-dependent autophagy is commenced through "Unc-51-like kinase" (ULK) complex comprising of numerous proteins: ULK1/2 (mammalian orthologs of yeast ATG1), FIP200 ("FAK-family interacting protein of 200 kDa"), ATG13, and ATG101. Activated ULK complex translocates to phagophore and leads to activation of class III "phosphatidylinositol 3-kinase" (PI3K) complex comprised of phosphatidylinositol 3-kinase Vps34 (VPS34), Beclin1, ATG14, and VPS15 proteins. These proceedings extend to autophagosome development following the enlargement and closing of the mature autophagosome. The ultimate stage in the degradation course is a combination of autophagosomes with lysosomes (Wong et al., 2013; Itakura et al., 2008).

3.4   REGULATION OF AUTOPHAGY

Autophagy is activated in reply to distinct strain and physiological circumstances. Major environmental modulators that induce autophagy are hyperthermia, food deprivation, and hypoxia (Nishida et al., 2009; Klionsky and Emr, 2000; Cuervo, 2004; the Chu, 2008). At the molecular stage, autophagy pathways are remarkably affected by factors that influence aging. Numerous factors, i.e., insulin/IGF-1, mTOR, DRAM & p53, and FOXO & ROS, which regulate autophagy, have been described in the following subsections.

3.4.1   INSULIN/IGF-1

The nutrient-responsive IGF-1/Insulin signaling pathway endorses reproductive growth, morphogenesis, and endurance. The mutant animals illustrate an elevated amount of autophagy in the cells related to morphogenesis. The distraction of the gene function of autophagy impedes morphogenesis and endurance. Several genes related to autophagy were found to persuade cell progression, which is generally facilitated through insulin/IGF-1 or TGF β signaling. Autophagy genes may control cell size through pathways related to growth modulator signaling. In the case of mammals, the liaison concerning autophagy and insulin/IGF-1 signaling seems to be closer (Meléndez et al., 2003; Yorimitsu et al., 2007).

3.4.2   M-TOR

Nutrient deficiency or medication using rapamycin stimulates autophagy. In the case of yeast, Atg13 is hyper-phosphorylated through rapamycin-sensitive "TOR kinase complex 1" (TORC1) and has an inferior attraction for Atg13 (Noda and Ohsumi, 1998). Moreover, TORC1 regulates the stimulation of numerous compounds that control processes such as "transcription" or "translation" of specific proteins via phosphorylation. TOR controls the stimulation of autophagy in assistance with protein kinase A and SCh9 nutrient-sensing pathways (Liang et al., 2007). In the case of mammals, mTOR seems to control autophagy in a manner analogous to that of yeast. Additionally, AMPK performing at upstream of TOR endorses autophagy, as reported in experiments on human cell lines and flies. Consequently, mTOR alongside with "insulin/IGF1 signaling" monitors autophagy at numerous stages. Normal cell growth necessitates a well equilibrium among a synthesis of protein/organelle and its destruction (Lippai et al., 2008). The investigation illustrates that the mammalian target of rapamycin (mTOR) acts as a destructive controller, and the degree of autophagy is controlled through proteins upstream of mTOR signaling such as "phosphate and tensin" homolog (PTEN), PDK1, TSC1/2, and Akt. PTEN and TSC1/2 positively control autophagy, while Akt obstructs it. Downstream targets of mTOR are S6 kinase and elongation factor-2 kinase (Scherz-Shouval and Elazar, 2007; Codogno and Meijer, 2005).

3.4.3   DRAM AND P53

The "p53 suppressor" is mutated in about 50% of cancers related to humans and provokes autophagy. It has been established that P53 performs as a crucial moderator for "damage-induced apoptosis" and has been revealed to generate autophagy in DRAM (damage-regulated autophagy modulator) dependent mode to accomplish a complete cell death in experiments on human cancer cell lines. DRAM is a lysosomal essential membrane protein, and an absolute target of p53-induces macroautophagy and facilitates in a buildup of autophagosomes. The p53 mediated apoptosis includes numerous chromatin-remodeling aspects (Codogno and Meijer, 2005; Tasdemir et al., 2008). For example, e2f1 contains transcriptional suppression of cell propagation as an element of constituent along with retinoblastoma complex. Autophagy genes might also be regulated through various factors concerned with the remodeling of chromatin. Current data illustrates that e2f1 reacts with the atg8, atg1, and DRAM regulatory regions in humans (Yorimitsu and Klionsky, 2005; Kumar and Cakouros, 2004).

3.4.4   FOXO AND ROS

Currently, it was reported that the transcriptional stage of numerous genes associated with autophagy had been augmented through the activation of FOXO. Various genres, such as Atg12, Atg8/LC3, Atg6, and Vps34 stimulate protein decomposition in deteriorating muscle cells, and astonishingly, controlling actions of FOXO on Atg12 and Atg8 appears to be straightforward (Polager et al., 2008). The chromatin remodeling factors deacetylate the transcription factors related to FOXO and endorse prolonged existence in experiments on worms, flies, and mammals (Wood et al., 2004).

Furthermore, "reactive oxygen species" (ROS) controls undernourishment stimulated autophagy. Current substantiation illustrates that autophagy-related gene 4 (ATG4), fundamental protease in the autophagy mechanism, was acknowledged as a straight target for ROS mediated oxidation. Accretion of ROS produced throughout numerous cellular functions primarily via respiration instigates an oxidative tension. The cells react to oxidative tension through the stimulation of several resistance mechanisms. Numerous investigations demonstrate that ROS performs as signaling molecules and are competent to stimulate autophagic progression and instigate successive damage of the affected cells. Autophagy seems to have a crucial role in the defensive response of cells to oxidative tension (Lee et al., 2008).

3.5   MECHANISMS FOR AUTOPHAGY DURING CANCER PROGRESSION

There are two ambiguous mechanisms for the autophagy process in cancer progression (Figure 3.5) (Mizushima, 2005).

Mechanism I	Mechanism II
⇩	⇩
• Autophagy removes destructed organelles or protein accretions • This further stimulates progression of programmed cell death in response to regorous damage of the cell	• Autophagy could be stimulated through ER tension and ROS and certain chemotherapeutic drugs e.g., cisplatin and doxorubicin. • Leads to clean up to ROS-damaged proteins from cancer stem cells.

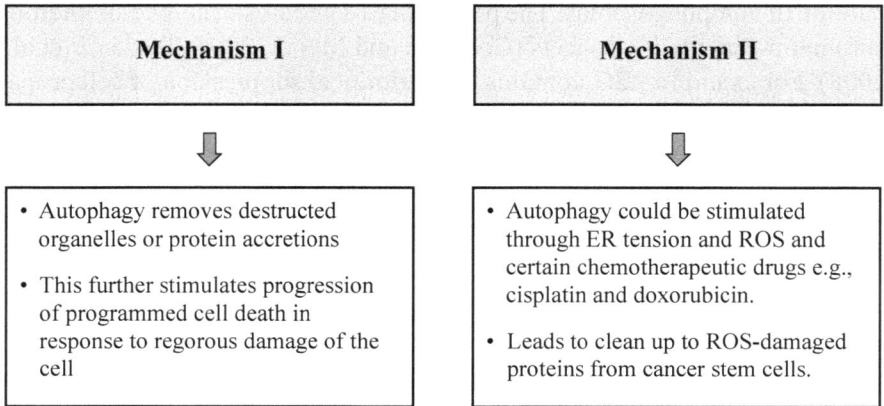

FIGURE 3.5   Mechanisms for autophagy in cancer progression.

3.6   PROS AND CONS OF AUTOPHAGY IN CANCER

Dual contradictory aspects of autophagy in progression of cancer have been represented in Table 3.1 (Brech et al., 2009).

TABLE 3.1   Pros and Cons of Autophagy in Cancer

Advantages	Disadvantages
Preserves stability of genome *via* scavenging the smashed peroxisomes and mitochondria	Imparts endurance mechanism for solid tumors with constrained blood perfusion
Tumor cell death induced through various therapies	Preclude chemo- and radiotherapy-induced apoptosis in tumors

3.7   AUTOPHAGY MODULATION FOR CANCER THERAPY

3.7.1   AUTOPHAGY INDUCERS

Certain cytotoxic therapeutic agents and irradiation have been revealed to persuade autophagy (Choi, 2012). Examples of anticancer drugs which could provoke autophagy have been detailed in Table 3.2.

3.7.2   AUTOPHAGY INHIBITORS

The pharmacological inhibitors of autophagy have been categorized into "early-stage" or "late-stage" inhibitors of the pathway as illustrated in Figure

3.6 (Rossi et al., 2008; Carew et al., 2011; Ruiz-Irastorza et al., 2010; Korolchuk et al., 2009; Ogata et al., 2006; Kouroku et al., 2007).

TABLE 3.2 Autophagy Inducer Drugs and Their Mechanism of Action

Mechanism of Action	Drug	References
TNF-related apoptosis-inducing ligand (TRAIL)	—	Amaravadi et al. (2007)
BCRABL tyrosine kinase inhibitor	Imatinib	Ertmer et al. (2007)
Anti-epidermal growth factor receptor, EGFR	Cetuximab	Li et al. (2010)
Proteosome inhibitors	—	Han et al. (2008)
HDAC inhibitors	Vorinostat and OSU-HDAC42	Han et al. (2008)
Regulation of mitochondrial stress sensor BNIP3 malignant glioma	Arsenic trioxide	Bursch et al. (1996)
Tamoxifen, cyclooxygenase inhibitors, and nelfinavir	—	Huang and Sinicrope, (2010); Gills et al. (2008)
Allosteric mTOR inhibitor	Rapamycin	Williams et al. (2008)
Selectively target mTORC1	Temsirolimus (CCI-779), everolimus (RAD-001), and deforolimus (AP-23573)	Williams et al. (2008)
Selective serotonin-norepinephrine reuptake inhibitor	Fluoxetine	Williams et al. (2008)
mTOR-independent pathway	Verapamil, minoxidil, and clonidine	Williams et al. (2008)

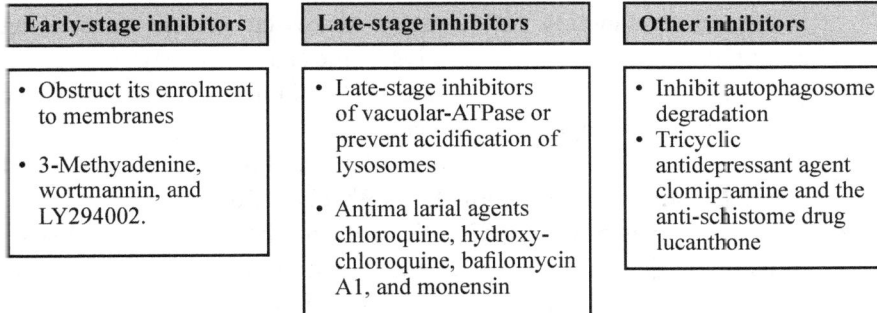

Early-stage inhibitors	Late-stage inhibitors	Other inhibitors
• Obstruct its enrolment to membranes • 3-Methyadenine, wortmannin, and LY294002.	• Late-stage inhibitors of vacuolar-ATPase or prevent acidification of lysosomes • Antima larial agents chloroquine, hydroxy-chloroquine, bafilomycin A1, and monensin	• Inhibit autophagosome degradation • Tricyclic antidepressant agent clomipramine and the anti-schistome drug lucanthone

FIGURE 3.6 Classification of autophagy inhibitors.

3.8   AUTOPHAGY INHIBITION IN CANCER THERAPY

Current cancer treatment options, i.e., inhibitors of angiogenesis, growth factor, and receptor enforce metabolic tension; consequently, autophagy inhibitors might be predominantly valuable. Yet traditional surgery, chemotherapy, and radiations disrupt tumors structural design and vascularization, subsequently, leading to higher susceptibility to metabolic tension and therapy using autophagy inhibitors. Autophagy inhibition may support apoptosis under nutrient depressed surroundings (Amaravadi et al., 2007).

3.9   NEW EFFECTIVE INHIBITORS OF AUTOPHAGY

Some of the potent inhibitors of autophagy are listed in Table 3.3:

- Hydroxychloroquine (HCQ) is approved clinically useful inhibitors of autophagy but it fails to reduce autophagy in acidic situations owing to its reduced cellular uptake and *in-vivo* activity (Shi et al., 2017).
- SBI-0206965 is a more potent small molecule which performs through inhibition of autophagy kinase ULK1 resulting in mortality of the tumor cells (Egan et al., 2015).
- Spautin-1 is innovative inhibitor of autophagy which instigates an augment in proteasomal decomposition of class III PI3 kinase complex. It supports the destruction of the PI3 kinase complexes through obstructing Ubiquitin-specific peptidase 10 (USP10) and USP13 (Shao et al., 2014).
- SAR405 is a potent inhibitor of kinases associated with the vacuolar protein sorting protein 18 (Vps18) and Vps34 leading to impairment in lysosomal function followed by distressed vesicle transferring among late endosome as well as lysosome (Pasquier, 2015).
- NSC185058 and NSC377071 are ATG4 inhibitors leading to the impediment of autophagy (Akin et al., 2014).
- Verteporfin acts as an early stage potent inhibitor of autophagy and restrains autophagosome formation (Wu et al., 2016).
- ROC325 is water-soluble dimeric molecule having improved scaffolds of HCQ and lucanthone. It demonstrated advanced lysosome autophagic inhibition in contrast to that of HCQ (Carew et al., 2011).

- Lys05 is a novel inhibitor of lysosomal autophagy which is water-soluble analog of HCQ and enhances anticancer effects of the inhibitors of tyrosine kinase.

TABLE 3.3   Newer Autophagy Inhibitors

Name	Target Point	Mechanism	References
3-Methyladenine	Phosphoinositide 3-kinase (PI3)	Inhibition of autophagosome formation	Wu et al. (2010)
Wortmannin	PI3-kinase		Hansen et al. (1995)
LY294002	PI3-kinase		Avni et al. (2012)
SBI-0206965	ULK1		Egan et al. (2015)
Spautin-1	USP10 and USP13		Liu et al. (2011)
SAR405	Vps18 and Vps34		Pasquier (2015)
NSC185058	ATG4		Akin et al. (2014)
Verteporfin	—	Autophagosome formation and accumulation	Wu et al. (2016)
ROC325	—	Lysosome	Carew et al. (2011)
Lys05	—		Brech et al. (2009)
Chloroquine	—		Cook et al. (2014)
Hydroxychloroquine	—		Cook et al. (2014)

3.10   CONCLUSION

As a cell-rejuvenator and metabolism maintenance of monitoring pathway, autophagy is mandatory for the customary process of cellular as well as organism physiology and health. HCQ's obstructing interaction with lysosome might be causing substandard lysosomes function, which has been identified to instigate lysosomal storage disease. Further, particular autophagy inhibitors are being acquired that could demonstrate to be superior at enhancing chemotherapy remedy in contrast to HCQ. Several imminent guidelines for the development of autophagy-associated cancer therapy comprise improved perception of the duplicitous function of autophagy in tumor survival, the advancement of a molecular marker for autophagic fluctuation in human tumors, the recognition of patient sub-populations that will be generally vulnerable to autophagy inhibition and enhanced perception of the interface of the immune system amid tumor cells.

KEYWORDS

- autophagy
- cancer therapy
- chaperone-mediated autophagy
- endoplasmic reticulum
- macroautophagy
- microautophagy

REFERENCES

Akin, D., Wang, S. K., Habibzadegah-Tari, P., Law, B., Ostrov, D., Li, M., Yin, X. M., Kim, J. S., Horenstein, N., & Dunn, Jr. W. A., (2014). A novel ATG4B antagonist inhibits autophagy and has a negative impact on osteosarcoma tumors. *Autophagy, 10*, 2021–2035.

Amaravadi, R. K., Yu, D., Lum, J. J., Bui, T., Christophorou, M. A., Evan, G. I., Thomas-Tikhonenko, A., & Thompson, C. B., (2007). Autophagy inhibition enhances therapy-induced apoptosis in a Myc-induced model of lymphoma. *J. Clin. Invest., 117*(2), 326–336.

Atlashkin, V., Kreykenbohm, V., Eskelinen, E. L., Wenzel, D., Fayyazi, A., & Fischer, V. M. G., (2003). Deletion of the SNARE vti1b in mice results in the loss of a single SNARE partner, syntaxin 8. *Mol. Cell. Biol., 23*, 5198–5207.

Avni, D., Glucksam, Y., & Zor, T., (2012). The Phosphatidylinositol 3-kinase (PI3K) inhibitor LY294002 modulates cytokine expression in macrophages via p50 nuclear factor κ inhibition, in a PI3K-independent mechanism. *Biochem. Pharmacol., 83*, 106–114.

Axe, E. L., Walker, S. A., Manifava, M., Chandra, P., Roderick, H. L., Habermann, A., Griffiths, G., & Ktistakis, N. T., (2008). Autophagosome formation from membrane compartments enriched in phosphatidylinositol 3-phosphate and dynamically connected to the endoplasmic reticulum. *J. Cell Biol., 182*, 685–701.

Brech, A., Ahlquist, T., Lothe, R. A., & Stenmark, H., (2009). Autophagy in tumor suppression and promotion. *Mol. Oncol., 3*, 366–375.

Bursch, W., Ellinger, A., Kienzl, H., Torok, L., Pandey, S., Sikorska, M., Walker, R., & Hermann, R. S., (1996). Active cell death induced by the anti-estrogens tamoxifen and ICI 164 384 in human mammary carcinoma cells (MCF-7) in culture: The role of autophagy. *Carcinogenesis, 17*, 1595–1607.

Carew, J. S., Espitia, C. M., Esquivel, 2nd J. A., Mahalingam, D., Kelly, K. R., Reddy, G., Giles, F. J., & Nawrocki, S. T., (2011). Lucanthone: A novel inhibitor of autophagy that induces cathepsin D-mediated apoptosis. *J. Biol. Chem., 286*(8), 6602–6613.

Choi, K. S., (2012). Autophagy and cancer. *Exp. Mol. Med., 44*, 109–120.

Chu, C. T., (2008). Eaten alive: Autophagy and neuronal cell death after hypoxia-ischemia. *A. J. Pathol., 172*(2), 284–287.

Codogno, P., & Meijer, A. J., (2005). Autophagy and signaling: Their role in cell survival and cell death. *Cell Death Differ., 12*, 1509–1518.

Cook, K. L., Warri, A., Soto-Pantoja, D. R., Clarke, P. A., Cruz, M. I., Zwart, A., & Clarke, R., (2014). Hydroxychloroquine inhibits autophagy to potentiate anti-estrogen responsiveness in ER+ breast cancer. *Clin. Cancer Res., 20*, 3222–3232.

Cuervo, A. M., (2004). Autophagy: In sickness and in health. *Trends Cell Biol., 14*(2), 70–77.

Darby, A., (2017). *The Autophagy Team.* Available online: https://www.med.uio.no/ncmm/english/news-and-events/profiles/autophagy-team.html (accessed on 23 July 2020).

Egan, D. F., Chun, M. G., Vamos, M., Zou, H., Rong, J., Miller, C. J., Lou, H. J., et al., (2015). Small molecule inhibition of the autophagy kinase ULK1 and identification of ULK1 substrates. *Mol. Cell, 59*, 285–297.

Ertmer, A., Huber, V., Gilch, S., Yoshimori, T., Erfle, V., Duyster, J., Elsässer, H. P., & Schätzl, H. M., (2007). The anticancer drug imatinib induces cellular autophagy. *Leukemia, 21*, 936–942.

Fujita, N., Itoh, T., Omori, H., Fukuda, M., Noda, T., & Yoshimori, T., (2008). The Atg16L complex specifies the site of LC3 lipidation for membrane biogenesis in autophagy. *Mol. Biol. Cell, 19*(5), 2092–2100.

Funderbur, S. F., Wang, Q. J., & Yue, Z., (2010). The Beclin1-VPS34 complex—at the crossroads of autophagy and beyond. *Trends Cell Biol., 20*, 355–362.

Geng, J., & Klionsky, D. J., (2008). The Atg8 and Atg12 ubiquitin-like conjugation systems in macroautophagy. *EMBO Reports, 9*(9), 859–864.

Gills, J. J., Lopiccolo, J., & Dennis, P. A., (2008). Nelfinavir, a new anticancer drug with pleiotropic effects and many paths to autophagy. *Autophagy, 4*(1), 107–109.

Han, J., Hou, W., Goldstein, L. A., Lu, C., Stolz, D. B., Yin, X. M., & Rabinowich, H., (2008). Involvement of protective autophagy in TRAIL resistance of apoptosis-defective tumor cells. *J. Biol. Chem., 283*(28), 19665–19677.

Hanada, T., Noda, N. N., Satomi, Y., Ichimura, Y., Fujioka, Y., Takao, T., Inagaki, F., & Ohsumi, Y., (2007). The Atg12-Atg5 conjugate has a novel E3-like activity for protein lipidation in autophagy. *J. Biol. Chem., 282*(52), 37298–37302.

Hansen, S. H., Olsson, A., & Casanova, J. E., (1995). Wortmannin, an inhibitor of phosphoinositide 3-kinase, inhibits transcytosis in polarized epithelial cells. *J. Biol. Chem., 270*, 28425–28432.

Hoyer-Hansen, M., & Jaattela, M., (2008). Autophagy: An emerging target for cancer therapy. *Autophagy, 4*(5), 574–580.

Huang, S., & Sinicrope, F. A., (2010). Celecoxib-induced apoptosis is enhanced by ABT-737 and by inhibition of autophagy in human colorectal cancer cells. *Autophagy, 6*(2), 256–269.

Ichimura, Y., & Komatsu, M., (2010). Selective degradation of p62 by autophagy. *Semin. Immunopathol., 32*(4), 431–436.

Itakura, E., Kishi, C., Inoue, K., & Mizushima, N., (2008). Beclin 1 forms two distinct phosphatidylinositol 3-kinase complexes with mammalian Atg14 and UVRAG. *Mol. Biol. Cell, 19*(12), 5360–5372.

Jager, S., Bucci, C., Tanida, I., Ueno, T., Kominami, E., Saftig, P., & Eskelinen, E. L., (2004). Role for Rab7 in maturation of late autophagic vacuoles. *J. Cell Sci., 117*, 4837–4848.

Kabeya, Y., Mizushima, N., Ueno, T., Yamamoto, A., Kirisako, T., Noda, T., Kominami, E., et al., (2000). LC3, a mammalian homolog of yeast Apg8p, is localized in autophagosome membranes after processing. *EMBO J., 19*(21), 5720–5728.

Kamada, Y., Yoshino, K., Kondo, C., Kawamata, T., Oshiro, N., Yonezawa, K., & Ohsumi, Y., (2010). TOR directly controls the Atg1 kinase complex to regulate autophagy. *Mol. Cell. Biol., 30*, 1049–1058.

Kimura, S., Noda, T., & Yoshimori, T., (2008). Dynein-dependent movement of autophagosomes mediates efficient encounters with lysosomes. *Cell Struct. Funct., 33*(1), 109–122.

Klionsky, D. J., & Emr, S. D., (2000). Autophagy as a regulated pathway of cellular degradation. *Science, 290*(5497), 1717–1721.

Klionsky, D. J., (2007). Autophagy: From phenomenology to molecular understanding in less than a decade. *Nat. Rev. Mol. Cell Biol., 8*(11), 931–937.

Korolchuk, V. I., Mansilla, A., Menzies, F. M., & Rubinsztein, D. C., (2009). Autophagy inhibition compromises degradation of ubiquitin-proteasome pathway substrates. *Mol. Cell, 33*(4), 517–527.

Kouroku, Y., Fujita, E., Tanida, I., Ueno, T., Isoai, A., Kumagai, H., Ogawa, S., et al., (2007). ER stress (PERK/eIF2alpha phosphorylation) mediates the polyglutamine-induced LC3 conversion, an essential step for autophagy formation. *Cell Death Differ., 14*(2), 230–239.

Kumar, S., & Cakouros, D., (2004). Transcriptional control of the core cell-death machinery. *Trends Biochem. Sci., 29*(4), 193–199.

Lee, I. H., Cao, L., Mostoslavsky, R., Lombard, D. B., Liu, J., Bruns, N. E., Tsokos, M., Alt, F. W., & Finkel, T., (2008). A role for the NAD dependent deacetylase Sirt1 in the regulation of autophagy. *Proc. Natl. Acad. Sci. U.S.A., 105*(9), 3374–3379.

Li, X., & Fan, Z., (2010). The epidermal growth factor receptor antibody cetuximab induces autophagy in cancer cells by down regulating HIF-1alpha and Bcl-2 and activating the beclin 1/hVps34 complex. *Cancer Res., 70*(14), 5942–5952.

Liang, J., Shao, S. H., Xu, Z. X., Hennessy, B., Ding, Z., Larrea, M., Kondo, S., et al., (2007). The energy sensing LKB1-AMPK pathway regulates p27kip1 phosphorylation mediating the decision to enter autophagy or apoptosis. *Nat. Cell Biol., 9*(2), 218–224.

Lippai, M., Csikos, G., Maroy, P., Lukacsovich, T., Juhasz, G., & Sass, M., (2008). SNF4Aγ, the Drosophila AMPK γ subunit is required for regulation of developmental and stress-induced autophagy. *Autophagy, 4*(4), 476–486.

Liu, J., Xia, H., Kim, M., Xu, L., Li, Y., Zhang, L., Cai, Y., et al., (2011). Beclin 1 controls the levels of p53 by regulating the deubiquitination activity of USP10 and USP13. *Cell, 147*, 223–234.

Maiuri, M. C., Tasdemir, E., Criollo, A., Morselli, E., Vicencio, J. M., Carnuccio, R., & Kroemer, G., (2009). Control of autophagy by oncogenes and tumor suppressor genes. *Cell Death Differ., 16*(1), 87–93.

Martens, S., & McMahon, H. T., (2008). Mechanism of membrane fusion: Disparate players and common principles. *Nat. Rev. Mol. Cell. Biol., 9*(7), 543–556.

Matsunaga, K., Morita, E., Saitoh, T., Akira, S., Ktistakis, N. T., Izumi, T., Noda, T., & Yoshimori, T., (2010). Autophagy requires endoplasmic reticulum targeting of the PI3-kinase complex via Atg14L. *J. Cell Biol., 190*(4), 511–521.

Meléndez, A., Tallóczy, Z., Seaman, M., Eskelinen, E. L., Hall, D. H., & Levine, B., (2003). Autophagy genes are essential for dauer development and life-span extension in *C. elegans*. *Science, 301*(5638), 1387–1391.

Mizushima, N., (2007). Autophagy: Process and function. *Genes Dev., 21*, 2861–2873.

Mizushima, N., Levine, B., Cuervo, A. M., & Klionsky, D. J., (2008). Autophagy fights disease through cellular self-digestion. *Nature, 28*(451), 1069–1075.

Nishida, Y., Arakawa, S., Fujitani, K., Yamaguchi, H., Mizuta, T., Kanaseki, T., Komatsu, M., et al., (2009). Discovery of Atg5/Atg7-independent alternative macroautophagy. *Nature, 461*(7264), 654–658.

Noda, T., & Ohsumi, Y., (1998). TOR, a phosphatidylinositol kinase homologue, controls autophagy in yeast. *J. Biol. Chem., 273*(7), 3963–3966.

Ogata, M., Hino, S., Saito, A., Morikawa, K., Kondo, S., Kanemoto, S., Murakami, T., et al., (2006). Autophagy is activated for cell survival after endoplasmic reticulum stress. *Mol. Cell. Biol., 26*(24), 9220–9231.

Okamoto, K., Kondo-Okamoto, N., & Ohsumi, Y., (2009). Mitochondria-anchored receptor Atg32 mediates degradation of mitochondria via selective autophagy. *Dev. Cell, 17*(1), 87–97.

Pasquier, B., (2015). SAR405, a PIK3C3/Vps34 inhibitor that prevents autophagy and synergizes with MTOR inhibition in tumor cells. *Autophagy, 11*, 725–726.

Polager, S., Ofir, M., & Ginsberg, D., (2008). E2F1 regulates autophagy and the transcription of autophagy genes. *Oncogene, 27*(35), 4860–4864.

Rossi, M., Munarriz, E. R., Bartesaghi, S., Milanese, M., Dinsdale, D., Guerra-Martin, M. A., Bampton, E. T., et al., (2009). Desmethylclomipramine induces the accumulation of autophagy markers by blocking autophagic flux. *J. Cell Sci., 122*(18), 3330–3339.

Ruiz-Irastorza, G., Ramos-Casals, M., Brito-Zeron, P., & Khamashta, M. A., (2010). Clinical efficacy and side effects of antimalarials in systemic lupus erythematosus: A systematic review. *Ann. Rheum. Dis., 69*(1), 20–28.

Scherz-Shouval, R., & Elazar, Z., (2007). ROS, mitochondria, and the regulation of autophagy. *Trends Cell Biol., 17*(9), 422–427.

Sekito, T., Kawamata, T., Ichikawa, R., Suzuki, K., & Ohsumi, Y., (2009). Atg17 recruits Atg9 to organize the pre-autophagosomal structure. *Genes Cells, 14*, 525–538.

Shao, S., Li, S., Qin, Y., Wang, X., Yang, Y., Bai, H., Zhou, L., Zhao, C., & Wang, C., (2014). Spautin-1, a novel autophagy inhibitor, enhances imatinib-induced apoptosis in chronic myeloid leukemia. *Int. J. Oncol., 44*, 1661–1668.

Shi, T. T., Yu, X. X., Yan, L. J., & Xiao, H. T., (2017). Research progress of hydroxychloroquine and autophagy inhibitors on cancer. *Cancer Chemother. Pharmacol., 79*, 287–294.

Simonsen, A., & Tooze, S. A., (2009). Coordination of membrane events during autophagy by multiple class III PI3-kinase complexes. *J. Cell Biol., 186*, 773–782.

Tasdemir, E., Maiuri, M. C., Galluzzi, L., Vitale, I., Djavaheri-Mergny, M., D'Amelio, M., Criollo, A., et al., (2008). Regulation of autophagy by cytoplasmic p53. *Nat. Cell Biol., 10*(6), 676–687.

Weidberg, H., Shvets, E., & Elazar, Z., (2011). Biogenesis and cargo selectivity of autophagosomes. *Annu. Rev. Biochem., 80*(1), 125–156.

Williams, A., Sarkar, S., Cuddon, P., Ttofi, E. K., Saiki, S., Siddiqi, F. H., Jahreiss, L., et al., (2008). Novel targets for Huntington's disease in an mTOR-independent autophagy pathway. *Nat. Chem. Biol., 4*(5), 295–305.

Wong, P. M., Puente, C., Ganley, I. G., & Jiang, X., (2013). The ULK1 complex sensing nutrient signals for autophagy activation. *Autophagy, 9*(2), 124–137.

Wood, J. G., Rogina, B., Lavu, S., Howitz, K., Helfand, S. L., Tatar, M., & Sinclair, D., (2004). Sirtuin activators mimic caloric restriction and delay ageing in metazoans. *Nature, 430*(7000), 686–689.

Wu, H. M., Shao, L. J., Jiang, Z. F., & Liu, R. Y., (2016). Gemcitabine-induced autophagy protects human lung cancer cells from apoptotic death. *Lung, 194*, 959–966.

Wu, Y. T., Tan, H. L., Shui, G., Bauvy, C., Huang, Q., Wenk, M. R., Ong, C. N., et al., (2010). Dual role of 3-methyladenine in modulation of autophagy via different temporal patterns of inhibition on class I and III phosphoinositide 3-kinase. *J. Biol. Chem., 285*, 10850–10861.

Yorimitsu, T., & Klionsky, D. J., (2005). Autophagy: Molecular machinery for self-eating. *Cell Death Differ., 12*, 1542–1552.

Yorimitsu, T., Zaman, S., Broach, J. R., & Klionsky, D. J., (2007). Protein kinase A and Sch9 cooperatively regulate induction of autophagy in *Saccharomyces cerevisiae*. *Mol. Biol. Cell, 18*(10), 4180–4189.

Zhong, Y., Wang, Q. J., Li, X., Yan, Y., Backer, J. M., Chait, B. T., Heintz, N., & Yue, Z., (2009). Distinct regulation of autophagic activity by Atg14L and Rubicon associated with beclin 1-phosphatidylinositol-3-kinase complex. *Nat. Cell Biol., 11*(4), 468–476.

Zhu, K., Dunner, Jr. K., & McConkey, D. J., (2010). Proteasome inhibitors activate autophagy as a cytoprotective response in human prostate cancer cells. *Oncogene, 29*(3), 451–462.

CHAPTER 4

Transthyretin Protein in Renowned Metastatic and Other Conditions

SANDEEP ARORA, TAPAN BEHL, and KIRANJEET KAUR

Chitkara College of Pharmacy, Chitkara University, Punjab, India

ABSTRACT

Cancer is a group of disorders involving rapid abnormal growth and division of cells in the body. It can be triggered on exposure to certain intoxicants like tobacco, alcohol radiations, but mainly mutations in genes lead to a rise in severe disorders of malignancies. Several therapeutic agents have been identified till date to suppress cancer and its progression. Transthyretin (TTR) is a protein in the serum and cerebrospinal fluid that moves the thyroid hormone thyroxine (T4) and retinol-binding protein-bound to retinol. The alterations in human TTR genes for their use in diagnosis as a biomarker in various types of cancer and management of diverse oncogenic disorders has been discussed in this review. TTR stabilizes protein production, which can be beneficial in suppressing the production of tumor cells producing proteins. Transthyretin is made up of the choroid plexus and can be used as an efficient immunohistochemical marker for the determination of choroid plexus papilloma as well as carcinomas. This leads to insignificant cell growth and further invasion of body tissues. Imposing of T4 binding protein strengthens transthyretin tetramer, hampering its neutrality to amyloid genic single units. Various active measures are under study to diminish and prevent the risk of cancer, and probably studying the TTRs can prove to be an efficient therapeutic approach.

4.1 INTRODUCTION

Transthyretin (TTR) is a protein in the serum and cerebrospinal fluid that moves the thyroid hormone thyroxine (T4) and retinol-binding protein-bound to retinol (Buxbaum and Reixach, 2009). It was initially known as Prealbumin, which was produced by the TTR gene (Herbert et al., 1986). It's fabricated predominantly in the liver, and some part of it is produced in the brain area named choroid plexus and also in the back of the eye called retina (Goodman, 1986). The name itself suggests about its transport properties, so the function of this protein is to haul hormone thyroxine and vitamin A, i.e., retinol, in the body. The transportation of thyroxine is perpetrated by TTR in the form of the tetramer, i.e., four units of protein get attached to one another. Likewise, for the transport of Retinol (Vitamin A) tetramer of TTR forms, which additionally gets attached with retinol-binding protein. TTR is a protein created by the TTR gene. Cancer is a group of disorders involving rapid abnormal growth and division of cells in the body. It can be triggered on exposure to certain intoxicants like tobacco, alcohol radiations, but mainly mutations in genes lead to a rise in severe disorders of malignancies. Several therapeutic agents have been identified till date to suppress cancer and its progression. In this chapter, the alterations in human TTR genes for their use in diagnosis as a biomarker in various types of cancer and management of diverse oncogenic disorders will be studied.

4.2   TRANSTHYRETIN AND CANCER

Cancer is a group of disorders that mainly comprise of uncontrolled and irrational growth and division of cells that further invade other regions of the body, worsening the condition of the patient. Consumption of tobacco and alcohol covers the major cause of cancer, but it may also be induced by exposure to certain environmental toxins, allergens, ionizing radiation, obesity, poor diet, etc. The causes may be genetically fostered as well, such as mutations in the genetic makeup of any individual. TTR protein's thorough nucleotide sequence was determined by Kanda et al. in 1974. The protein comprises of analogous 127 amino acids systematized in tetramer with a molecular mass of about 14 kDa. The monomer of TTR molecule contains eight β-strands characterized as A-H and E, F has a short helix. Two antiparallel four-stranded b-sheets consisting of DAGH and CBEH strands, respectively, form a wedge-shaped b-barrel, in which b-strands are arranged. Two TTR molecules form dimer by attaching end-to-end, balanced by antiparallel H-bonds between H-H and F-F strands (Kingsbury et al., 2007). TTR dimer has a marked concave shape, comprised of two eight stranded sheets. Total body potassium and total body nitrogen and levels are expressed in blood concentration reflecting transthyretin in embryonic growth in adult life. The body's nitrogen balance is copied by serum TTR concentration so precisely that it is applied as an indicator of malnutrition and inflammation in various cases. The concentrations of TTR serve as a potential biomarker in the detection of ovarian cancer as well. This has proved to be a great hallmark in the treatment and management of ovarian cancer as the survival rate of patients suffering with it is very low (10–30%) (Schweigert and Sehouli, 2005).

TTR stabilizes protein production, which can be beneficial in suppressing the production of tumor cells producing proteins. The levels of retinol, triiodothyronine, thyroxine, and retinol-binding protein in the circulating fluid are checked by protein TTR as indicated by Episkopou et al. in 1993. On account of TTR being a transporter of retinol and thyroxine, two analogs of T4 attach with the central cavity of the TTR molecule and contribute to the stability of TTR tetramer production of hence slowing the process of dissociation. Rodents have an enhanced rate of transthyretin than primates indicated in terms of evolution (Dorus et al., 2004). Amyloidotic polyneuropathy, amyloidotic vitreous opacities, euthyroid hypertyrosinemia, cardiomyopathy, meningocerebrovascular amyloidosis, oculoleptomeningeal amyloidosis, carpal tunnel syndrome, etc., diseases are caused by the transfiguration of proteins. TTR could be an organic detoxing agent, because the T4 linking plot coheres minuscule molecules with replaced aromatic rings bound by connectors of various chemical conformation, including structures such as stilbenes, flavones, benzoxazoles, tetrahydroquinolines, etc.

Developing proofs describe that WT transthyretin could additionally have a defensive outcome in senile dementia via combining with the amyloid genic Ab-amyloid peptide (Wisniewski et al., 1995). Nerve physiology and increased nerve regeneration are influenced by this protein in the mouse. In the peripheral nervous system of convalescent with TTR-FAP, there is a deposition of altered TTR conglomerates (Westermark and Pathol, 1998). Transformation of TTR causes amyloidosis because of extracellular precipitation of amyloid fibrils established by genesis and misfolding of proteins that lead to compromised organ function. The volume of serum TTR enhances till adolescence and becomes stable till 60 years of life, and then diminishes with the increase in age. Serum TTR functions as a serviceable clinical marker of acute systemic disorder mostly to under-nutrition and infections, because of selectivity to painfulness and nutritional status (Lumeij, 2008). Disorders related to TTR are hereditary amyloid polyneuropathy (FAP) and cardiomyopathy (Connors et al., 2011). Hereditary amyloid polyneuropathy is an inherited autosomal governing disorder that happens due to the accumulation of amyloid aggregates of TTR; the focus is mostly on infected peripheral nerves. Portugal faced this anomaly first, in victim anguishing from inherent amyloidosis caused by peripheral polyneuropathy and autonomic dysfunction (Benson, 2013). In the process of accumulation, the rate terminating of amyloid fibril formation is caused by TTR tetramer segregation, whilst a biased misfolding of the single unit must occur to incite amyloid genesis. The significance of this disorder is manifested in sexual impotence, dyshidrotic, alternating diarrhea and constipation, urinary incontinence, and orthostatic hypotension. Ataxia, seizures, dementia, convulsion, spastic paralysis, visual deterioration, and hemorrhage could be the end. Mutations cause disability to the architecture of TTR protein. Hence conformational changes occur that lead to the distinction of the tetramers into fractionated unfolded forms, which gets self-aggregated into amyloid fibrils. The stability of TTR is affected by both temperature and pressure (Schwarzman et al., 1994). The levels of TTR can also be used in the detection of lung cancer, and patients suffering with lung cancer and lung infection can be easily differentiated. Patients victimized with cancer of lungs exhibited augmented concentrations of TTR in the pleural effusion and serum. TTR has been synthesized in lungs, and on certain infection, their levels fall due to malproduction of TTR, but in cases of lung cancer, the concentrations of TTR rise remarkably and also migrate to fulfill deficient TTR needs enabling better resolution between lung cancer and lung infection (Ding et al., 2014).

A condition of eosinophilic, homogeneous, congophilic characters getting in the cardiac atria and ventricles is known as senile cardiac amyloidosis (SCA). Other parts, like lungs, guts, etc., also have been impacted by these aggregations, and are called senile systemic amyloidosis (SSA) (González-López et al., 2015). Congestive heart failure and arrhythmias are end results of this disease. Atrial and ventricular accumulation occurs as well. The progenitor of both the amyloid aggregation is different. Atrial amyloid aggregates are established from atrial natriuretic factor (ANF), while ventricular aggregates occur from the serum protein TTR. TTR is also connected with autoimmune disorders. IA, i.e., Juvenile idiopathic arthritis, is a very general pediatric rheumatological situation (Gaspari et al., 2011). It is an autoimmune condition. JIA has affected around three lakh youngsters in the United States manifestations comprise persistent joint pain, inflammation, and rigidity that can remain for a handful of months to a lifespan and has no remedy for it. TTR can also be used efficiently in demolishing symptoms of cancer and impart relief to the patient by successfully arresting cell growth and prevent tumor growth and malignancy. The second most leading cause of cancer death in colorectal carcinoma (CRC). With the help of the SELDI-TOF-MS technique, the levels of TTR protein and C3a-desArg in the serum of patients can be identified, which leads to an advanced diagnosis of colorectal cancer and better therapeutic opportunities (Fentz et al., 2007).

For controlling indications and convolutions, therapies like biologic response modifiers and anti-inflammatory drugs (NSAIDs) are used. The predisposition of TTR to accumulate, for a little enhancement in TTR genesis or half-life, easily gets the protein out of solution (Page and Henry, 2000). Also, this protein has molecular protection, which is an antigenic target for B and T cell immune responses. Amyloid aggregates of TTR originated in the synovial membrane of these victims (Lester and Susan, 2010). It is ventured that joints get affected by familial amyloidosis, whose other symptoms are JIA. The amplified viscosity of a synovial fluid is due to enhancement in concentration and aggregation of TTR. Inflammation also fastens the genesis of reactive oxygen species (ROS), further increasing TTR aggregation (Stadtman, 1995). Protein aggregation is caused by the antigen-presenting cells causes by phagocytosis; the outcome is that there is potential growth in the antigenic load and number of MHC II epitopes. Amyloid formation and direct complement activation are incited by protein accumulation. Depletion in serum TTR concentration is comparable with other patients having various TTR alterations related to FAC or FAP as reported in presymptomatic black American bearer (Lundblad, 2005). The greater fraction of the protein is fabricated in the liver due to the minor susceptibility of non-mutant TTR to misfold as compared to other mutant cells. It is complex to understand why serum TTR concentrations are diminished in convalescent with TTR amyloidosis with alteration and not in persons accumulated with the tissue of the non-mutant protein. With aging, possibility is there that the intensified serum IL-6 volume visible in senior people might be accountable for the common curtailment in serum TTR. Right now, there is no established treatment for TTR-familial amyloidosis (Sekijima, 2015). Various conventional chemotherapeutic agents are under use, which successfully manage symptoms of cancer. TTR can be used alone or in combination with conventional therapies to prohibit cancer growth. In this chapter, we introduce TTR as an emerging therapy in the management of cancer via misfolding of proteins and its ability to prevent disease by adapting to protein homeostasis and ameliorating the network of cancer growth.

Only symptomatic relief is provided by available two treatments which treat TTR-FAP due to unusual or non-operating proteins. Liver transplantation (LT) was the first curative commencement to eradicate TTR-FAP, hence helped in removing the etiological factor TTR mutant by liver. This leads to the removal of 98% mutated TTR, resulting in the success of this therapy, yet it continued to have some drawbacks such as persistent amyloid fibril exposure from wild-type (WT) TTR, which leads to ailment advancement in some convalescent. A mutant TTR tetramer was substituted with an indigenous allele having enhanced stability and less amyloid genic properties by doing orthotropic LT utilizing givers carrying two WT TTR genes to terminate the increase of polyneuropathy in convalescent with TTR-FAP as reported by Holmgren et al. (1994). Although, LT is a life-threatening methodology needing immunosuppressive treatment forever and has bounded relevancy to a cautiously designated section of particularly Val30Met convalescent (non-elderly) with the premature-stage disease, and superior nutritional stature (Gomes, 2011). Other therapeutic pathways are hence also relevant apparent. Wild type TTR can dissociate, misfold, and aggregate, producing point mutations within it which destabilize the mutant TTR subunit comprising tetramer and facilitate dissociation that is more facile and/or misfolding and amyloidogenesis. TTR also binds to beta-amyloid protein and prevents its natural tendency to accumulate into the plaques serving beneficial effects in the early stages of Alzheimer's disease and enables the cell to rid itself from toxic protein.

4.3   USES OF TAFAMIDIS

TTR is made up of the choroid plexus and can be used as an efficient immunohistochemical marker for the determination of choroid plexus papillomas as well as carcinomas. This leads to insignificant cell growth and further invasion of body tissues. Imposing of T4 binding protein strengthens TTR tetramer, hampering its neutrality to amyloid genic single units. Imprecisely, 50% of TTR transmitting in lifeblood is deficient of a confined ligand (Diao et al., 2010). All these monitored facts provide a strong hypothesis on the evolution of little molecule ligands, which stick to the predominantly uninhabited T4 binding sites. When cancer is initiated, no symptoms are detected earlier. Although non-steroidal anti-inflammatory drugs are related with cardiac and renal side effects, the use of benzoxazole carboxylic acids came to light. Hence, there is an obligation that can alter the development of this disease. Tafamidis has surfaced as the latest benchmark for the treatment of patients with TTR-FAP as approved in several countries in Latin America and the Asia-Pacific and the European Union (Bulawa et al., 2012).

Deceleration of disease advancement in convalescent heterozygous for the V30M TTR alteration was displayed by Tafamidis meglumine (F×1006A), having currently accomplished phase 2/3 trials in the remedy of TTR-FAP and it was suitable for fortifying the two most remarkable alteration, V122I TTR and Val30Met, in a similar way as it stabilized WT TTR, including thirty other amyloid genic types of TTR. The pace of tetramer segregation at physiological pH is reduced dose-dependently by Tafamidis, which is thoroughly attached to plasma proteins along with glucuronidation being the chief metabolic mechanism; the main flowing configuration in plasma is originator compound.

One dose of 20 mg of Tafamidis was instantaneously absorbed in normal subjects. 2.0 hr was the precisely recorded median time (Tmax) to attain the maximum concentration (Cmax) (Coelho et al., 2013). Absorption of Tafamidis is diminished once taken along with food, but overall absorption is not affected. Evidence of a deficiency of metabolic induction or blockade due to Tafamidis was reported as the Pharmacokinetic stipulations that were comparable after one or continuous dosing. The mean half-life of precisely 59 h makes the termination slow. Steady-state was effectuated from day fourteen, at a daily dose of 20 mg Tafamidis for 14 days, with Cmax and Cmin at 2.7 and 1.6 lg/mL, respectively. Kinetic perpetuality was provided to avoid recurrence of disease. Tafamidis coheres specifically and with negative collaboration with the two ordinarily uninhabited thyroxine-linking areas of the tetramer, and kinetically neutralizes TTR. The dissociative activation barrier, which is the rate-limiting step in amyloid genesis, is enhanced by Tafamidis. Also, fibrils are usually found in perceivable pathology in many amyloid diseases. Hence has some evidence of a possibility of the pathway of amyloid fibril formation, showing nonfibril transitions, that are etiological factors of proteotoxicity (Barroso et al., 2014).

Since various epigenetic modifications can be established in patients with cancers, the manifestation of DNA repair genes and proteins reduced involvement of particular importance. Such alterations happen in the early stages of cancer progression and cause genetic instability. The repair of DNA is suppressed. Hence, for ideal therapy, preference is given to pausing the amyloid genic cascade at an early stage—that is, the scale-controlling stage of the process that is presumed to be the shattering of tetramers to monomers. Progress of clinical trials on Tafamidis was based on the speculation that TTR neutralization would result in undiminished amyloid aggregates along with decreased neuro-degeneration (Ueda, 2014). Inter-allelic trans suppression, averted by FAP commencement, and Tafamidis

TTR union enhances the energy barrier for tetramer detachment, hindering fibril generation for mutating in physiologic situations. Clinical potency was shown by kinetic stabilizer in phase 2/3 clinical test of patients Tafamidis in V30M TTR-FAP convalescent. Convalescent administered with Tafamidis had 52% low neurologic perversion, 53% and 80% conservancy of big- and compact-nerve fiber action, and augmented nutritional rank. All this helped in raised quality of life as compared to victims acquiring placebo and this was due to TTR neutralization, efficiency, and harmlessness of the therapy (Lozeron et al., 2013).

4.4   TAFAMIDIS IN JUVENILE IDIOPATHIC ARTHRITS (JIA)

Various active measures are undertaken to diminish and prevent the risk of cancer. Risk factors are hard to determine based on a compact number of convalescents treated with tafamidis. Symptoms of underlying disease constitute 5% of the adverse effects. With the clinical investigation process in midway for TTR-FAC, Tafamidis is the solo certified pharmacotherapy for the cure of initial TTR-FAP on the basis of tolerability outline and patients for prolonged use, and so it has many profits in convalescent with TTR amyloidosis. Determining disease in convalescents at a premature stage for the onset of tafamidis treatment precedent to the considerable aggregation of amyloid in the organs and nerves is of high value. A conclusion was drawn that TTR is the main factor to transfer diverse molecules in bloodstream and cerebral spinal liquid, and aggregation of TTR leads to JIA, from the latest research for anomalous assembling of proteins in the blood and synovial fluid of JIA convalescent. It was reported that JIA patients have much-increased concentrations of TTR and antibodies against TTR as compared with the control subjects (Peeters et al., 2017). This new research proved its efficiency to augment the quality of life for children suffering with Juvenile Idiopathic Arthritis, and the UK has around 15,000 patients enrolled in trials. JIA ruins about three lakhs lives of children in the United States. A genetic testing of individuals suffering with cancer is also highly recommended.

Evidences consist of chronic joint pain, abscess, and rigidity, remaining for some months or a lifetime. The cure is not possible. Therapies like NSAIDs indicate and avoid aggravation. France was the 1st country in September 2011 to certify Tafamidis as medicine for convalescent with stage one TTR-FAP to reduce illness development (Merlini et al., 2013). Therapy has to be started and observed by a skillful doctor. Every six-month, an overall multisystem pathway is utilized, and opinion is generated to continue with Tafamidis and finding a new drug consisting of LT. Judgments to alter therapy are decided on a rise in pathologic stage and developed Val30Met TTR-FAP, and it could not terminate disease development such as NIS and disability. Tafamidis is utilized for a nonsurgical remedy probability or TTR-FAP (Ericzon et al., 2015). Tafamidis will presumably find a more important use as a drug capable of postponing or arresting TTR-FAP expression by reducing abnormal and irrational cell growth as much as possible in the future. However, this will be possible only on its proper use at the correct time.

KEYWORDS

- **atrial natriuretic factor**
- **familial amyloid polyneuropathy**
- **liver transplantation**
- **senile cardiac amyloidosis**
- **senile systemic amyloidosis**
- **transthyretin**
- **wild-type**

REFERENCES

Barroso, F., et al., (2014). Long term effects of tafamidis treatment on transthyretin familial amyloid polyneuropathy (TTR-FAP): Interim results from the F×1A-303 study. *Eur. J. Neurol.*, 21–81.

Benson, M. D., (2013). *Emery and Rimoin's Principles and Practice of Medical Genetics* (6ᵗʰ edn., pp. 1–18). 79.2.1.2.

Bulawa, C. E., Connelly, S., De Vit, M., Wang, L., Weigel, C., Fleming, J. A., Wilson, I. A., et al., (2012). Tafamidis, a potent and selective transthyretin kinetic stabilizer that inhibits the amyloid cascade. *Proceedings of the National Academy of Sciences*, 109(24), 9629–9634.

Buxbaum, J. N., & Reixach, N., (2009). Transthyretin: The servant of many masters, *Cell Mol Life Sci.*, 66, 3095–3101.

Coelho, T., Maia, L. F., Da Silva, A. M., Cruz, M. W., Planté-Bordeneuve, V., Suhr, O. B., Labaudiniere, R., et al., (2013). Long-term effects of tafamidis for the treatment of transthyretin familial amyloid polyneuropathy. *Journal of Neurology*, 260(11), 2802–2814.

Connors, L. H., Doros, G., Sam, F., Badiee, A., Seldin, D. C., & Skinner, M., (2011). Clinical features and survival in senile systemic amyloidosis: comparison to familial transthyretin cardiomyopathy. *Amyloid.*, 18(1), 157–159.

Diao, H., Xiao, S., Cui, J., Chun, J., Xu, Y., & Ye, X., (2010). Progesterone receptor-mediated up-regulation of transthyretin in preimplantation mouse uterus. *Fertility and Sterility*, *93*(8), 2750–2753.

Ding, H., Liu, J., Xue, R., Zhao, P., Qin, Y., Zheng, F., & Sun, X., (2014). Transthyretin as a potential biomarker for the differential diagnosis between lung cancer and lung infection. *Biomedical Reports*, *2*(5), 765–769.

Dorus, S., Vallender, E. J., Evans, P. D., Anderson, J. R., Gilbert, S. L., Mahowald, M., et al., (2004). Accelerated evolution of nervous system genes in the origin of Homo sapiens. *Cell*, *119*(7), 1027–1040.

Episkopou, V., Maeda, S., Nishiguchi, S., Shimada, K., Gaitanaris, G. A., Gottesman, M. E., & Robertson, E. J., (1993). Disruption of the transthyretin gene results in mice with depressed levels of plasma retinol and thyroid hormone. *Proceedings of the National Academy of Sciences*, *90*(6), 2375–2379.

Ericzon, B. G., Wilczek, H. E., Larsson, M., Wijayatunga, P., Stangou, A., Pena, J. R., et al., (2015). Liver transplantation for hereditary transthyretin amyloidosis: After 20 years, still the best therapeutic alternative. *Transplantation*, *99*(9), 1847–1854.

Fentz, A. K., Spörl, M., Spangenberg, J., List, H. J., Zornig, C., Dörner, A., et al., (2007). Detection of colorectal adenoma and cancer based on transthyretin and C3a-desArg serum levels. *PROTEOMICS-Clinical Applications*, *1*(6), 536–544.

Gaspari, S., Marcovecchio, M. L., Breda, L., & Chiarelli, F., (2011). Growth in juvenile idiopathic arthritis: The role of inflammation. *Clinical and Experimental Rheumatology-Incl Supplements*, *29*(1), 104.

Gomes, R. A., (2011). *Beyond Genetic Factors in Familial Amyloidotic Polyneuropathy: Protein Glycation and the Loss of Fibrinogen's Chaperone Activity.*

Gonzalez-Lopez, E., Gallego-Delgado, M., Guzzo-Merello, G., De Haro-Del, M. F. J., Cobo-Marcos, M., Robles, C., et al., (2015). Wild-type transthyretin amyloidosis as a cause of heart failure with preserved ejection fraction. *European Heart Journal*, *36*(38), 2585–2594.

Goodman, D. S., (1986). Statement regarding nomenclature for the protein known as prealbumin, which is also (recently) called transthyretin, Springer, Boston, MA. In: *Amyloidosis* (pp. 287–288).

Herbert, J., Wilcox, J. N., Pham, K. T. C., Fremeau, R. T., Zeviani, M., Dwork, A., et al., (1986). Transthyretin: A choroid plexus-specific transport protein in human brain: The (1986). S. Weir Mitchell Award. *Neurology*, *36*(7), 900–900.

Holmgren, G., Costa, P. M., Andersson, C., Asplund, K., Steen, L., Beckman, L., et al., (1994). Geographical distribution of TTR met30 carriers in northern Sweden: Discrepancy between carrier frequency and prevalence rate. *Journal of Medical Genetics*, *31*(5), 351–354.

Kanda, Y., Goodman, D. S., Canfield, R. E., & Morgan, F. J., (1974). The amino acid sequence of human plasma prealbumin. *Journal of Biological Chemistry*, *249*(21), 6796–6805.

Kingsbury, J. S., Theberge, R., Karbassi, J. A., Lim, A., Costello, C. E., & Connors, L. H., (2007). Detailed structural analysis of amyloidogenic wild-type transthyretin using a novel purification strategy and mass spectrometry. *Analytical Chemistry*, *79*(5), 1990–1998.

Lester, M. D., & Susan, C., (2010). PhD. In: *Manual of Pathological Surgery, Bone, and Joints.*

Lozeron, P., Theaudin, M., Mincheva, Z., Ducot, B., Lacroix, C., & Adams, D., (2013). French Network for FAP (CORNAMYL). Effect on disability and safety of Tafamidis in late onset of Met30 transthyretin familial amyloid polyneuropathy. *European Journal of Neurology*, *20*(12), 1539–1545.

Lumeij, J. T., (2008). *Clinical Biochemistry of Domestic Animals* (6th edn.). Avian Clinical Biochemistry.

Lundblad, R. L., (2005). Considerations for the use of blood plasma and serum for proteomic analysis. *The Internet Journal of Gastroenterology*, 1.

Merlini, G., Plante-Bordeneuve, V., Judge, D. P., Schmidt, H., Obici, L., Perlini, S., et al., (2013). Effects of tafamidis on transthyretin stabilization and clinical outcomes in patients with non-Val30Met transthyretin amyloidosis. *Journal of Cardiovascular Translational Research*, *6*(6), 1011–1020.

Page, J., & Henry, D., (2000). Consumption of NSAIDs and the development of congestive heart failure in elderly patients: An under-recognized public health problem. *Arch Intern. Med., 160*, 777–784.

Peeters, J., Boltjes, A., Vervoort, S., Coffer, P., Vastert, B., Van, W. F., Van, L. J., et al., (2017). Epigenetic profiling of juvenile idiopathic arthritis (JIA) synovial fluid monocytes points towards a role for monocytes in bone damage. 111 River ST, Hoboken 07030-5774, NJ USA: Wiley. In: *Arthritis and Rheumatology* (Vol. 69, pp. 200–201).

Schwarzman, A. L., Gregori, L., Vitek, M. P., Lyubski, S., Strittmatter, W. J., Enghilde, J. J., et al., (1994). Transthyretin sequesters amyloid beta protein and prevents amyloid formation. *Proceedings of the National Academy of Sciences*, *91*(18), 8368–8372.

Schweigert, F. J., & Sehouli, J., (2005). Transthyretin, a biomarker for nutritional status and ovarian cancer. *Cancer Research*, *65*(3), 1114.

Sekijima, Y., (2015). Transthyretin-type cerebral amyloid angiopathy: A serious complication in post-transplant patients with familial amyloid polyneuropathy. *J. Neurol. Neurosurg. Psychiatry, 86*, 124.

Stadtman, E. R., (1995). The status of oxidatively modified proteins as a marker of aging. In: Esser, K., & Martin, G. M., (eds.), *Molecular Aspect of Aging* (pp. 129–143).

Ueda, M., & Ando, Y., (2014). Recent advances in transthyretin-amyloidosis therapy. *Transl. Neurodegener., 3*, 19.

Westermark, P., & Pathol, A. J., (1998). *The Pathogenesis of Amyloidosis: Understanding General Principles, 152*, 1125–1127.

Wisniewski, E., et al., (1995). Fibrillogenesis of Alzheimer's amyloid peptides and apolipoproteins E. *Biochem., 306*, 599–604.

CHAPTER 5

Role of CXCR4 Receptor Protein in Cancer Development and Therapies

SANDEEP ARORA and K. A. SHAIMA

Chitkara College of Pharmacy, Chitkara University, Punjab, India

ABSTRACT

CXCR4 is a chemokine receptor. Chemokines are 8 to 12 KD polypeptides (a linear organic polymer which consists of a large number of amino-acid residues bonded together in a chain, forming part of (or the whole of) a protein molecule) that contain two internal disulfide loops. There are 11 distinct receptors for CC chemokines (CCR1-CCR11) and 6 receptors for CXC chemokines (CXCR1-CXCR6). Chemokine receptors are expressed on the leucocytes with the greatest number of distinct chemokine receptors seen on the T cells. Receptors show cellular expression patterns and chemokines overlapping specificity within each subfamily that determines which cell type responds to which chemokines.

5.1 INTRODUCTION

CXCR4 is one of the chemokine receptors. Chemokines are a large family of structurally homologous cytokines (proteins secreted by the cells of innate and adaptive immunity) that regulate leukocytes movement and migration of leukocytes from blood to tissues. Chemokine receptors are part of a super-family of class A seven-transmembrane guanine nucleotide-binding protein, or G protein-coupled receptors (GPCRs). Chemokine receptors are the binding site for chemokines, and they produce desired effects in the human body (Table 5.1) (Zlotnik et al., 2000).

TABLE 5.1 Chemokine Receptor and its Function

Chemokine Receptor	Ligand (Chemokine)		Function
	Original Name	Systematic Name	
CXCR4	SDF-1	CXCL 12	1. Mixed leucocyte recruitment
			2. HIV Coreceptor

5.2 STRUCTURE OF HUMAN CXCR4

All chemokines are 8 to 12 KD polypeptides that contain two internal loops of disulfide. On the basis of location and number of N terminal cysteine residue, chemokines are classified following families (Murphy et al., 2000).

Families of chemokines:

1. **CC Chemokines:** Cysteine residues are adjacent.
2. **CXC Chemokines:** Cysteine residues are separated by one amino acid.

In inflammation:

*   *CXC chemokines act mainly on neutrophils.
*   *CC chemokines act mainly on monocytes, lymphocytes, and eosinophils.

There have been eleven different CC chemokine (CCR1-CCR11) as well as 6 CXC chemokine (CXCR1-CXCR6) receptors. Chemokine receptors are expressed on the leucocytes with the greatest number of distinct chemokine receptors that are part of T cells. Receptors show cellular expression patterns and chemokines overlapping specificity within each subfamily that determines which cell type responds to which chemokines.

Chemokine receptors exhibit structural characteristics with α helical domain transmembranes. This characteristic is seen in other receptors that are coupled to trimeric guanosine triphosphate (GTP)-binding protein (G proteins), and such receptors belong to the family of G protein-coupled receptors (GPCRs). While occupied by ligand, these receptors act as GTP exchange proteins, catalyzing the replacement of bound guanosine diphosphate (GDP) by GTP. Various cellular enzymes and cellular locomotion get stimulated by these forms of G protein that are associated with GTP. Chemokine receptors may get quickly down-regulated (the process of reducing or suppressing a response to a stimulus) by chemokines exposure. So this could likely be the mechanism for terminating receptors (Balkwill, 2004).

Human CXCR4 can bind to various ligands. The molecule is described as similar to a wine glass wedged in the cell membrane with the ligand-binding site as the glass opening 10. Figure 5.1 shows two molecules of CXCR4 contributing to the formation of a ligand-binding site which is fully occupied by the CVX15 peptide. CXCR4 is made up of 63% alpha-helices, 4% beta-sheets, and 33% random coils, and contains 502 residues in its homodimeric state. It has a molecular weight of 113,782.06 Da and an isoelectric point (pI) of 8.47. The main fold of CXCR4 contains seven transmembrane alpha-helices connected by six loops. Three loops are extracellular while the other three are intracellular. The first two extracellular domains and their associated loops do not seem to serve a functional purpose. The N-terminal domain is specific for ligand binding and the C-terminal domain is in the cytoplasm. The protein shares certain structural properties that are characteristic of chemokine receptors. The extracellular portion has a net negative charge under physiological conditions, while the intracellular portion has many serine and threonine residues which act as sites for phosphorylation. Further, chemokine receptors are classified in part by a short basic third intracellular loop, a short N-terminus, and a cysteine in each of the four extracellular domains (Zlotnik, 2006).

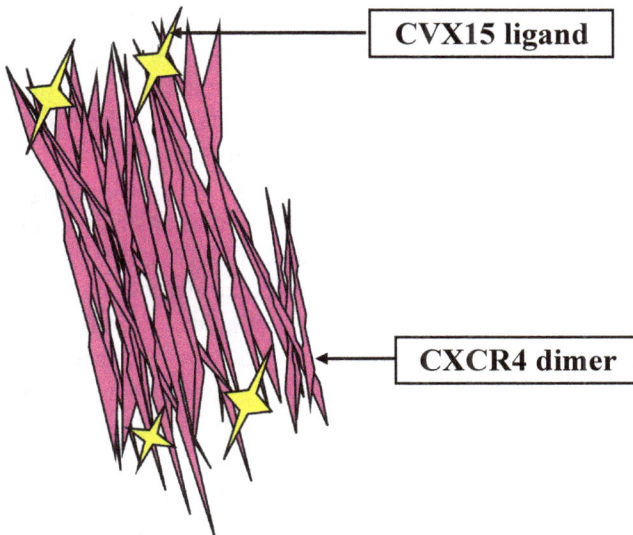

FIGURE 5.1   CXCR4 binding with CVX15 ligand.

5.3   AGONISTS FOR CXCR4 RECEPTOR

There are three endogenous proteins that bind to CXCR4 (Zou et al., 1998).

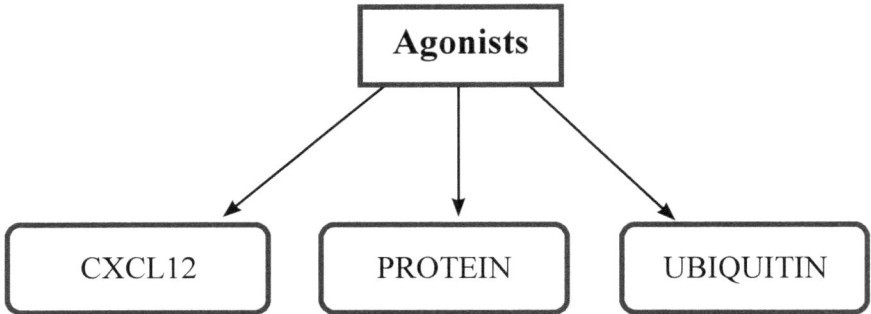

```
              ┌─────────────────┐
              │    Agonists     │
              └─────────────────┘
            ↙          ↓          ↘
┌──────────────┐ ┌──────────────┐ ┌──────────────┐
│   CXCL12     │ │   PROTEIN    │ │  UBIQUITIN   │
└──────────────┘ └──────────────┘ └──────────────┘
```

5.3.1   CHEMOKINE CXCL12

Binding of the CXCL12 ligand to CXCR4 increases intracellular calcium ion (Ca^{2+}) levels and reduces cellular cyclic adenosine monophosphate (cAMP) production. The mechanism for intracellular signaling of chemokine receptors is complex. The receptors are coupled with a heterotrimeric G protein by their C-terminal domain. After binding with the chemokine, signaling from CXCR4 causes a dissociation of the G protein into two distinct subunits, each of which activates effectors. The effectors then act as signal transducers and physiological process regulators. Researchers believe that the chemokine activation of GPCRs takes place at two sites. The first site is the N-terminal domain of the receptor and the second site is the N-terminal domain of the chemokine. After binding at both sites, the G-protein signal pathway is activated. The first site, the extracellular N-terminal domain of CXCR4, must undergo sulfonation at Tyr-7, Tyr-12, and Tyr-21. This post-translational modification is critical to high-affinity binding of the receptor to CXCL12, but is less important for binding of the receptor to HIV gp120. Two other methods of post-translational modification are present in CXCR4. Glycosylation, which occurs at Asn-11, Ser-18, and Asn-176 (zoomed in), seems to have no specific function for the protein. Phosphorylation at the following sites affects the modulation of CXCR4 signaling and receptor desensitization: Ser-319, Ser-321, Ser-324, Ser-325, Ser-330, Ser-339, Ser-348, and Ser-351. The ligand-binding pocket in CXCR4 is created in part by two disulfide bonds, between Cys-28 and Cys-274, and Cys-109 and Cys-186. The basic residue Lys-1 in CXCL12, a critical site for receptor activation, is thought to interact with the acidic residuesAsp-187,

Glu-288, and Asp-97 of CXCR4. Additionally, the sequence DRYLAIVHA is found between Asp-33 and Ala-140. Some version of this sequence is found in the second intracellular loop of all chemokine receptors and is critical to the binding of G proteins.

5.3.2   UBIQUITIN

Ubiquitin may be another natural ligand for the CXCR4 receptor. Ubiquitin is a natural component of plasma which acts as a post-translational protein modifier, and its extracellular functions have only recently been investigated. Patient treatment with ubiquitin is linked to a decrease in inflammation and organ injury. The ubiquitin and CXCR4 complex causes a cellular response similar to that induced by the CXCL12 and CXCR4 complex, namely increased Ca^{2+} levels and a reduction of cAMP levels.

CXCR4 is found in cells from more than 23 types of cancer. It is thought to promote metastasis, angiogenesis, and tumor growth, furthering the disease. In areas of the tumor, growth CXCR4 is found both on the surface and inside of cells and its physiological migration induces tumor proliferation. The cell migration is greatly influenced by lipid rafts, which are membrane regions enriched in lipids, as well as other transmembrane proteins. It is possible that these molecules in the membrane may interfere with the chemokine-receptor interactions through an antagonist approach. Certain transmembrane proteins lead to the blockage of the CXCL12/CXCR4 binding site, resulting in a reduction of tumor growth and angiogenesis.

5.3.3   PROTEIN GP120

Envelope glycoprotein GP120 (or gp120) is a glycoprotein exposed on the surface of the HIV envelope. The 120 represents its molecular weight of 120 kDa. Gp120 plays a critical role in attachment to specific cell surface receptors and thus facilitating viral entry into the cell. Viral entry is started when the strain binds to CD4 and promotes a conformational change in the HIV subunit gp120. The conformational change exposes the V3 loop of the virus, thus causing a second conformational change in gp120 by interacting with the chemokine receptor. This conformational change directs viral entry into the cell membrane of the host cell.

5.4   ANTAGONIST FOR THE CXCR4/CXCL12 COMPLEX (ABBAS ET AL., 2000)

The structure and function of CXCR4 show great promise in the therapeutic drug industry. Approximately 40% of globally distributed medications are designed to control GPCRs. Drug-like molecules are blocking the formation of natural receptor-ligand complexes. With a reduction in such complexes, there should be a reduction in metastasis or viral entry into host cells. However, little progress has been made in the field of x-ray structures of drug-receptor complexes associated with CXCR4. Despite this setback, there are many drugs currently in development that target the chemokine receptor, and advances in bioinformatics and computer modeling are crucial to their development.

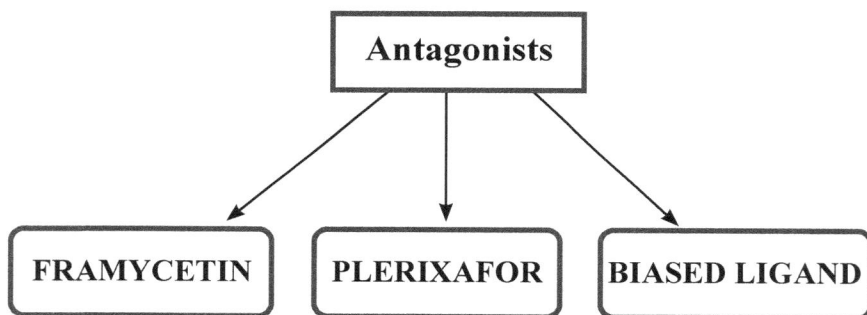

```
                    ┌─────────────────┐
                    │   Antagonists   │
                    └─────────────────┘
         ┌──────────────────┼──────────────────┐
         ▼                  ▼                  ▼
┌─────────────────┐ ┌─────────────────┐ ┌─────────────────┐
│   FRAMYCETIN    │ │   PLERIXAFOR    │ │  BIASED LIGAND  │
└─────────────────┘ └─────────────────┘ └─────────────────┘
```

5.4.1   FRAMYCETIN

Framycetin acts as an antagonist for the CXCR4/CXCL12 complex. It is used to treat bacterial eye infections.

5.4.2   PLERIXAFOR

Plerixafor will block the CXCR4/CXCL12 complex and is used as a hematopoietic stem cell mobilizer. The drug regulates the release of stem cells from the bone marrow into the blood for the treatment of multiple myeloma and non-Hodgkin lymphoma. These produced stem cells may be collected to replace cells that are destroyed by chemotherapy.

5.4.3   BIASED LIGAND

Biased ligand activates only one of the two pathways associated with CXCR4. Biased ligands are advantageous because they can induce desired therapeutic effects while not affecting pathways which may be associated with side effects.

5.5   LOCATION

Currently, there are 19 known human chemokine receptors, which are found in leukocytes and human tissue. Chemokine receptors are present in the following cells (Zou et al., 1998):

- hematopoietic cells;
- endothelial cells;
- epithelial cells;
- hepatocytes;
- neurons; and
- astrocytes.

5.6   PHYSIOLOGICAL ACTIONS (MURPHY ET AL., 2000)

1.   **Anti-Inflammatory Function:**

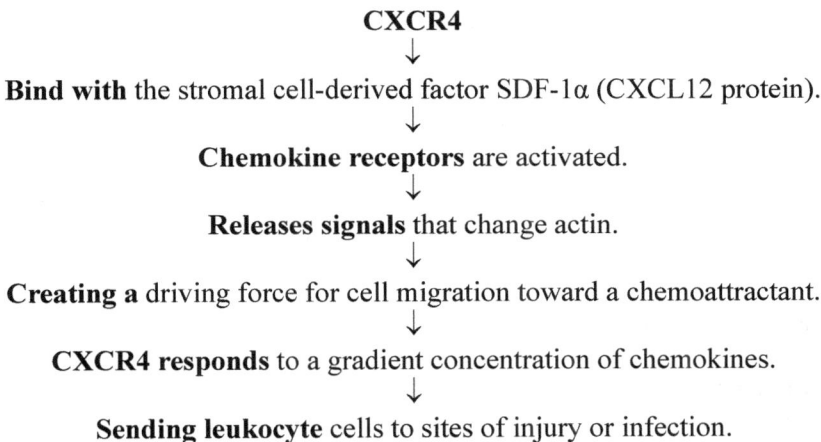

CXCR4
↓
Bind with the stromal cell-derived factor SDF-1α (CXCL12 protein).
↓
Chemokine receptors are activated.
↓
Releases signals that change actin.
↓
Creating a driving force for cell migration toward a chemoattractant.
↓
CXCR4 responds to a gradient concentration of chemokines.
↓
Sending leukocyte cells to sites of injury or infection.

2. **HIV Entry:** In order to reach the cell, HIV requires attaching to a chemokine co-receptor. One of several key co-receptors associated in HIV entry is CXCR 4. The development of a complex CD4-gp120 induces conformative modifications within viral envelope, which enables this to connect with CCR5 or CXCR4.
3. **Angiogenesis:** In tumorigenesis, the CXCL12-CXCR4 axis plays a crucial role in facilitating angiogenesis as well as tumor cell migration towards metastatic sites.
4. **Tumor Growth and Metastasis:** The signaling axis of the CXCR4-CXCL12 chemokine maintains tumor cell proliferation and regulates distant metastasis development.
5. **Development of Nervous System Inflammation:** In leukocytes as well as tumor cells, CXCR4 is a key mediator for cell migration. Throughout evolution with functional origins in the formation of several organ systems, including the immune as well as central nervous systems (CNS), CXCR4 is the evolutionarily conserved chemokine receptor.

5.7   CXCR4 IN DISEASE STATES (ZLOTNIK ET AL., 2000)

5.7.1   CXCR4 AND DEVELOPMENTAL DEFECTS

CXCR4 is articulated by cells of the immune systems and CNS. It binds with CXCL12 also called stromal development factor 1 (SDF1) in the extracellular matrix. This particular binding is important in early embryonic development stages of vascular, nervous, hematopoietic, and cardiac systems. Bone marrow defects and cardiac dysfunction may be caused with errors in the CXCR4/CXCL12 interaction during embryonic stage. Moreover, this interaction is equally concerned during the mature phase of life, where it is important for the direction of hematopoietic precursor cells in the bone marrow.

5.7.2   CXCR4 AND HIV

Acquired immune deficiency syndrome (AIDS) is a disease caused by human immunodeficiency virus (HIV). The interaction between lentivirus and the human cell is the etiology behind AIDS. Here a compromised immune system plants the host susceptible to opportunistic, viral, and bacterial infections.

HIV virus is using the receptors such as CXCR4 and CCR5 for the entering into host T cells. CXCR4 is the key receptor facilitating viral entry for the HIV strain HIV2. CXCR4 can function as a co-receptor for T-cell line-adapted HIV-1 viral entry into CD4$^+$ host cells, and is the main receptor for some HIV-2 isolates. Approximately half of the AIDS population experiences a physiological co-receptor switch from R5 HIV-1, a strain which uses CCR5, to X4 HIV-1, a strain which uses CXCR4. This transition to the X4 strain usually leads to advancement of AIDS, and therefore correlates to a worse prognosis. This is because the R5 strain can infect both T cells and macrophages, but the X4 strain can infect T cells only due to the coexpression of CD4 and CXCR4 and is essentially required. Viral entry is started when the strain binds to CD4 and causes a conformational change in the HIV subunit gp120. The conformational change exposes the V3 loop of virus, which interacts with chemokine receptor to cause a second conformational change in gp120. This second conformational change directs viral entry into the host cell membrane. G-protein signaling appears to be absent from this mechanism.

5.7.3   CXCR4 AND WHIM SYNDROME

WHIM syndrome is defined as group of immunodeficiency disorders comprising hypogammaglobulinemia, infection, warts, Myelokathexis syndrome (neutrophils are retained in bone marrow). CXCR4 mutations is the main reason for this syndrome, where the carboxy terminus is shortened by cutting off the residues between the 10th and 19th, causing the receptor to continue in an activated state. There is more prone to occur in bacterial and viral infections in patients with this rare disorder. The development of warts is due to human papillomavirus infection. A reduction in gamma globulins leads to reduced immunity.

5.7.4   CXCR4 AND CANCER

CXCR4 has been identified as imparting the main role in cancer, including lung, breast colon, ovary, bone marrow, and bladder. The oncogenic cell retaining in tissues that are more in CXCL12 and enables growth and metastasis of tumors because the receptor in cancer cell interacts with CXCL12(as in normal cells). In some tumors, the reason for metastasis is found to be the overexpression of CXCR4 receptor. Worse prognosis is one of the disadvantages in Lung and breast cancer patients with overexpressed CXCR4.

5.8 DISCUSSION

Upon binding with CXCR4, SDF-1α and ubiquitin increase intracellular Ca^{2+} levels and reduce cAMP production. This results in the migration of leukocytes to damaged areas of the body and acts as a critical immune response. However, binding with the receptor can also have deleterious effects to humans. The immune response can cause tumor growth and metastasis in cancer patients, and the HIV-1 protein can enter a host cell upon binding with the receptor. Many other molecules act as antagonists, blocking the natural binding of CXCR4. These antagonists have prospective use as therapeutic drug agents, and are currently under development in labs worldwide. As more information on the structure and function of CXCR4 becomes known, many new therapeutic strategies will be unlocked. CXCR4 is part of the exciting and ever-growing field of GPCR research.

5.9 SUMMARY

To understand the structure and interactions of CXCR4 is absolutely important for successful drug development. The emerging role of CXCR4 inhibitors in novel therapeutics for the treatment of the diseases should be documented.

KEYWORDS

- acquired immune deficiency syndrome
- cyclic adenosine monophosphate
- guanosine diphosphate
- guanosine triphosphate
- human immunodeficiency virus
- stromal development factor 1

REFERENCES

Abbas, A. K., & Lichtman, A. H., (2000). *Cellular and Molecular Immunology* (Vol. 255, p. 467). China: Saunders.

Balkwill, F., (2004). Cancer and the chemokine network. *Nat. Rev. Cancer, 4*(7), 540–550.

Murphy, P. M., Baggiolini, M., Charo, I. F., Hebert, C. A., Horuk, R., Matsushima, K., Miller, L. H., et al., (2000). International union of pharmacology. XXII. Nomenclature for chemokine receptors. *Pharmacol. Rev., 52*(1), 145–176.

Zlotnik, A., & Yoshie, O., (2000). Chemokines: A new classification system and their role in immunity. *Immunity, 12*(2), 121–127.

Zlotnik, A., (2006). Involvement of chemokine receptors in organ-specific metastasis. *Contrib. Microbiol., 13*, 191–199.

Zou, Y. R., Kottmann, A. H., Kuroda, M., Taniuchi, I., & Littman, D. R., (1998). Function of the chemokine receptor CXCR4 in hematopoiesis and in cerebellar development. *Nature, 393*(6685), 595–599.

CHAPTER 6

C3D Complement System in Immunotherapy-Based Cancer Treatment

SANDEEP ARORA, NIDHI GARG, and POOJA SHARMA

Chitkara College of Pharmacy, Chitkara University, Punjab, India

ABSTRACT

Despite the major advances in the understanding of the immunological basis of cancer, cancer is still a serious public health issue that causes many deaths around the world. Most of the cancer patients do not show a response to the treatment and die from metastatic disease. In addition to being a component of innate immunity and an ancient defense mechanism against invading pathogens, complement activation also participates in the adaptive immune response, inflammation, hemostasis, embryogenesis, and organ repair and development. Complement activation end products and their receptors mediate cell-cell interactions that regulate several biological functions in the extravascular tissue. As a result, complement activation in the tumor microenvironment enhances tumor growth and increases metastasis. In this review, we discuss the immune and non-immune functions of complement proteins and the tumor-promoting effect of complement activation. This review discusses these issues with a view to inspiring the development of new agents that could be useful for the treatment of cancer.

6.1 INTRODUCTION

Cancer can be defined as a serious public health issue that causes many deaths around the world (Alwan et al., 2010). In females, breast cancer is very common, and in males, mouth cancer is very common (WHO, 2008). The most frequently detected cancers caused in females are breast cancer and in males is lung cancer (WHO, 2004). Despite major development in the chemotherapeutic management of the disease, most of the cancer patients do not show response to the treatment and die from metastatic disease. There are severe side effects associated with cancer chemotherapy. Extraordinary effectiveness has been shown by some rationally targeted therapies (Liu, 2009). The immune modulation of cancer therapies has also been conducted (Arnold, 2004; Janeway, 1989).

The unfamiliar microorganisms and other detrimental material congregated in the body of humans are cleared by our immune system. Innate immunity and acquired immunity are the two main parts of the immune system which complement each other. The response of the immune system, which proceeds rapidly and is able to condemn peculiar matter without a precursory association with the conquering creatures, can be defined as an innate immunity response. Removal of internal debris engendered by mutilated cells or tissues can also be done by it. B and T lymphocytes comprise the acquired immunity. Specificity and immunological memory are the two important features of the acquired immunity. An acquired immune response is very distinct against the attacker. The most important element of innate immunity is the C system. Cells that cause phagocytoses like macrophages, cytokines, and natural killer cells work beside this system. C1q, after getting bound to immune complexes, triggers the C pathway (Kawai and Akira, 2010).

Tumor cells are recognized as foreign before the stimulation of cytolytic effector mechanisms. Genetic mutations and other alterations take place in the process of malignant transformation. For host immune reactions, these antigens serve as target tumor-antigens. The extent of keeping emerging tumors away is not known. The immune system possesses the power to ambush the cells of the tumor. Not only the immune machinery but the complement (C) system is efficacious in the eradication of tumor cells. But the immune attack must be properly targeted and triggered for the eradication of tumor cells.

6.2   THE COMPLEMENT (C) SYSTEM

The above system plays a very vital character in the mediation of inflammatory responses and in the elimination of foreign pathogens. Protection of the individuals from a variety of microbial infections is done by the C system. Biological 'self' from 'non-self' is recognized by the C system. The activation of C is aimed against the accepted targets. Protein-protein interactions are responsible for the activation of the C system by generating amplified activation reactions. C regulators regulate the activation of the complement because an immoderate, unconstrained activation may cause harm to autologous cells, more than the required consumption of C components and to inflammation. Many features of inflammation and tissue damage are caused by the C system. The target structures get opsonized, by the invigoration of C products like C1q, C4b, etc. C-receptors and Fc-receptors remark the surface placed C3b, its immobilized form, and immunoglobulins. The recognition causes the exhilaration of phagocytes and the inundation of targets.

The cleavage of C3 and C5 by C3/C5 convertases is a very important step in activating the C. C3a, and C5a are bioactive molecules which are proficient in acting as anaphylatoxins and chemotoxins (Köhl, 2007). The enhancement in vascular permeability and smooth muscle cell contraction also through them (Wills-Karp, 1999). The antibody-mediated humoral B cell immune is directed by C3d. C3b (CR1) and C3d (CR2) receptors are expressed by B cells. The brink for the triggering and development of B cells falls gradually in the presence of C. Antibody responses are induced by C.

6.3 PATHWAYS OF COMPLEMENT ACTIVATION

Immunoglobulins (IgG, IgM) activate the classical pathway (CP) in case they are bound to a suitable target surface. CRP and the complexes formed between the polyanion and polycation activate the CP.

Activation of complement pathways
• Classical
• Alternative
• Lectin

Autoactivation of the alternate pathway (AP) of C occurs at a decreased level in plasma. In the case of encountering a peculiar surface, the activation proceeds and becomes boosted with the help of an affirmative feedback loop (Hu et al., 1995).

The inceptive signals and the triggering paths are not the same among the three pathways, but the generation of C3b remains the same. The three activation routes integrate into a typical terminal pathway (TP) after C5 cleavage. In the triggering, management, and authorization of C, 35 proteins are involved. C proteins, which act in plasma, are 18 in number, membrane-bound regulators are four in number, regulators which act in the fluid phase are seven in number, and six C receptors are held to cell membranes. The role played by the five FH-related proteins is still not understood (Center et al., 2011; Vera-Llonch et al., 2006).

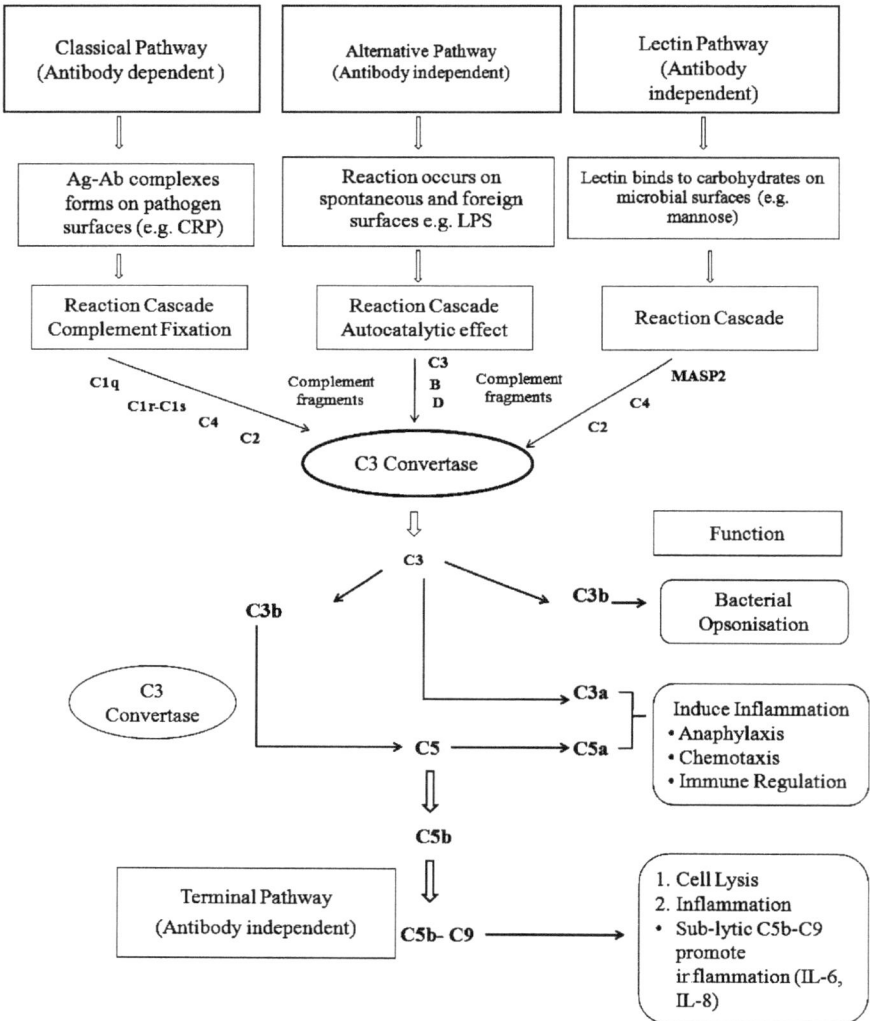

FIGURE 6.1   Various pathways of compliment activation

6.3.1 CLASSICAL PATHWAY (CP)

CP activation is commenced when C1q binds to the Fc. In the binding of C1r and C1s molecules to C1q, C1 complex is formed. Therefore, C1s splinters C4 and C2 by acting as an active enzyme. The binding of the 25-product formed by cleavage to C4b to cell surface leads to the formation of the C4bC2 complex (Ricklin et al., 2010). Amplification is caused by the formation of further C3b via the AP.

Factors causing CP activation
• C-reactive protein
• Serum amyloid P component
• Cardiolipin

6.3.2 ALTERNATIVE PATHWAY (AP)

Activation of AP occurs in plasma at a short rate because of the extemporaneous hydrolysis of C3 to C3 (H_2O). C3b molecules bind covalently to adjacent activating surfaces, if unveiled groups like hydroxyl or amino groups are present. C3 molecules are cleaved to C3b fragments by C3 convertase which in turn leads to binding to neighboring areas and behaves as small units for C3 or C5 convertases. Convertase is sustained by properdin. Properdin acts as a positive C regulator. Monocytes and neutrophils are responsible for synthesizing properdin at the sites of inflammation (Holers, 2014; Merle et al., 2015).

6.3.3 LECTIN PATHWAY (LP)

This pathway is generated when one of the mannose-binding lectins gets binded to targeted carbohydrates (Takahashi et al., 2006). It forms an enzyme complex (Haurum et al., 1993).

6.3.4   TERMINAL PATHWAY (TP)

C5, C6, C7, C8, and C9 proteins comprise the TP. C5 convertases generate C5b which can cohere to C6 and C7 in the aqueous phase. C7 molecule can bind the hydrophobic complex to cell membranes. The confining of C8 and C9 molecules from the aqueous phase occurs by C5b-7 complex and initiation of formation of the membrane attack complex occurs (Haurum et al., 1993; Kawasaki et al., 1978). A transmembrane pore is generated when the complement membrane attack complex is formed (Estabrook et al., 2004). Osmotic cell lysis may occur.

6.4   COMPLEMENT REGULATION

Here, 11 out of 40 proteins regulate the triggeration whereas properdin acts as an inhibitor. The regulators consist of both the cellular membrane-bound and regulators of the aqueous phase.

6.4.1   MEMBRANE REGULATORS OF COMPLEMENT

To prevent C, all host cells revealed to C require advanced protection procedures. Specific membrane inhibitors which restrict the activity of C protect human cells against C-mediated damage are present (Berends et al., 2015; Jore et al., 2016).

Various proteins which restrict activity of C protect human cells
• Complement Receptor Type 1 (CR1; CD35
• Membrane Cofactor Protein (MCP; CD46)
• Decay Accelerating Factor (DAF; CD55)
• Protectin (CD59)

6.4.2   SOLUBLE COMPLEMENT REGULATORS

Soluble C regulators hinder the excessive C activation. C1 inhibitor (C1INH) and C4b-binding protein (C4bp) occur as foremost distinguished soluble regulators of CP. C1r and C1s serine esterases are inactivated by C1INH. MASP serine proteases of the LP are also inhibited.

C3b and C4b are inactivated by Factor I. The regulation of AP is done by FH and FHL-1. The activation of TP is prevented by Vitronectin and clusterin. There is prevention of lodging of C5b-7 to the target cell membrane (Scharfstein et al., 1978).

6.4.3   FACTOR H (FH)

Soluble FH controls the C activation in the fluid phase. The liver, monocytes, and macrophages synthesize Factor H (FH). The essential steps in AP activation are controlled by FH. The binding of FH to host cells causes AP downregulation. AP activation is limited when FH interacts with the C3b-polyanion complex. Serious consequences can occur by lack of FH, as the protection of basement membranes (BM) of kidney glomeruli depends on FH. C regulators DAF and MCP are lacked in BM. C-mediated membranoproliferative glomerulonephritis can be caused by FH deficiency (Villiers et al., 1983; Dahlback et al., 1983).

Sites for FH binding
• SCRs1-4
• SCRs8-15
• SCRs19-20

6.5   COMPLEMENT ACTIVATION IN CANCER CELLS

Procurement in genetic and epigenetic alterations accompanies the malignant transformation. Cell-surface proteins, glycosylation, and phospholipids patterns are changed (Jemal et al., 2010). Innate and adaptive immune mechanisms are able to recognize cancer-related membrane modifications and the host is protected against cancer (Vathipadiekal et al., 2012). Elimination, equilibrium, and escape are the three phases in immune editing theory (Berkenblit and Cannistra, 2005). Tumor cells enter an equilibrium period if they are able to pass the phase of elimination. There is no evidence if the complement can eliminate nascent tumors. The triggeration of complement in people affected with cancer has been reported in many clinical studies. The expansion of complement pursuit occurring in cancer patients is the other evidence of complement activation. C5 is deposited and the active product C5a is generated. The major promoter in triggering of complement on immunized TC-1 cervical cancer cells is the CP (Sasaroli et al., 2009). The elements of the CP are deposited by the follicular and MALT lymphomas (Meyer and Rustin, 2000) and in affected people with persistent lymphocytic leukemia, the alterations of this pathway have been described (His et al., 2011). The alternative pathway is actuated by lymphoma and myeloma cells (Delecluse, 1997).

In patients with colorectal cancer, the lectin pathway (LP) is increased (Swerdlow et al., 2016). An eccentric antigenic identity and a typical profile are possessed by each tumor. A variety of activation pathways occur due to complement recognition molecules and regulators. Complement activation pathways make the things more difficult. By the action of the extrinsic pathway, C5a is produced by the lung cancer cells in the absence of serum (Swerdlow et al., 2008).

Various markers such as complement components and their triggering products are being initiated (Swerdlow et al., 2008). Elevated measure of complement proteins and activation specks are present in lung cancer patients (Swerdlow et al., 2008; Takahashi et al., 2006). Increased complement levels correlate with lung tumor size (Meyer and Rustin, 2000). In people affected with other tumors, complement-related proteins are increased (Delecluse et al., 1997; Swerdlow et al., 2008, 2016). In patients with persistent lymphocytic leukemia, a positive association is noticed among the endurance time and the commencing pursuit of the CP (Colomo et al., 2004).

6.5.1   PROMOTION OF CANCER GROWTH BY COMPLEMENT

The complement system recognizes the cancer cells which are related with an effector pursuit that destroys cells of the tumor. Various strategies are being developed to elevate complement activation in the ambiance of therapy of the immune system. Growth is stimulated by the complement when cells are served with little congregation of antitumor antibodies (Dougan and Dranoff, 2009). Complement elements recognize cancer cells and create a selective pressure. In a syngeneic mouse model of cervical cancer, the role of complement in cancer was proposed. Impaired tumor growth is caused by complement deficiencies (Colomo et al., 2004). This seminal observation is seen in mouse models. Significant reduction in tumor progression occurs when tumor cells overexpress C5a. Tumor growth is regulated by the complement activation.

6.5.2 ROLE OF COMPLEMENT SYSTEM IN TUMOR-ASSOCIATED INFLAMMATION

Harmful stimuli are removed from the organism by inflammation. Tumor immune surveillance is caused by persistent inflammation. Mycobacterium bovis triggers inflammation which impairs bladder cancer progression. Antitumor T-cell responses cause permeation of various leukocytes (Dougan and Dranoff, 2009).

Multiple hallmarks are caused by tumor-associated inflammation. Defense against neoplastic cells is caused by acute responses; neoplastic transformation is caused by sustained inflammation. The possibility of having lung cancer can be due to exposure to tobacco smoke, radon, and asbestos. Complement plays an important role in inflammation. Strong immune effectors like anaphylatoxins C5a and C3a are generated by complement breakdown reactions. Potent chemoattractants are anaphylatoxins. In the pathogenesis of some chronic inflammatory diseases, deregulated complement activity is involved (Ribas, 2012). Altered cells are identified by complement in cancer.

The expression of TGF-β is stimulated by the complement activity. Pro- and antitumor effects are displayed by TGF-β. Activation of the complement plays a crucial role in the stromal accumulation of cytokines and growth factors. The plasticity of tumors in adapting to different physiological conditions is an important feature. Hypoxia is related to inflammation of the tumor (Ricklin et al., 2010). Complement activity is increased in hypoxic conditions due to breakdown in FH (Markiewski and Lambris, 2009), and as a result, C5a and other proinflammatory molecules are generated.

KEYWORDS

- alternate pathway
- basement membranes
- C1 inhibitor
- C4b-binding protein
- classical pathway
- factor H
- immunoglobulins G
- lectin pathway
- terminal pathway

REFERENCES

Alwan, A., et al., (2010). Monitoring and surveillance of chronic non-communicable diseases: Progress and capacity in high-burden countries. *The Lancet, 376*, 1861–1868.

Arnold, L., Henry, A., Poron, F., Baba-Amer, Y., Van, R. N., Plonquet, A., Gherardi, R. K., & Chazaud, B., (2007). Inflammatory monocytes recruited after skeletal muscle injury switch into anti-inflammatory macrophages to support myogenesis. *J. Exp. Med., 204*, 1057–1069.

Berends, E. T. M., Gorham, R. D., Ruyken, M., et al., (2015). Molecular insights into the surface-specific arrangement of complement C5 convertase enzymes. *BMC Biol., 13*, 9.

Berkenblit, A., & Cannistra, S. A., (2005). Advances in the management of epithelial ovarian cancer. *J. Reprod. Med., 50*, 426–438.

Castillo, J. J., Winer, E. S., Stachurski, D., et al., (2010). Clinical and pathological differences between human immunodeficiency virus-positive and human immunodeficiency virus-negative patients with plasmablastic lymphoma. *Leukemia and Lymphoma, 51*(11), 2047–2053.

Center, M., Siegel, R., & Jemal, A., (2011). *American Cancer Society Global Cancer: Facts and Figures*.

Colomo, L., Loong, F., Rives, S., et al., (2004). Diffuse large B-cell lymphomas with plasmablastic differentiation represent a heterogeneous group of disease entities. *American Journal of Surgical Pathology, 28*(6), 736–747.

Dahlback, B., (1983). Purification of human C4b-binding protein and formation of its complex with vitamin K-dependent protein S. *Biochem. J., 209*, 847–856.

Delecluse, H. J., Anagnostopoulos, I., Dallenbach, F., et al., (1997). Plasmablastic lymphomas of the oral cavity: A new entity associated with the human immunodeficiency virus infection. *Blood, 89*(4), 1413–1420.

Dougan, M., & Dranoff, G., (2009). Immune therapy for cancer. *Annu. Rev. Immunol., 27*, 83–117.

Estabrook, M. M., Jack, D. L., Klein, N. J., & Jarvis, G. A., (2004). Mannose-binding lectin binds to two major outer membrane proteins, opacity protein, and porin, of *Neisseria meningitidis*. *J. Immunol., 172*(6), 3784–3792.

Ezzati, M., Lopez, A. D., Rodgers, A. A., & Murray, C. J., (2004). *Comparative Quantification of Health Risks: Global and Regional Burden of Disease Attributable to Selected Major Risk Factors*. World Health Organization.

Haurum, J. S., Thiel, S., Haagsman, H. P., Laursen, S. B., Larsen, B., & Jensenius, J. C., (1993). Studies on the carbohydrate-binding characteristics of human pulmonary surfactant-associated protein A and comparison with two other collections: Mannan-binding protein and conglutinin. *Biochem. J., 293*(Pt 3), 873–878.

Holers, V. M., (2014). Complement and its receptors: New insights into human disease. *Annu. Rev. Immunol., 32*, 433–459.

Hsi, E. D., Lorsbach, R. B., Fend, F., & Dogan, A., (2011). Plasmablastic lymphoma and related disorders. *American Journal of Clinical Pathology, 136*(2), 183–194.

Hu, Y., Benedict, M. A., Wu, D., Inohara, N., & Nunaez, G., (1995). Bcl-xL interacts with Apaf-1 and inhibits Apaf-1-dependent caspase-9 activation. *Proc. Natl. Acad. Sci. U.S.A., 95*, 4386–4391.

Janeway, C. A. Jr., (1989). Approaching the asymptote: Evolution and revolution in immunology. *Cold Spring Harb. Symp. Quant. Biol., 54*, 1–13.

Jemal, A., Siegel, R., Xu, J., & Ward, E., (2010). Cancer statistics, 2010. *CA Cancer J. Clin., 60*, 277–300.

Jore, M. M., Johnson, S., Sheppard, D., et al., (2016). Structural basis for therapeutic inhibition of complement C5. *Nat. Struct. Mol. Biol., 23*, 378–386.

Kawai, T., & Akira, S., (2010). The role of pattern-recognition receptors in innate immunity: Update on toll-like receptors. *Nat. Immunol., 11*, 373–384.

Kawasaki, T., Etoh, R., & Yamashina, I., (1978). Isolation and characterization of a mannan-binding protein from rabbit liver. *Biochem. Biophys. Res. Commun., 81*(3), 1018–1024.

Köhl, J., & Wills-Karp, M., (2007). Complement regulates inhalation tolerance at the dendritic cell/T cell interface. *Mol. Immunol., 44*(1–3), 44–56.

Liu, F. S., (2009). Mechanisms of chemotherapeutic drug resistance in cancer therapy: A quick review. *Taiwanese Journal of Obstetrics and Gynecology, 48*(3), 239–244.

Markiewski, M. M., & Lambris, J. D., (2009). Is complement good or bad for cancer patients?: A new perspective on an old dilemma. *Trends Immunol., 30*, 286–292.

Mathers, C., (2008). *The Global Burden of Disease: 2004 Update*. Geneva, World Health Organization.

Merle, N. S., Church, S. E., Fremeaux-Bacchi, V., & Roumenina, L. T., (2015). Complement system part I-molecular mechanisms of activation and regulation. *Front Immunol., 6*, 262.

Meyer, T., & Rustin, G. J., (2000). Role of tumor markers in monitoring epithelial ovarian cancer. *Br. J. Cancer, 82*, 1535–1538.

Ribas, A., (2012). Tumor immunotherapy directed at PD-1. *N Engl. J. Med., 366*, 2517–2519.

Ricklin, D., Hajishengallis, G., Yang, K., & Lambris, J. D., (2010). Complement: A key system for immune surveillance and homeostasis. *Nat Immunol., 11*(9), 785–797.

Sasaroli, D., Coukos, G., & Scholler, N., (2009). Beyond CA125: The coming of age of ovarian cancer biomarkers. Are we there yet? *Biomark. Med., 3*, 275–288.

Scharfstein, J., Ferreira, A., Gigli, I., et al., (1978). Human C4-binding protein: Isolation and characterization. *J. Exp. Med., 148*, 207–222.

Swerdlow, S. H., Campo, E., Harris, N. L., et al., (2008). *Who Classification of Tumors of Haematopoietic and Lymphoid Tissues.* Lyon, France: IARC Press.

Swerdlow, S. H., Campo, E., Pileri, S. A., et al., (2016). The 2016 revision of the world health organization classification of lymphoid neoplasms. *Blood, 127*(20), 2375–2390.

Takahashi, K., & Ezekowitz, R. A., (2005). The role of the mannose-binding lectin in innate immunity. *Clin. Infect. Dis., 41*(7), S440–S444.

Takahashi, K., Ip, W. E., Michelow, I. C., & Ezekowitz, R. A., (2006). The mannose-binding lectin: A prototypic pattern recognition molecule. *Curr. Opin. Immunol., 18*(1), 16–23.

Vathipadiekal, V., Saxena, D., Mok, S. C., Hauschka, P. V., Ozbun, L., & Birrer, M. J., (2012). Identification of a potential ovarian cancer stem cell gene expression profile from advanced stage papillary serous ovarian cancer. *PLoS One, 7*, e29079.

Vera-Llonch, M., Oster, G., Hagiwara, M., & Sonis, S., (2006). Oral mucositis in patients undergoing radiation treatment for head and neck carcinoma: Risk factors and clinical consequences. *Cancer: Interdisciplinary International Journal of the American Cancer Society, 106*(2), 329–336.

Villiers, M. B., Reboul, A., Thielens, N. M., et al., (1983). Purification and characterization of C4-binding protein from human serum. *FEBS Letters, 132*, 49–53.

Wills-Karp, M., (1999). Immunologic basis of antigen-induced airway hyperresponsiveness. *Annu. Rev. Immunol., 17*(9), 255–281.

CHAPTER 7

BH3 Mimetics

SANDEEP ARORA, SUKHBIR SINGH, and NEELAM SHARMA

Chitkara College of Pharmacy, Chitkara University, Punjab, India

ABSTRACT

Apoptosis is the mortality of cells that take place as evolutionally conserved practice and controlled stage of an organism's growth, tissue homeostasis, and act as resistance to oncogenic alteration. This chapter summarizes the role of BH3 domains in the apoptosis pathway during cancer disease as well as strategies for the design of BH3 mimetic and their underlying principle for targeting tumors. Previously characterized BH3 mimetic, i.e., ABT-737 and ABT-263 (navitoclax), obatoclax (GX15-070), gossypol family, and S1 are briefly described in this chapter. Several new putative BH3 mimetic, i.e., ABT-199 (venetoclax), BIM SAHB (BIM Stabilized α-helix of BCL-2 domains), MIM 1, BAM 7, BI-97D6, S1 derivative, BH3-M6, poly-quinoline derivatives, and marinopyrrole-A (maritoclax) are briefly detailed in this chapter.

7.1 INTRODUCTION

Apoptosis is the mortality of cells that take place as evolutionally conserved practice and controlled stage of an organism's growth, tissue homeostasis and act as resistance to oncogenic alteration (Hanahan and Weinberg, 2000; Johnstone et al., 2002). Modification in the fundamental mechanism of apoptosis causes cancerous growth. For example, mutations in the p53 tumor suppressor gene abolish p53 triggered apoptosis and overexpression of anti-apoptotic proteins; for instance, Bcl-2 (B-cell lymphoma-2) and Bcl-X instigate cancer disease. One of the most auspicious tactics to prevent cancer is through restraining cancerous cell endurance employing compounds which imitate pro-apoptotic (promoting apoptosis) Bcl-2 homology 3 (BH3) domains and neutralize anti-apoptotic Bcl-2 super-family proteins (Vogelstein and Kinzler, 2004; Vogelstein et al., 2000; Reed, 2003). Bcl-2 proteins are over-expressed in numerous cancer disorders and perform significant functions in controlling apoptosis. This over-expression of these proteins is linked to the augmented resistance of anticancer drugs and the survival of tumor cells. An orally bioavailable, selective small-molecule BH3 mimetic have great potential in pro-apoptotic and anti-neoplastic activities.

7.2   ROLE OF BH3 DOMAINS IN APOPTOSIS PATHWAY DURING CANCER DISEASE

Bcl-2 programmed in individuals via BCL2 gene has been one of the founding types of the Bcl-2 super-family proteins which control apoptosis through either preventing ("anti-apoptotic") or encouraging ("pro-apoptotic") apoptosis (Figure 7.1).

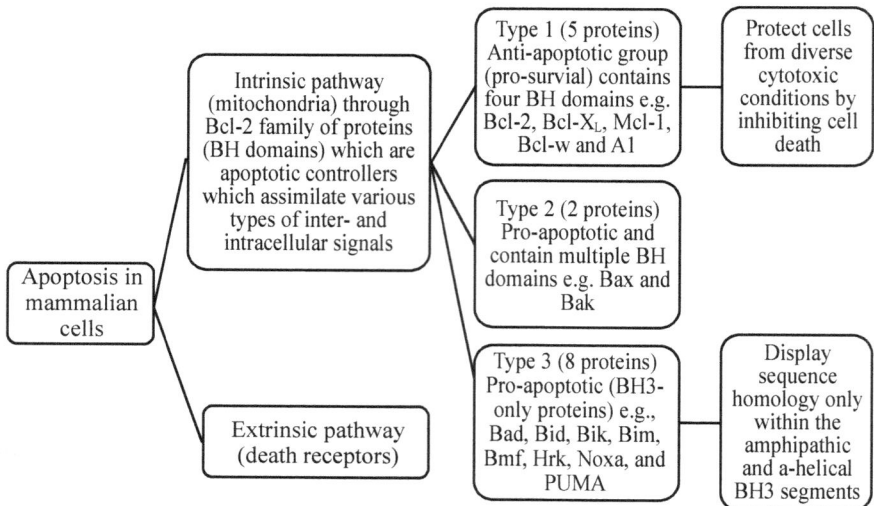

FIGURE 7.1   Bcl-2 family of regulator proteins, which controls apoptosis.

BH3 domains are crucial inhibitors of anti-apoptotic Bcl-2 family members, and hence, BH3 mimetic-induced killing could be a tool for cancer disease treatment (Danial and Korsmeyer, 2004; Adams and Cory,

2007; Huang and Strasser, 2000). Mechanism of action of BH3 domains in the apoptosis pathway involves the interaction of endoplasmic reticulum (ER) with Beclin 1/BCL-2, which leads to inhibition of anti-apoptotic Bcl-2 family members resulting in cancer cell apoptosis (Rebecca et al., 2013).

7.3   BENCHMARK FOR ANTICANCER ACTIVITY OF BH3 DOMAINS

Protein-protein interactions mediate the balance between pro-apoptotic and anti-apoptotic Bcl2 members, which is a key determinant for the destiny of the cells either to stay alive or to decease (Danial and Korsmeyer, 2004). It has been demonstrated through structural investigations that BH1, BH2, and BH3 domains of the anti-apoptotic proteins bend up into a globular sphere zone having a lipophilic or hydrophobic peripheral cavity (Sattler et al., 1997). Binding of α-helical BH3, domains of pro-apoptotic proteins to lipophilic cavity deactivate anti-apoptotic proteins (Petros et al., 2000). During normal cell conditions, initial concentrations of anti-apoptotic proteins restrain Bax and Bak (type 2 proteins) to be stimulated. Under the cancerous condition, the response of the apoptotic signals is received, leading to activation of BH3-only proteins (type 3 proteins) which bind to the hydrophobic cavities of anti-apoptotic proteins in a competitive manner (type 1 proteins) via the BH3 domains and displaces Bax and Bak which further form multimers and permeabilize the mitochondrial outer membrane. This leads to the break-down of the membrane potential of mitochondria, discharge of apoptogenic proteins of mitochondria, for instance, "cytochrome C," "SMAC/Diablo" and "AIF," and triggering of caspases (Figure 7.2) (Cheng et al., 2001; Danial and Korsmeyer, 2004; Zong et al., 2001; Green and Kroemer, 2004; Wang, 2001; Certo et al., 2006; Kim et al., 2006).

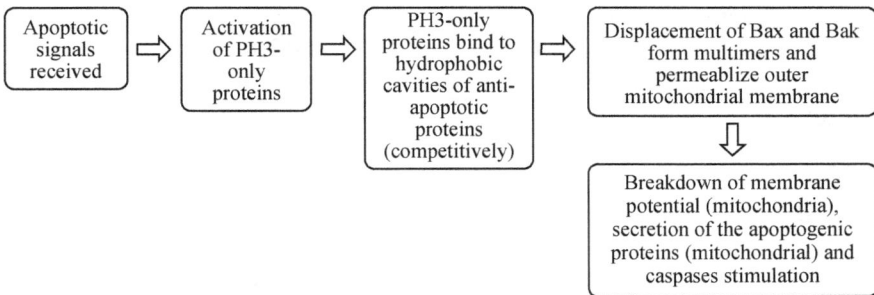

FIGURE 7.2   Mechanism of action of BH3 domains.

7.4   STRATEGIES FOR DESIGN OF BH3 MIMETIC

Advanced knowledge of competitive binding of the "pro-apoptotic" proteins with "anti-apoptotic" proteins helps in accessing the specific interactions of the BH3 domains and hydrophobic cavities of the "anti-apoptotic" proteins, which lead to the design and development of BH3 mimetic. Preferential competitive interaction of the "pro-apoptotic" proteins (type 3) with "anti-apoptotic" proteins (type 1) has been depicted in Table 7.1 (Chen et al., 2005; Kuwana et al., 2005).

TABLE 7.1   Competitive Binding of "Pro-Apoptotic" with "Anti-Apoptotic" Proteins

Pro-Apoptotic Proteins	Anti-Apoptotic Proteins
PUMA and Bim	Bcl-2, Bcl-X_L, Mcl-1, Bcl-w, and A1
Bad and Bmf	Bcl-2, Bcl-X_L, Bcl-w
Bik, Bid, and Hrk	Strongly bind to Bcl-w, Bcl-X_L, and A1, Weakly bind to Bcl-2 and Mcl-1
Noxa	Mcl-1 and A1

7.5   UNDERLYING PRINCIPLE FOR TARGETING TUMORS WITH BH3 MIMETIC

Agents mimicking the BH3 domains (BH3 mimetic) probably impart a stage of choosiness compared to the cancerous cells. BH3 domain sequences containing peptides possibly would imitate functions of BH3-only proteins and might be studied as leading pharmacological compounds (Shangary and Johnson, 2002). Larger BH3 peptides consisting of greater than fourteen amino acids could preserve α-helical assembly as well as several pharmacological activities (Letai et al., 2002; Shangary et al., 2004). Analogous to the BH3-only proteins, BH3 peptides bring about the oligomerization of Bax and Bak (type 2 proteins), permeabilization of the outer membrane of mitochondria, and secretion of cytochrome C (Chen et al., 2005; Kuwana et al., 2005; Letai et al., 2002).

7.6   DRAWBACKS OF BH3 MIMETIC AND THEIR MODIFICATIONS

Applications of BH3 peptides as pharmacologically active compounds have demonstrated restricted critical pharmaceutical characteristics, i.e., deprived cellular permeability, low solubility, poor bioavailability, and metabolic un-stability *in-vivo* (Denicourt and Dowdy, 2004). These limitations can be overcome through modification as illustrated in Table 7.2 (Shangary and Johnson, 2003; Walensky et al., 2004).

TABLE 7.2   BH3 Modification Approaches for Superior Properties

Characteristics	Methodology	References
Intracellular uptake enhancement	Labeling with peptide transduction domains from human immunodeficiency virus-1 (HIV-1) TAT protein or *Drosophila antennapedia* protein	Shangary and Johnson (2003)
Improved pharmacological properties	Modification of Bid BH3 peptide through the chemical fundamental to preserve its α-helical conformation	Walensky et al. (2004)

7.7   PREVIOUSLY CHARACTERIZED BH3 MIMETIC

Small-molecule organic inhibitor of Bcl-2 and Bcl-XL, which acts as BH3 mimetics, seems to grasp exclusive assurance to target the Bcl-2 protein super-family. Owing to profound lipophilic cavities on the exterior of Bcl-XL, it produces substantial inhibitory superficially targeting to Bcl-XL (Petros et al., 2000). Therapeutic significance of the proteins of Bcl-2 super-family motivated substantial concern in discovering small organic compounds competent of interacting with Bcl-2 and/or Bcl-X, preventing their "anti-apoptotic" activity and consequently, augmenting the process of apoptosis (Reed and Pellecchia, 2005; Belmar and Fesik, 2015).

Few natural or synthetic small-molecule inhibitors of BCL-2, i.e., HA14-1, antimycin A demonstrated either cytotoxicity or meager pharmaceutical attributes or unsuccessful in binding with the lipophilic cavity of BCL-2 proteins or encourage BAK/BAX-dependent apoptosis (Lessene et al., 2008; Baell and Huang, 2002). An antagonist of numerous pro-survival BCL-2 proteins which were either published or have been advanced to the clinical stages has been comprehensively reviewed in this chapter (Reed and Pellecchia, 2005; Lessene et al., 2008; Azmi et al., 2011; Khaw et al., 2011; Billard, 2012; Quinn et al., 2011; Belmar and Fesik, 2015). Their descriptions and chemical structures are presented in Table 7.3 and Figure 7.3, respectively.

TABLE 7.3 Features of Previously Developed BH3 Mimetic

Name and Chemical Class	Targets	Therapeutic Uses	Clinical Status	References
ABT-737 (Small organic molecule)	Bcl-X$_L$, Bcl-2, Bcl-w	Cervical, lymphoma, leukemia, myeloma, lung, and breast cancer	Preclinical	Kojima et al. (2006); Kuroda et al. (2006); Konopleva et al. (2006); Deng et al. (2007); Moore et al. (2007)
ABT-263 (Navitoclax) (Orally bioavailable analog of ABT-737)	Bcl-X$_L$, Bcl-w, Bcl-2	Hodgkin lymphoma	Phase I/II	Billard (2013); www.clinicaltrials.gov
HA14-1 and derivatives	Bcl-2	Colon, glioma, glioblastoma, leukemia, myeloma, and prostate cancer	Preclinical	Sinicrope et al. (2004); Hao et al. (2004); Manero et al. (2006); An et al. (2007); Oliver et al. (2007); www.clinicaltrials.gov
Antimycin A and its derivatives	Bcl-2, Bcl-X$_L$	Leukemia and cervical cancer	Preclinical	Tzung et al. (2001); Wang et al. (2005); Schwartz et al. (2007)
GX015-070 (Obatoclax) (Derivative of natural progidiosin)	Bcl-2, Bcl-X$_L$, Mcl-1	Leukemia, myeloma, lymphoma, and lung cancer	Phase I/II	Perez-Galan et al. (2007); www.clinicaltrials.gov
ApoG2 (Apogossypol and TW-37) (Plant-derived polyphenol)	Bcl-2, Bcl-X$_L$, Mcl-1	Leukemia, non-Hodgkin's lymphoma, head and neck, lung, and prostate cancer	Phase I/II	Van Poznak et al. (2001); Oliver et al. (2004); Becattini et al. (2004); Verhaegen et al. (2006); www.clinicaltrials.gov

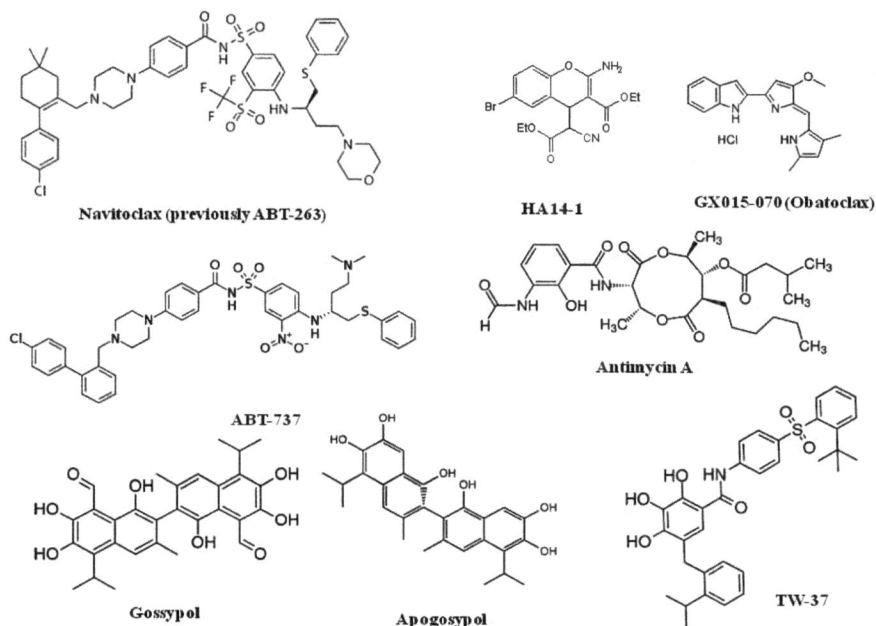

FIGURE 7.3 Chemical structures of various previously developed BH3 mimetics.

7.7.1 ABT-737 AND ABT-263 (NAVITOCLAX)

ABT-737, as well as its orally bioavailable analog ABT-263 (Navitoclax), are the preliminary BH3 mimetics (Oltersdorf et al., 2005; Tse et al., 2008; Van Delft et al., 2006). The features of ABT-737 and ABT-263 (Navitoclax) are mostly similar, excluding their pharmacokinetic characteristics. ABT-737 and navitoclax illustrate noteworthy pro-apoptotic and anticancer properties only under conditions that MCL-1 is not expressed or weakly expressed (Khaw et al., 2011; Van Delft et al., 2006).

7.7.2 OBATOCLAX (GX15-070)

It is a synthetic analog of natural product prodigiosin and interacts with all the pro-survival BCL-2 proteins although with little potency (Nguyen et al., 2013). This could bring out apoptosis as well as surmount the drug resistance of the cancerous cells to ABT-737 which is unable to interact with MCL-1 protein (Vogler et al., 2009; Albershardt et al., 2011; Billard, 2012).

7.7.3   GOSSYPOL FAMILY

Gossypol is a polyphenolic aldehyde derivative obtained from plants. This assumed pan-BH3 mimetic interacts with BCL-X, BCL-2, and MCL-1 with mild potency. Gossypol derivatives: apogossypol and apogossypolone (ApoG2) which do not have aldehyde structure have reduced toxicity are presently under preclinical stage, whereas benzoyl sulfonideanalog TW37 is under phase I/II clinical trials (Azmi et al., 2011; Quinn et al., 2011; Kitada et al., 2003; Arnold et al., 2008). Fascinatingly, a current report exposed that ApoG2 can activate mitochondrial mechanism of apoptosis in primary chronic lymphocytic leukemia (CLL) (Billard, 2012).

7.7.4   S1

It is a small organic molecule compound which functions as an alternative prompt BH3-only protein NOXA, consequently, resulting in BAK release (Albershardt et al., 2011; Zhang et al., 2011; Zhong et al., 2012).

7.8   IDENTIFICATION OF NEW PUTATIVE BH3 MIMETICS

Several new putative BH3 mimetics have been recently discovered through structure-based drug design, computational modeling, and high-throughput screening of natural compounds and synthetic libraries. These newly recognized molecules were projected to act as BH3 mimetics and direct BAX stimulators. Their structures are presented in Figure 7.4 (Billard, 2013).

7.8.1   ABT-199 (VENETOCLAX)

It is synthetic derivative of navitoclax (ABT-263), orally bioavailable, and substantially exclusive inhibitor of Bcl-2 and stimulates apoptosis dependent on BAX/BAK to treat Hodgkin lymphoma. Bcl-2 protein gets hyper expressed in certain tumors and therefore, its inhibition becomes necessary for controlling apoptosis (Billard, 2013).

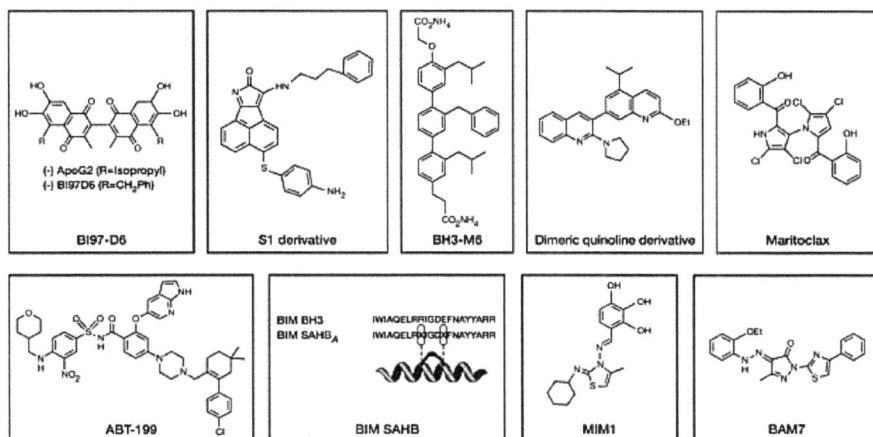

FIGURE 7.4   Structures of new putative compounds as BH3 mimetics.

7.8.2   BIM SAHB (BIM STABILIZED A-HELIX OF BCL-2 DOMAINS)

LaBelle and colleagues characterized pharmacologic perspective of BIM SAHB which is proficient in engaging five major pro-survival BCL-2 proteins to prompts BAK/BAX-associated cytochrome C release in mitochondria for curing leukemia.

7.8.3   MIM 1

It is an innovative, small-molecule organic selective inhibitor of Mcl-1 which acts by interacting with lipophilic cavity of Mcl-1 to stimulate apoptosis mediated by BAX/BAK. It has thiazol scaffold replaced with methyl, cyclohexylimino, and benzenetriol functional groups.

7.8.4   BAM 7

It is a direct BAX stimulator that selectively binds with the BAX trigger spot has been recently identified by Gavathiotis and colleagues. It has a pirazolonemoiety substituted by various functional groups and stimulates activation of BAX and apoptosis mediated by BAX in cells lacking of BAK-for treatment of leukemia.

7.8.5   BI-97D6

This is novel compound which belongs to gossypol family which illustrated diminutive cytotoxicity for BAK/BAX-lacking cells which indicated that predominantly, it has BAX/BAK pathway dependent mechanism of action (Billard, 2013).

7.8.6   S1 DERIVATIVE

It is a series of substituted S1 (S1 derivatives) which targets BCL-2, BCL-X, and MCL-1 with 9- to 35-times higher potency than S1 and prompts an improved pro-apoptotic action in malignant cell lines compared to S1 (Song et al., 2013).

7.8.7   BH3-M6

It is a small synthetic molecule containing moieties that imitate the structure and conformation of chief amino acids in the BH3 helix. Computational docking investigations recommended that it can interact with BCL-X, BCL-2, and MCL-1 (Billard, 2013; Kazi et al., 2011).

7.8.8   POLY-QUINOLINE DERIVATIVES

These are synthetic derivatives of polyquinoline (dimeric derivatives of quinoline). These compounds diminish the binding of BIM to pro-survival proteins and stimulate apoptosis dependent on BAX/BAK in human malignant lymphoid cells (Billard, 2013; Saugues et al., 2012).

7.8.9   MARINOPYRROLE-A (MARITOCLAX)

This is derived from marine streptomycetes species. It gets bind to MCL-1 to acquire apoptosis in leukemia or lymphoma cell lines (Billard, 2013; Hugues et al., 2008; Doi et al., 2012).

7.9   OTHER BH3 MIMETIC

Walensky et al. primarily produced a sequence of SAHB intended to target members of pro-survival BCL-2 super-family proteins. These hydrocarbon-scaffold peptides derivatives were stable, cell-permeable, and resistant to protease (Table 7.4).

TABLE 7.4   Other Mimetics and Their Targets

Class	Targets
SAHBA (modeled on BH3-only protein BID)	Bcl-2 and Bcl-X$_L$ Induces BAX/ BAK-dependent apoptosis
NOXA-like BH3 mimetics [BIMS2A (variation of the BIM BH3 region) and MCL-1 SAHB (obtained by modification of BH3 domain of MCL-1)]	Mcl-1

7.10   CONCLUSION

This chapter described a variety of identified BH3 mimetic and illustrated current findings in this era. Previously characterized BH3 mimetic includes ABT-737 and ABT-263 (navitoclax), obatoclax (GX15-070), gossypol family, and S1. Several new putative BH3 mimetic includes ABT-199 (vene-toclax), BIM SAHB (BIM Stabilized α-helix of BCL-2 domains), MIM 1, BAM 7, BI-97D6, S1 derivative, BH3-M6, poly-quinoline derivatives, and marinopyrrole-A (maritoclax).

KEYWORDS

- **anti-neoplastic**
- **apogossypolone**
- **apoptosis**
- **B-cell lymphoma-2**
- **BH3 mimetic**
- **pro-apoptotic**

REFERENCES

Adams, J. M., & Cory, S., (2007). The Bcl-2 apoptotic switch in cancer development and therapy. *Oncogene, 26*, 1324–1337.

Albershardt, T. C., Salerni, B. L., Soderquist, R. S., Bates, D. J. P., Pletnev, A. A., Kisselev, A. F., & Eastman, A., (2011). Multiple BH3 mimetics antagonize anti-apoptotic MCL-1 protein by inducing the endoplasmic reticulum stress response and up-regulating BH3-only protein NOXA. *J. Biol. Chem., 286*, 24882–24895.

An, J., Chervin, A. S., Nie, A., Ducoff, H. S., & Huang, Z., (2007). Overcoming the radio resistance of prostate cancer cells with a novel Bcl-2 inhibitor. *Oncogene, 26*, 652–661.

Arnold, A. A., Aboukamel, A., Chen, J., Yang, D., Wang, S., Al-Katib, A., & Mohammad, R. M., (2008). Preclinical studies of apogossypolone: A new nonpeptidic pan small molecule inhibitor of Bcl-2, Bcl-XL, and Mcl-1 proteins in follicular small cleaved cell lymphoma model. *Mol. Cancer, 7*, 20.

Azmi, A. A., Wang, Z., Philip, P. A., Mohammad, R. M., & Sarkar, F. H., (2011). Emerging Bcl-2 inhibitors for the treatment of cancer. *Expert Opin. Emer. Drugs, 16*, 59–70.

Baell, J. B., & Huang, D. C. S., (2002). Prospects for targeting the Bcl-2 family of proteins to develop novel cytotoxic drugs. *Biochem. Pharmacol., 64*, 851–863.

Becattini, B., Kitada, S., Leone, M., Monosov, E., Chandler, S., Zhai, D., Kipps, T. J., et al., (2004). Rational design and real time, in-cell detection of the pro-apoptotic activity of a novel compound targeting Bcl-X(L). *Chem. Biol., 11*, 389–395.

Belmar, J., & Fesik, S. W., (2015). Small molecule Mcl-1 inhibitors for the treatment of cancer. *Pharmacol. Ther., 145*, 76–84.

Billard, C., (2012). Design of novel BH3 mimetics for the treatment of chronic lymphocytic leukemia. *Leukemia, 26*, 2032–2038.

Billard, C., (2013). BH3 mimetics: Status of the field and new developments. *Mol. Cancer Ther., 12*(9), 1691–1700.

Certo, M., Del, G. M. V., Nishino, M., Wei, G., Korsmeyer, S., Armstrong, S. A., & Letai, A., (2006). Mitochondria primed by death signals determine cellular addiction to anti-apoptotic BCL-2 family members. *Cancer Cell, 9*, 351–365.

Chen, S., Dai, Y., Harada, H., Dent, P., & Grant, S., (2007). Mcl-1 down-regulation potentiates ABT-737 lethality by cooperatively inducing Bak activation and Bax translocation. *Cancer Res., 67*, 782–791.

Cheng, E. H., Wei, M. C., Weiler, S., Flavell, R. A., Mak, T. W., Lindsten, T., & Korsmeyer, S. J., (2001). BCL-2, BCL-X(L) sequester BH3 domain-only molecules preventing BAX-and BAK-mediated mitochondrial apoptosis. *Mol. Cell, 8*, 705–711.

Danial, N. N., & Korsmeyer, S. J., (2004). Cell death. Critical control points. *Cell, 116*, 205–219.

Deng, J., Carlson, N., Takeyama, K., Dal, C. P., Shipp, M., & Letai, A., (2007). BH3 profiling identifies three distinct classes of apoptotic blocks to predict response to ABT-737 and conventional chemotherapeutic agents. *Cancer Cell, 12*, 171–185.

Denicourt, C., & Dowdy, S. F., (2004). Medicine: Targeting apoptotic pathways in cancer cells. *Science, 305*, 1411–1413.

Doi, K., Li, R., Sung, S. S., Wu, H., Liu, Y., Manieri, W., Krishnegowda, G., et al., (2012). Discovery of marinopyrrole A (maritoclax) as a selective Mcl-1 antagonist that overcomes ABT-737 resistance by binding to and targeting Mcl-1 for proteasomal degradation. *J. Biol. Chem., 287*, 10224–10235.

Green, D. R., & Kroemer, G., (2004). The pathophysiology of mitochondrial cell death. *Science, 305*, 626–629.

Hanahan, D., & Weinberg, R. A., (2000). The hallmarks of cancer. *Cell, 100*, 57–70.

Hao, J. H., Yu, M., Liu, F. T., Newland, A. C., & Jia, L., (2004). Bcl-2 inhibitors sensitize tumor necrosis factor-related apoptosis-inducing ligand-induced apoptosis by uncoupling of mitochondrial respiration in human leukemic CEM cells. *Cancer Res., 64*, 3607–3616.

Huang, D. C., & Strasser, A., (2000). BH3-only proteins-essential initiators of apoptotic cell death. *Cell, 103*, 839–842.

Hugues, C. C., Prieto-Davo, A., Jensen, P. R., & Fenical, W., (2008). The marinopyrroles, antibiotics of an unprecedented structure class from a marine *Streptomyces sp. Org. Lett., 10*, 629–631.

Johnstone, R. W., Ruefli, A. A., & Lowe, S. W., (2002). Apoptosis: A link between cancer genetics and chemotherapy. *Cell, 108*, 153–164.

Kazi, A., Sun, J., Doi, K., Sung, S. S., Takahashi, Y., Yin, H., Rodriguez, J. M., et al., (2011). The BH3 a-helical mimic BH3-M6 disrupts Bcl-X, Bcl-2, Bad, or Bim and induces apoptosis in a Bax- and Bim-dependent manner. *J. Biol. Chem., 286*, 9382–9392.

Khaw, S. L., Huang, D. C. S., & Roberts, A. W., (2011). Overcoming blocks in apoptosis with BH3-mimetic therapy in hematological malignancies. *Pathology, 43*, 525–535.

Kim, H., Rafiuddin-Shah, M., Tu, H. C., Jeffers, J. R., Zambetti, G. P., Hsieh, J. J., & Cheng, E. H., (2006). Hierarchical regulation of mitochondrion-dependent apoptosis by BCL-2 subfamilies. *Nat. Cell Biol., 8*, 1348–1358.

Kitada, S., Leone, M., Sareth, S., Zhai, D., Reed, J. C., & Pellecchia, M., (2003). Discovery, characterization, and structure-activity relationships studies of pro-apoptotic polyphenols targeting B-cell lymphocyte/leukemia-2 proteins. *J. Med. Chem., 46*, 4259–4264.

Kojima, K., Konopleva, M., Samudio, I. J., Schober, W. D., Bornmann, W. G., & Andreeff, M., (2006). Concomitant inhibition of MDM2 and Bcl-2 protein function synergistically induce mitochondrial apoptosis in AML. *Cell Cycle, 5*, 2778–2786.

Konopleva, M., Contractor, R., Tsao, T., Samudio, I., Ruvolo, P. P., Kitada, S., Deng, X., et al., (2006). Mechanisms of apoptosis sensitivity and resistance to the BH3 mimetic ABT-737 in acute myeloid leukemia. *Cancer Cell, 10*, 375–388.

Kuroda, J., Puthalakath, H., Cragg, M. S., Kelly, P. N., Bouillet, P., Huang, D. C., Kimura, S., et al., (2006). Bim and Bad mediate imatinib-induced killing of Bcr/Abl+ leukemic cells, and resistance due to their loss is overcome by a BH3 mimetic. *Proc. Natl. Acad. Sci. U.S.A., 103*, 14907–14912.

Kuwana, T., Bouchier-Hayes, L., Chipuk, J. E., Bonzon, C., Sullivan, B. A., Green, D. R., & Newmeyer, D. D., (2005). BH3 domains of BH3-only proteins differentially regulate Bax-mediated mitochondrial membrane permeabilization both directly and indirectly. *Mol. Cell, 17*, 525–535.

Lessene, G., Czabotar, P. E., & Colman, P. M., (2008). Bcl-2 family antagonists for cancer therapy. *Nat. Rev., 7*, 989–1000.

Manero, F., Gautier, F., Gallenne, T., Cauquil, N., Gree, D., Cartron, P. F., Geneste, O., et al., (2006). The small organic compound HA14-1 prevents Bcl-2 interaction with Bax to sensitize malignant glioma cells to induction of cell death. *Cancer Res., 66*, 2757–2764.

Moore, V. D. G., Brown, J. R., Certo, M., Love, T. M., Novina, C. D., & Letai, A., (2007). Chronic lymphocytic leukemia requires BCL2 to sequester prodeath BIM, explaining sensitivity to BCL2 antagonist ABT737. *J. Clin. Invest., 117*, 112–121.

Nguyen, M., Marcellus, R. C., Roulston, A., Watson, M., Serfass, L., Madiraju, S. R. M., Goulet, D., et al., (2007). Small molecule obatoclax (GX15-070) antagonizes MCL-1 and overcomes MCL-1-mediated resistance to apoptosis. *Pro. Natl. Acad. Sci. U.S.A., 104,* 19512–19517.

Oliver, C. L., Bauer, J. A., Wolter, K. G., Ubell, M. L., Narayan, A., O'Connell, K. M., Fisher, S. G., et al., (2004). *In vitro* effects of the BH3 mimetic, (−) gossypol, on head and neck squamous cell carcinoma cells. *Clin. Cancer Res., 10,* 7757–7763.

Oliver, L., Mahe, B., Gree, R., Vallette, F. M., & Juin, P., (2007). HA14-1, a small molecule inhibitor of Bcl-2, bypasses chemoresistance in leukemia cells. *Leuk. Res., 31,* 859–863.

Oltersdorf, T., Elmore, S. W., Shoemaker, A. R., Armstrong, R. C., Augeri, D. J., Belli, B. A., Bruncko, M., et al., (2005). An inhibitor of Bcl-2 family proteins induces regression of solid tumors. *Nature, 435,* 677–681.

Perez-Galan, P., Roue, G., Villamor, N., Campo, E., & Colomer, D., (2007). The BH3-mimetic GX15-070 synergizes with bortezomib in mantle cell lymphoma by enhancing noxa-mediated activation of Bak. *Blood, 109,* 4441–4449.

Petros, A. M., Nettesheim, D. G., Wang, Y., Olejniczak, E. T., Meadows, R. P., Mack, J., Swift, K., et al., (2000). Rationale for BclxL/Bad peptide complex formation from structure, mutagenesis, and biophysical studies. *Protein Sci., 9,* 2528–2534.

Quinn, B. A., Dash, R., Azab, B., Sarkar, S., Das, S. K., Kumar, S., Oyesanya, R. A., et al., (2011). Targeting Mcl-1 for the therapy of cancer. *Expert Opin. Investig. Drugs, 20,* 1397–1411.

Rebecca, M., Tsao, W., Faust, N., & Xu, L., (2013). *Drug Resistance and Molecular Cancer Therapy: Apoptosis versus Autophagy, Apoptosis* (pp. 155–196). Justine Rudner, IntechOpen.

Reed, J. C., & Pellecchia, M., (2005). Apoptosis-based therapies for hematologic malignancies. *Blood, 106,* 408–418.

Reed, J. C., (2003). Apoptosis-targeted therapies for cancer. *Cancer Cell, 3,* 17–22.

Sattler, M., Liang, H., Nettesheim, D., Meadows, R. P., Harlan, J. E., Eberstadt, M., Yoon, H. S., et al., (1997). Structure of Bcl-xL-Bak peptide complex: Recognition between regulators of apoptosis. *Science, 275,* 983–986.

Saugues, E., Debaud, A. L., Anizon, F., Bonnefoy, N., & Moreau, P., (2012). Synthesis and biological activities of polyquinoline derivatives: New Bcl-2 family protein modulators. *Eur. J. Med. Chem., 57,* 112–125.

Schwartz, P. S., Manion, M. K., Emerson, C. B., Fry, J. S., Schulz, C. M., Sweet, I. R., & Hockenbery, D. M., (2007). 2-Methoxy antimycin reveals a unique mechanism for Bcl-xL inhibition. *Mol. Cancer Ther., 6,* 2073–2080.

Shangary, S., & Johnson, D. E., (2002). Peptides derived from BH3 domains of Bcl-2 family members: A comparative analysis of inhibition of Bcl-2, Bcl-x(L) and Bax oligomerization, induction of cytochrome c release, and activation of cell death. *Biochemistry, 41,* 9485–9495.

Shangary, S., Oliver, C. L., Tillman, T. S., Cascio, M., & Johnson, D. E., (2004). Sequence and helicity requirements for the pro-apoptotic activity of Bax BH3 peptides. *Mol. Cancer Ther., 3,* 1343–1354.

Sinicrope, F. A., Penington, R. C., & Tang, X. M., (2004). Tumor necrosis factor related apoptosis-inducing ligand-induced apoptosis is inhibited by Bcl2 but restored by the small molecule Bcl-2 inhibitor, HA 14-1, in human colon cancer cells. *Clin. Cancer Res., 10,* 8284–8292.

Song, T., Li, X., Chang, X., Liang, X., Zhao, Y., Wu, G., Xie, S., et al., (2013). 3-thiomorpholin-8oxo-8H-acenaphto [1,2-b] pyrrole-9-carbonitrile (S1) derivatives as pan-Bcl-2-inhibitors of Bcl-2, Bcl-x, and Mcl-1. *Bioorg. Med. Chem., 21*, 11–20.

Tse, C., Shoemaker, A. R., Adickers, J., Chen, J., Jin, S., Johnson, E. F., Marsh, K. C., et al., (2008). ABT-263: A potent and orally bio-available Bcl-2 family inhibitor. *Cancer Res., 68*, 3421–3428.

Tzung, S. P., Kim, K. M., Basanez, G., Giedt, C. D., Simon, J., Zimmerberg, J., Zhang, K. Y., & Hockenbery, D. M., (2001). Antimycin A mimics a cell-death-inducing Bcl-2 homology domain 3. *Nat. Cell Biol., 3*, 183–191.

Van, D. M. F., Wei, A. H., Mason, K. D., Vandenberg, C. J., Chen, L., Czabotar, P. E., Willis, S. N., et al., (2006). The BH3 mimetic ABT-737 targets selective Bcl-2 proteins and efficiently induces apoptosis via Bak/Bax if Mcl-1 is neutralized. *Cancer Cell, 10*, 389–399.

Van, P. C., Seidman, A. D., Reidenberg, M. M., Moasser, M. M., Sklarin, N., Van, Z. K., Borgen, P., et al., (2001). Oral gossypol in the treatment of patients with refractory metastatic breast cancer: A phase I/II clinical trial. *Breast Cancer Res. Treat., 66*, 239–248.

Verhaegen, M., Bauer, J. A., Martin, D. L. V. C., Wang, G., Wolter, K. G., Brenner, J. C., Nikolovska-Coleska, Z., et al., (2006). A novel BH3 mimetic reveals a mitogen-activated protein kinase-dependent mechanism of melanoma cell death controlled by p53 and reactive oxygen species. *Cancer Res., 66*, 11348–11359.

Vogelstein, B., & Kinzler, K. W., (2004). Cancer genes and the pathways they control. *Nat. Med., 10*, 789–799.

Vogelstein, B., Lane, D., & Levine, A. J., (2000). Surfing the p53 network. *Nature, 408*, 307–310.

Vogler, M., Weber, K., Dinsdale, D., Schmitz, I., Schulze-Osthoff, K., Dyer, M. J., & Cohen, G. M., (2009). Different forms of cell death induced by putative BCL2 inhibitors. *Cell Death Diff., 16*, 1030–1039.

Walensky, L. D., Kung, A. L., Escher, I., Malia, T. J., Barbuto, S., Wright, R. D., Wagner, G., et al., (2004). Activation of apoptosis *in vivo* by a hydrocarbon-stapled BH3 helix. *Science, 305*, 1466–1470.

Wang, H., Li, M., Rhie, J. K., Hockenbery, D. M., Covey, J. M., Zhang, R., & Hill, D. L., (2005). Preclinical pharmacology of 2-methoxyantimycin A compounds as novel antitumor agents. *Cancer Chemother. Pharmacol., 56*, 291–298.

Wang, X., (2001). The expanding role of mitochondria in apoptosis. *Genes Dev., 15*, 2922–2933.

Zhang, L., Ming, L., & Yu, J., (2007). BH3 mimetics to improve cancer therapy; mechanisms and examples. *Drug Resist. Updat., 10*, 207–217.

Zhang, Z., Song, T., Zhang, T., Gao, J., Wu, G., An, L., & Du, G., (2011). A novel BH3 mimetic S1 potently induces Bax/Bak-dependent apoptosis by targeting both Bcl-2 and Mcl-1. *Int. J. Cancer, 128*, 1724–1735.

Zhong, J. T., Xu, Y., Yi, H. W., Su, J., Yu, H. M., Xiang, X. Y., Li, X. N., et al., (2012). The BH3 mimetic S1 induces autophagy through ER stress and disruption of Bcl-2/Beclin 1 interaction in human glioma U251 cells. *Cancer Lett., 323*, 180–187.

Zong, W. X., Lindsten, T., Ross, A. J., MacGregor, G. R., & Thompson, C. B., (2001). BH3-only proteins that bind pro-survival Bcl-2 family members fail to induce apoptosis in the absence of Bax and Bak. *Genes Dev., 15*, 1481–1486.

CHAPTER 8

Spherical Nucleic Acid Platform-Based Drug Delivery for Brain Cancer and Improved Blood-Brain Barrier Crossing for Alzheimer's and Other Diseases

SANDEEP ARORA, SAURABH GUPTA, and SUKHBIR SINGH

Chitkara College of Pharmacy, Chitkara University, Punjab, India

ABSTRACT

Billions of dollars have been invested in the genetic coding therapeutic application of gene silencing in humans since the last 10 years after the Nobel Prize-winning discoveries of RNA interference (RNAi). Today, positive results for the treatment of age-related neuro-muscular degeneration and respiratory syncytial virus were obtained from ongoing clinical trials. Nevertheless, following these early successes, the widespread use of RNAi therapy for disease prevention and treatment requires the creation of medically relevant, safe, and effective vehicles for drug delivery. Spherical nucleic acid (SNA) constructs promise new single-entity gene control materials capable of knocking down both cellular transfection and gene, but so far, they are promiscuous structures with excellent genetic but poor cellular and molecular selectivity. Based on their enhanced cell absorption, SNAs have become a potentially useful tool in biological applications, stability, biocompatibility, and flexible surface functionality. This viewpoint describes the synthetic methods used to prepare these SNAs, accompanied via a review of their distinctive properties and molecular and cellular level explaining theoretical and experimental models. Key examples of advances in technology made it possible in the area of chemistry, cellular and molecular level diagnosis, regulation of gene expression, and sequential coding; the science of medicine and materials are also discussed.

8.1   INTRODUCTION

Glioma is the primary and most prominent brain tumor, distinguished to date by extremely infiltrative existence, low tumor, and very poor clinical outcome. Despite significant advances in surgical techniques, radiotherapy, and chemotherapy, the effectiveness of these therapies remains low until this tumor's prognosis. Depending on the level of malignancy, the World Health Organization (WHO) classified gliomas as gliomas of low grade (grade I and grade II) and gliomas of high grade (grade III and grade IV). Grade I tumors show the best prognosis and are relatively benign. Tumors of Grade II include many anaplastic cells and may progress to tumors of a higher grade. Tumors of grade III show a high degree of anaplasia and mitotic activity and are often lethal rapidly. Grade IV astrocytoma or multiforme glioblastoma (GBM) is the most aggressive type of glioma. This is a tumor that is highly anaplastic and malignant and is almost always lethal due to its resistance to radiotherapy and chemotherapy when altering the cell wall of microflora (Louis et al., 2007; International Health Organization, IARC, 2012).

Tremendous technological developments have been identified in the area of cancer therapy in recent decades. Researchers have sought to efficiently deliver therapeutic agents to the tumor area and reduce the accumulation of unwanted drugs in normal brain and peripheral tissues. In recent decades, effective guided drug delivery systems have gained significant attention for brain tumors. Because brain tumors have many distinguishing characteristics from peripheral tumors due to their complicated oncogenesis (Figure 8.1A, B), consideration must be given to many factors for successful brain tumor-targeted drug delivery such as blood-brain barrier (BBB), blood-brain tumor barrier (BBTB), and a relatively weak Enhanced Permeation and Retention (EPR) effect (Sanai et al., 2008).

Nanotechnology keeps on offering essentially diverse approaches to brain cancer cure and other neurological disorders. In general, spherical nucleic acids (SNAs), functionalized nanoconjugates those are gold-based with tightly packed, highly directed antisense DNA or siRNA antisense oligonucleotides (ASOs) are one of the most well-known and capable platforms for controlling nanoscale genes ASOs can reduce protein translation by either blocking steric translation or recruiting RNase H endonuclease. The former technique involves a sequence-specific manner of binding of ASOs to objected mRNA in the cytoplasm, thereby protecting the translation of mRNA ribosomal (In Figure 8.1A). The latter includes RNase H-dependent breakdown, where RNase H founds RNA-DNA heteroduplex, selectively breaks the RNA strand, and releases the intact strands of DNA (Figure 8.2) (Cerritelli et al., 2009).

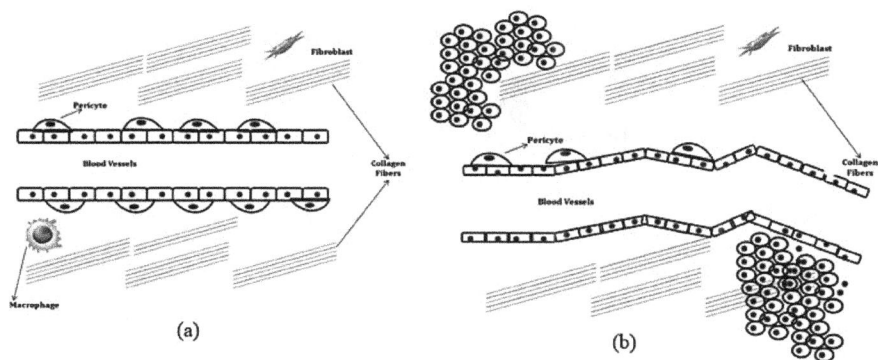

FIGURE 8.1 A and B structural variations that cause interstitial fluid pressure between normal tissue and tumor tissue. (A) Healthy tissues contain rectangular blood vessels lined with a smooth layer of endothelial cells with pericytes that preserve the vessel's internal integrity.

Given these cellular mechanisms facilitating highly specific therapeutic modulation of genetic expression, once nucleic acids are systemically delivered, a variety of obstacles to successful transmission are encountered, reducing theirs in vivo usefulness. Oligonucleotides those are not modified undergo quick renal clearance, are subject to serum cleavage by RNAs and DNAs, and exhibit incompetent target tissue absorption. Furthermore, oligonucleotides those are not modified do not cross the cell membranes efficiently and have been shown to cause a cellular immune response (Stegh et al., 2008; Boveri et al., 2015; Leachman et al., 2009). These in vivo obstacles to the delivery of oligonucleotides have delayed the transition into the clinic of nucleic acid-based therapies and forced the use of oligonucleotide carrier systems such as nanoparticles, dendrimers, liposomes, etc. (Fabian et al., 2010; Kanasty et al., 2012).

Within nanomaterials, SNAs (Figure 8.3) are a desirable group of Singular entity species in which medicinal oligonucleotides can be engineered and synthesized to function either through the RNAi or the antisense pathway. SNAs that consisting of a range of oligonucleotides (e.g., DNA, siRNA, microRNA, or locked nucleic acid (LNA)), peptide nucleic acid (PNA) and a range of nanoparticular core forms like gold (Au), silver (Ag), iron oxide (Fe_3O_4), silver, silica (SiO_2), quantum dots (QDs) (CdSe, CdSe/ZnS), core-shell ($Au@SiO_2$), and liposomes usually ranging from 10 to 50 nm (Young et al., 2012; Banga et al., 2014).

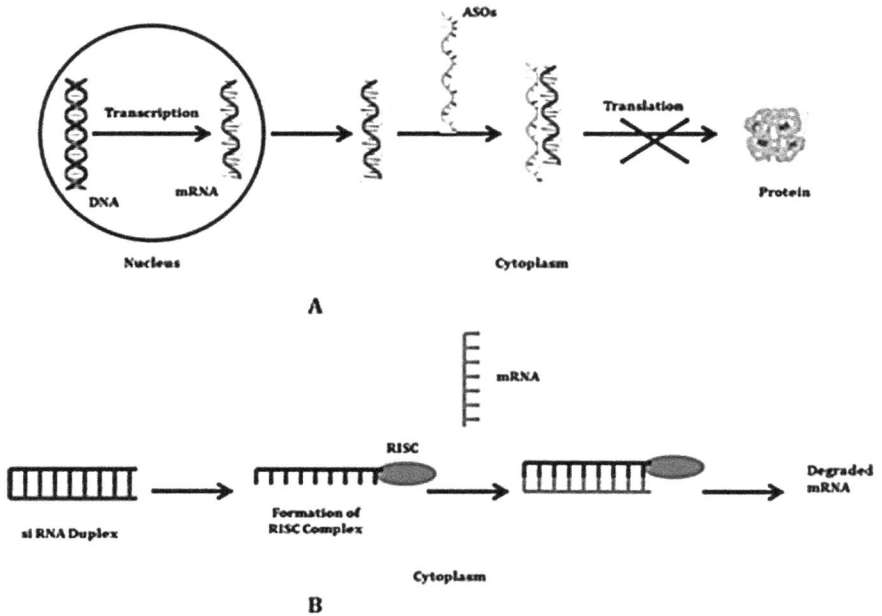

FIGURE 8.2 Different mechanisms of antisense oligonucleotide (ASOs) intracellular action and small interfering RNAs (siRNAs) intracellular action. (A) Action mechanism for ASOs that bind complementary mRNA and induce translation inhibition or recruitment of RNase H to cleave the moiety of RNA within a duplex of RNA-DNA; (B) Action mechanism for siRNAs, including RISC which means RNA induced silencing complex formation and consequent depletion of target mRNA.

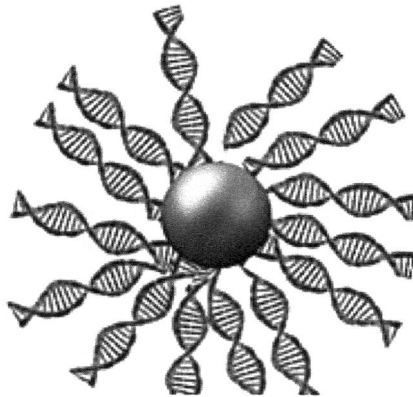

FIGURE 8.3 Spherical nucleic acid (SNA) conjugates with gold.

In 1996, a synthetic process was developed with tightly functionalized and directed nucleic acids strongly covalently bound to their surfaces to prepare polyvalent nucleic acid-nanoparticle conjugates, spherical nanostructures. Such structures represent the first well-characterized types of conjugates of SNA and were originally designed with shells of gold and DNA (Giljohann et al., 2009).

They also have different properties from those of both the nanoparticles (NPs) and the DNA they come from. In many significant and, in some cases, commercially viable applications, these materials have been used since the initial work; in addition, the use of well-characterized nanostructures as new labels for in vitro biodetection schemes and intracellular assays has catalyzed global interest, as well as active cell transfection materials; therapeutic and regulation of gene expression. Subsequent studies showed that two functions were fulfilled by inorganic NPs:

- They have novel chemical and physical characteristics (for, e.g., plasmonic, catalytic, scattering, and quenching) that are particularly significant in product plan and probe plan contexts; and
- They serve as a scaffold to assemble and organize oligonucleotides into a dense structure that produces many of their functional characteristics.

Significantly, new research has revealed that one could use the gold core as a scaffold, then cross-link the DNA at the particle base and dissolve the gold to establish a new coreless type of SNAs with several distinctive properties of the original gold nanoparticles (AuNP) conjugates, including cooperative hybridization and trimming of complementary nucleic acids. This research illustrated one of the basic characteristics of SNAs, namely that many of these nanostructures' properties are derived from a dense layer of directed nucleic acids and are core-independent. Because there is still more to be understood from using these materials, an important objective of this point of view is to encourage future research into spherical and other structures based on 3D nucleic acids.

8.1.1   INTRACELLULAR UPTAKE OF SPHERICAL NUCLEIC ACID (SNA) NANOPARTICLE CONJUGATES

Usually, cationic carriers are needed to be used intracellular nucleic acid delivery as agents of gene expression regulation. SNAs are polyanionic entities that are covalently bound to the surface of the nanoparticles and can penetrate effectively through the process of endocytosis. SNAs are single-entity agents in biological settings that possess different chemical and physical characteristics. Without the use of ancillary transfection reagents, nearly any type of cell is easily absorbed in high quantities. These trigger a minimal immune response (i.e., 25-fold reduced immune response compared to delivery of cationic carriers) and show increased stability in solution compared to free oligonucleotides (Fabian et al., 2010). Chung Hang J. and Choia et al. studied the intracellular absorption of Cyanine 5 (Cy5)-labeled single-stranded oligonucleotides and Cy5-SNAsmade from Cy5-ssDNAs of the same sequence covalently attached to the surface of 10 nM spherical AuNP on endothelial cells of the mouse C166. Their finding showed that no substantial uptake of Cy5-labeled single-stranded oligonucleotides could be observed in Cy5-SNAs after 2 hours of incubation. Inductively combined plasma mass spectrometry (ICP-MS), confocal imaging, and TEM data collectively demonstrate three key events describing SNAs endocytosis:

1. Binding to the cell membrane;
2. Uptake via invaginations;
3. Sorting into early endosomes.

Our findings show that SNAs have rapid cellular uptake kinetics and intracellular transport due to the presence of the NP center, while linear oligonucleotides do not. In addition, due to the 3D structure of oligonucleotides, SNAs can interact more significantly with cell surface receptors (scavenger receptors (SRs)) than linear oligonucleotides (Barnaby et al., 2014; Chunj et al., 2013).

8.1.2 SURFACE LIGAND FOR NANOPARTICLES AS AN EMERGENCE OF DNA

The ligands tied to the surface of an NP (the ligand shell) are mainly responsible for managing the overall chemistry of an NP and its stability in complex media. Usually, these molecules are designed with a head group moiety appropriate for attachment of interest to the NP and a tail group extending into the solution, helping to maintain colloidal stability and regulating particle reactivity. The structures synthesized in the original work consisted of tightly functionalized 13 nm gold cores with a DNA surface shell coordinated to the gold via sulfur groups; they were the first well-characterized SNA-NP conjugates. At the same time, Alivisatos and colleagues developed techniques for preparing monovalent types of smaller particles (2 nm) with the aim of using DNA templates to organize individual particles on such templates in a controllable manner. Such systems have led to fascinating developments in their own right, including the creation of a plasmon ruler theory, but the structure and properties of the SNA do not conjoin analogs, which are the object of this perspective. The main difference between linear nucleic acids and SNAs is that SNAs are small oligonucleotide dense, directed spherical arrays. While the majority of nucleic acid types depend on the hybridized duplex as the basic structural unit that defines their overall shape, SNAs can be made from single- and double-stranded nucleic acids, and the inorganic core structure defines their orientation. SNA nanostructures are also distinct from field-based artificial structures, also referred to as "DNA nanotechnology and origami," in which DNA recognition properties are used to assemble duplexes into rationally engineered forms. The physical SNA structures mentioned herein are synthesized irrespective of nucleic acid sequence and hybridization; they are developed by chemical bonds, not recognition processes.

8.1.3 STRUCTURAL CONSIDERATIONS OF SNA-NP CONJUGATES AND SNA

SNA nanostructures are chemically very complex and can have significantly different properties depending on the components and their position in such structures. For example, they have higher binding constants for their complements than free strands of the same sequence, display cooperative links, and subsequent quick transitions of melting are resistant to nuclease degradation, and are worth transfecting cell lines without the need for physical or chemical transfection processes. While these materials also possess an inorganic nucleus in the outer region of the nanostructure, the emerging properties unique to SNAs are largely derived from the density and orientation of oligonucleotides. Lastly, prototype nucleic acids could provide additional functions, all of which can be used in the production of gene-controlled molecular diagnostic systems and structures as well as product synthesis. The core material is an essential factor of layout for SNA conjugates. The oligonucleotide shell's properties are now well understood and highly predictable based on its structure, an additional way to modify SNA conjugates 'actions by selecting the core material. To date, the majority of studied conjugates have been Au NP core functionalized with alkyl thiolated oligonucleotides bound to the 3' or 5' end of the molecule through an Au-S connection. Au NPs have been Chosen as initial core product candidates because they are easily synthesized with a variety of particle diameters, have plasmon resonances with high extinction coefficients, can be easily controlled with a wide range of chemical reagents, and have well-defined catalytic effects. Once replaced with a thick monolayer of DNA, these molecules, in addition to all SNAs, demonstrate extremely useful properties in applications of molecular diagnosis, therapy, and materials. The oligonucleotides composed of SNAs are made of three main components: a moiety of particle attachment (in the case of structures centered on particles), a more spaced region, and a programmable recognition region. This category is an integral part of the SNA process, and each unit is the focus of numerous studies. A typical attachment group for Au NPs is a single propyl-or hexyl thiol group that can be incorporated by traditional amidite phosphorus chemistry (usually at 5' or 3' ends, but can be incorporated throughout the series in theory). The lack of side reactions to gold for thiol adsorption allows the functionalization cycle to continue as long as needed, resulting in very high densities of oligonucleotides on the surfaces of Au NP. A standard conjugate stability test involves an examination of the oligonucleotide displacement level with the dithiothreitol disulfide reduction agent. The second segment of the sequence of oligonucleotides, the spacer band, moves the recognition region away from the surface of Au NP and may consist of DNA bases (e.g., T10 or A10) or other artificial groups such as polyethylene glycol (PEG) units. The strand identification portion is ultimately tailored for each investigation or practical use and is usually the active segment available for additional base-pairing with other strands of interest (e.g., connecting strands with sticky ends, target strands in detection assays, or complementary strands for siRNA formation).

This section can be made up of any such component that can be combined with traditional nucleic acids (DNA or RNA) by phosphoramidite chemistry. Complex metals such as analogs of cis-diamminedichloroplatinum(II) and chelates with gadolinium, have been combined with conjugates to create powerful drug delivery vehicles and contrasting agents for magnetic resonance imaging (MRI). Regarding environmental monitoring purposes, chemical tags such as alkynes and azides have been used to label specimens for the detection of copper ions. Antibodies are co-adsorbed on the particle surface with the oligonucleotides to create multifunctional samples used in protein detection assays. The high stability of nucleic acid-modified nanostructures in aqueous media can be used to solubilize drugs, such as paclitaxel, by binding to the conjugate. In addition, these are chemically flexible structures that allow one to use the SNA platform to prepare multifunctional materials.

8.1.4 CONTROLLING THE SNA CONJUGATES DENSITY

Initial studies with DNA-Au NPs have shown the potential for using SNA conjugates across a large number of disciplines. Nonetheless, the first findings of these structures touched upon a decade and a half of the ongoing research that branched from material synthesis to fundamental studies in assembly, diagnosis, and therapy based on DNA-NP. The application of these conjugates to such fields was based on their high stability and unique characteristic, which depends directly on the NP surface structure and density of the monolayer oligonucleotide. It was, therefore, necessary to understand the important synthetic parameters to produce fairly well-defined conjugates with properties optimized for planned use. The variables regulating the loading of oligonucleotides were analyzed in-depth for this reason. These include the reaction solution's salt concentration, the NP's size, and shape, the bases nearest to the surface of the molecule, sonication or heating, and the chemical attachment moiety's name. The maximum DNA surface density depends on the molecule's size and shape. For spherical particles, smaller particles may support higher densities, far larger than those obtained on planar surfaces. For example, 10 nm particles will typically support 2.0×10^{13} oligos/cm while 5.8×10^{12} oligos/cm surface coverage for the same sequence oligonucleotides assembled under the same conditions on a macroscopic planar gold layer. This effect decreases as the particles increase in steric and electronic repulsion constraints and thus reduce them, allowing for higher surface densities of DNA. Eventually, a mathematical model developed by Hill et al. showed that natural loading for anisotropic particles such as gold nanorods and triangular prisms could be predicted reliably by combining experimental density values for curved and flat surfaces.

8.1.5 COOPERATIVE CONJUGATIONS OF HIGH-DENSITY SNA

Based on the nucleic acid sequence, SNAs are entities with extremely tailorable identification characteristics. In relation to the assembly through linker strings that occur through the region of DNA sequence recognition, it is possible to hybridize specific particles. As individual building blocks, one can learn about the SNA-NP conjugates, each with a special identity determined by their sequence. Through creating particle-DNA and linker, the NPs are mixed, resulting in a polymeric macroscopic assembly. Due to the fact that the particles are held together by means of DNA connections and their cores do not interact or fuse, the DNA-NP conjugates can be separated from the aggregate by heating the duplexes or by increasing the solution's salt concentration. As temperature rises above the melting point (Tm), DNA duplexes undergo predictable "melting" dehybridization. The same applies to SNA conjugates; however, their multi-purpose binding behavior is very different from linear duplexes. Surprisingly, there is no limited cooperative binding for canonical DNA binding. The SNA structure can also access DNA binding modes which depend on G-quadruplex formation. One would normally expect one melting transformation from the two sequences, 5'-CCCC-3' and 5'-GGGGG-3'. Nevertheless, as the G-rich sequence can form quadruplexes, functionalized particles, two melting transitions are shown with these strings. This also has implications for sequence design; SNAs should not be synthesized with G-based oligonucleotides. DNA bases are to DNA strands in some ways as DNA strands are to SNA conjugates. This hierarchy makes it possible to use fascinating 3D hybridization modes that are not anticipated if the dynamics of single linear strands are only viewed in isolation. Such aspects are incredibly important, and researchers can only realize new ways of making macroscopic materials from these nano-scale building blocks by understanding such fundamental multi-purpose interactions of SNAs.

8.1.6 NANOPARTICLE ASSEMBLY AND CRYSTALLIZATION PROGRAMMED WITH SPHERICAL AND OTHER NANOSTRUCTURES 3D NUCLEIC ACID

The SNA conjugate is a flexible chemically configurable synthon which can be used to build higher-ordered materials, specifically colloidal crystals. In addition, Initial work demonstrated that linker strings can be used to combine various particle structures into polymeric materials with peculiar properties resulting from the position of particles in these assemblies. The changes in properties that followed these assembly activities became the basis for many modern diagnostic systems based on the nucleic acid. In contrast to testing applications, recent work started to show how colloidal crystals with short-range order can be forced to assemble these particles, where interparticle ranges can be amplified by linking length.

Further research has demonstrated the ability to construct complex discrete structures such as asymmetrically functionalized particles and clusters assembled in a programmable way. A key idea was that the weak linking connections of short DNA connector sequences coupled with the multi-purpose mutual binding observed for SNA conjugates allow the system to auto-correct defects and turn it into an energetically desired crystalline configuration from the initial disordered aggregate. Particularly, a large number of links can keep the aggregate together, but they can hybridize and dehybridize dynamically because they are poor individually. Thus, the thermal energy required to move from a disordered structure to an ordered structure is provided by annealing the aggregate at a temperature slightly below its melting temperature. The NP superlattices produced by using SNA conjugates possess a very high level of crystalline order, as expressed by small-angle X-ray scattering (SAXS). SAXS is the primary characterizing method for such structures because these superlattices typically only occur under conditions where DNA duplexes are stable, i.e., aqueous saline solution. A resin-embedding method for the visualization of NP superlattices was developed by transmission electron microscopy (TEM) as a secondary structural characterization technique to supplement SAXS. Such early studies demonstrated the use of DNA to build highly ordered NP superlattices as a robust and programmable assembly device and further revealed the potential applications of materials enabled by the unique features of SNA conjugates. This system has evolved into one that offers a high predictability rate based on a set of newly introduced design rules. The seven laws, outlined below but discussed elsewhere in depth, are as follows:

1. For a system where all SNA-Au NPs have the same hydrodynamic radii, the most stable crystal structure maximizes all possible forms of DNA hybridization interactions; the SNA-Au NP in the thermodynamic material increases the number of closest neighbors it can shape DNA connections.

2. If two lattices have similar energy stabilization, the rates of DNA connector and rehybridization are slowed down and the kinetic product that forms.

3. The SNA-Au NP hydrodynamic radii conjugate their assembly and packing actions somewhat than the volume of the Au NPs or the size of the oligonucleotides.

4. The size ratio and DNA connector ratio between particles determine the thermodynamically preferred crystal structure for binary systems.

5. The same thermodynamic material is generated by two systems with the same size ratio and DNA connector ratio.
6. In nanoparticle superlattices, Hollow SNAs can be used as spacer components to reach non-accessible symmetries with core-filled structures.

These six laws were used to create more than 50 SNA-Au NP superlattices with nine distinct crystallography symmetries based on experiments and model phase diagrams. Superlattices are synthesized with close-packed hexagonal (hcp), cesium chloride (CsCl), AB2 (isostructural aluminum diboride), AB3 (isostructural Cr3Si), AB6 (isostructural alkali-fullerene complex Cs6C60), sodium chloride (NaCl) and simple cubic (sc) symmetry in addition to fcc and bcc lattices. With the exception of hcp, it is assumed that all are thermodynamic products produced near the beginning of the melting process by temperature annealing of the programmed structures. The rules are similar to Pauling's rules in deciding the packing nature of complex ionic solids for greater predictability and durability, but in many respects due to the ease with which DNA interactions can be programmed.

8.1.7 SPHERICAL CONJUGATES TO OTHER DIFFERENT FORMS OF 3D NUCLEIC ACIDS (3D-NA)

Besides properties depend on some physical and optical properties depend on the form of nanoparticles, and some are exceptional to anisotropic NPs (e.g., rods, prisms, cubes). For, e.g., these structures 'The resonance of plasmons depends heavily on its form and aspect ratio'. The different characteristics of anisotropic NPs have been extensively discussed elsewhere; here we will focus exclusively on the emerging features of anisotropic particles functionalized by DNA in the creation of non-sphere 3D-NA. Due to the often different conditions of anisotropic particle synthesis from those of spherical nanostructures, DNA surface immobilization must be adapted to each of these particle types. For example, In the presence of the capping agent cetyltrimethylammonium bromide (CTAB), most anisotropic Au nanostructures are synthesized. Because CTAB is a positively charged surfactant, it combines and sequesters the DNA efficiently to prevent adsorption to the Au NP layer. Therefore, iterative centrifugation and washing steps must be used to remove it before DNA functionalization can occur analogously to the functionalization of spherical Au NPs. Non-spherical 3D nucleic acid nanostructures give access to NP superlattices with greater structural complexity than isotropic

NPs in the field of material synthesis and programmed colloidal crystal-lization. The integration of the principle of NP type into the DNA-based assembly method exerts a kind of "nanoparticle valence" where directional hybridization interactions between particles permit for the formation of one, two, and three-dimensional superlattices that would be hard, if not impos-sible, to synthesize with other assembly or lithography processes. Such spatial interactions occur as DNA base-pairing between anisotropic particles is preferred along pathways that promote face-to-face parallel interactions between particles. Ultimately, attempts to face-selectively functionalize particles with various oligonucleotides will increase noticeably to regulate the valence, the synthetic tunability of this process, and the flexibility of the kinds of materials and crystals that can be developed.

8.2 PHARMACEUTICAL APPLICATION OF SPHERICAL NUCLEIC ACID (SNA)

8.2.1 CANCER THERAPY

Zheng Jing et al. prepared nanoparticles combined with SNAs by hybridiza-tion reactions, creating a long fragment of DNA polymer like the shell of nanoparticles. Their result shows cellular uptake regulation of nucleolin-binding aptamer, possessing high drug charging, specificity, and delivering DOX to CEM cells selectively. This strategy could develop new drugs, improve existing drugs, and provide drugs for cancer therapy (Zheng et al., 2013).

8.2.2 SIRNA DELIVERY

RNA interference (RNAi) was recognized internationally in 1998 when Fire, Mello, and colleagues reported the potential of double-stranded RNA to suppress gene expression in the nematode worm *Caenorhabditis elegans*. Tuschl and colleagues published their successful proof-of-principle experiment three years later showing that sequence-specific gene knockdown in a mamma-lian cell line could be achieved by synthetic small interfering RNA (siRNA). Soon afterward, the first successful use of siRNA for gene silencing in mice was achieved for a target of hepatitis CIn addition; synthetic siRNAs have already been documented to be capable of knocking down targets in various in vivo diseases, including hypercholesterolemia, hepatitis B virus (HBV), human papillomavirus, ovarian cancer, and bone cancer. To incorporate these developments in a clinical setting, it is necessary to develop safe and effective delivery systems. Although' naked' chemically modified siRNA has shown efficacy in certain physiological settings such as the brain and lung, most tissues in the body require an additional delivery system to allow transfection. This is because of naked siRNA which is subject to endogenous enzyme degradation and is too big (~13 kDa) to cross cell membranes and too negatively charged.

8.2.3 SILENCE NEURONAL GENE EXPRESSION IN THE BRAIN

Ravi et al. developed a method for implying siRNA in lipid nanoparticles (LNPs) to effectively silence the expression of neuronal genes in cell culture by intracranial brain injection. Our finding is that these LNPs are processed in an apolipoprotein E-dependent manner by neurons, resulting in very effective cell culture uptake (100%) with little noticeable toxicity. *In vivo* injections of intracortical or intracerebroventricular (ICV) siRNA-LNP resulted in the knockdown of target genes either in isolated areas around the injection site or in wider areas following ICV injections without obvious toxicity or immune reactions from LNPs. Active targeted knockdown was demonstrated by demonstrating that intracortical delivery of siRNA to GRIN1 (NMDAR subunit GluN1 encoding) selectively decreased in vivo synaptic NMDAR currents relative to Currents in synaptic AMPA receptors. Therefore, siRNA delivery of LNP quickly manipulates the expression of proteins involved *in vivo* neuronal processes, possibly allowing gene therapies to develop for neurological disorders (Rungta et al., 2013).

8.2.4 RNAI-BASED THERAPY FOR GLIOBLASTOMA

Jensen et al. (2013) established that Glioblastoma brain tumors are extremely hard to kill as they usually recur following surgical, chemical, and biological attacks. Now, Jensen and colleagues identify a new nanoparticle conjugate that has the capability of passing the BBB, reaching the tumor, and targeting a recognized oncogene, breaking down the cancer-promoting signals and inducing glioma cell apoptosis. The nanoparticles, known as SNAs, are densely packed siRNA around a gold heart. In this case, the oncogene Bcl2L12 was targeted by the siRNA to prevent gene expression in human glioma cell lines and tumor neurospheres derived from the patient. The SNA nanoparticles quickly accumulated in the brain—primarily in the tumors—demonstrating their ability to cross the BBB when administered systemically to mice. Then animals with human brain tumors are treated with the SNAs infected with siRNA.

8.2.5 LIPOSOMAL SPHERICAL NUCLEIC ACIDS (SNAS)

For novel metal-free liposomal SNAs, Mirkin A. Chad et al. developed a scalable synthetic path. It is possible to rapidly assemble these structures from readily available, non-toxic starting materials. The architecture of the SNA not only stabilizes these small liposomal structures but also enables SKOV3-3 cells to internalize them. Therefore, these structures show promise as new biocompatible gene regulation constructs exhibiting many of the attractive properties of the more traditional SNAs based on AuNP (Banga et al., 2014).

8.2.6 POLYVALENT NUCLEIC ACID NANOSTRUCTURES (PNANS)

Mirkin A. Chad et al. have developed a new classification of polyvalent nucleic acid nanostructures (PNANs), consisting only of cross-linking and directed nucleic acids. It has been shown that these particles, without the need for a cationic polymer co-carrier, can impact on high cell uptake and regulation of gene. The PNANs also show binding cooperative behavior and properties of nuclease resistance (Cutler et al., 2011).

8.2.7 ANTIBODY-LINKED CELLULAR TARGETING

Mirkin A. Chad et al. documented the development and created a new SNA nucleic acid-antibody conjugate showing exceptional Cell line selectivity with antibody-recognized receptors showed that such structures demonstrate cell type selectivity relative to analog antibiotics in terms of their absorption and significantly greater gene knockdown in cells over target antigen expression (Zhang et al., 2012).

8.2.8 AMYLOID-B 1–40 FOR ALZHEIMER'S

Mackic B. Jasmina et al. stated that a soluble monomeric made up of amyloid β (1–40) peptide (sAβ 1–40) in Alzheimer's bloodstream is present and can contribute to neurotoxicity if it crosses the brain's capillary endothelium, including the BBB *in vivo*. This work uses an in vitro model of human BBB to describe the endothelial binding and transcytosis of a synthetic peptide homologous to human sAβ 1–40. I sAβ 1–40 which was time dependent on the brain microvascular endothelial cell monolayer, polarized to the apical side, and saturable with constants of high and low-affinity dissociation of 7.8±1.2 and 52.8±6.2 nM, respectively. Anti-RAGE (receptor for advanced glycation products) antibody (63%) and acetylated low-density lipoproteins (33%) inhibited the binding of I sAβ 1–40. In accordance with these results, RAGE or macrophage SR transfected cultured cells, type A, showed I sAβ 1–40 binding and internalization. I sAβ 1–40 transcytosis was time-and temperature-dependent, asymmetrical from the apical to basolateral side, saturable with a Michaelis constant of 45±9 nM, and partially resistant to RAGE blockade (36%) but not to SR blockade. We conclude that RAGE and SR mediate on the apical side of human BBB binding of sAβ 1–40 and that RAGE is also involved in sAβ 1–40 transcytosis (Shibata et al., 2000).

8.3   OTHER APPLICATIONS OF SNAS

8.3.1   DIAGNOSTICS

It was immediately recognized during the early studies of the SNA-Au NP conjugates that their reversible melting behavior over a wide temperature range and their subsequent hybridization-dependent optical changes could be useful for high-selectivity (vide infra) detection platforms. SNA nanostructures have since been used to build a wide variety of molecular diagnostic systems for a number of analytes in vitro and intracellular. These include colorimetric solution-based and chip-based scanometric systems for targets based on nucleic acid, DNA, small molecule, and metal ion (vide infra). The utility of SNA structures in diagnostic applications derives in part from both the SNA's polyvalent oligonucleotide shell properties and the inorganic core's physical and chemical properties. Such two components together generate probes that offer significant advantages over molecular equivalents. Strategies have been implemented that rely on more sophisti-cated SNA conjugates, such as the biobarcode assay. These assays layout an NP probe with "barcode" DNA strands that are hybridized to an SNA conjugate functionalized with strands complementing the barcode sequence as well as an antibody for an antigen of interest (for example, PSA). In the barcode assay, instead of directly detecting antigen molecules, signal amplification is achieved by releasing barcode DNA strings, post antigen sequestration, and isolation, accompanied by scanometric assay detection. More amplification of the signal is possible with the use of polymerase chain reaction (PCR) to increase barcode DNA copies, although the PCR-less technique with larger AuNPs (30 nm) has been shown to effectively detect PSA at attomolar concentrations. Variants of this procedure were used to study medical disease conditions, including Alzheimer's disease and cancer of the prostate.

8.3.2   REGULATION OF GENE EXPRESSION

Regulation of gene expression by means of artificial oligonucleotides has led to significant breakthroughs in knowing intracellular activity and can contribute to viable treatment choices for genetic-based diseases such as many forms of cancer and neurological disorders. Nevertheless, the transmission of synthetic nucleic acids to disease sites and across membranes of the cell remains a major obstacle for therapies for gene regulation (antisense DNA and si-RNA). The environment has, in fact, made a network of protection against foreign nucleic acids. Since nucleic acids are positively charged, for example, they cannot go without difficulty across the cell membrane that is negatively charged. Therefore, nucleases are quickly killed, and cells activate the innate immune response. Traditionally, Researchers recommended that protein purification agents like cationic polymers, liposomes, and modified viruses be used to move nucleic acids through the negatively charged cell membrane to protect them from enzymatic damage. Unfortunately, due to their inability to degrade spontaneously, extreme immunogenicity, and high concentration toxicity, these methods are not appropriate for systemic release. The most commonly used chemicals, cationic polymers complex, and neutralize the nucleic acid component, allowing the hybrid material to fuse cell membranes. 140 SNA constructs include an alternative in this aspect because of their large negative load; they were found to join cells in very high numbers without the ancillary need (zeta potential < -30 mV). 15 SNA-NP conjugates have a particular set of intracellular features, such as high binding coefficients for complementary DNA and RNA (vide supra), nuclease resistance, limited immune response, no observed toxicity, and highly effective gene-regulating abilities. Once, the 3D structure of the densely packed, strongly oriented oligonucleotide shell on the particle surface derives all of these properties (Stegh et al., 2008, 2010).

For the field of gene regulation, the high cell SNA internalization is encouraging; however, their indiscriminate adoption may present challenges for *in vivo* targeting. In reality, they are suitable for local delivery implementations where targets can be accomplished at the genetic level in their current state of development. Not like chemotherapy, in which all cells may be susceptible to drug cytotoxic effects, SNAs target only cancer cell gene expression profiles. Nevertheless, the nucleic acid shell's chemical tailorability gives an ideal scaffold for chemical change. For example, through modified bases and bioconjugation, one can consider the covalent attachment of shell peripheral guided moieties. These approaches together provide a blueprint for creating a broad range of new SNA-based therapeutic candidates (Boveri et al., 2005).

8.3.3 COMBINED DIAGNOSTICS INTRACELLULAR AND IMAGING

SNAs also contribute to methods and services for intracellular diagnosis and imaging. It is possible to attach fluorophore tags to them, making it easy to identify and image particles in cells. However, by adding gadolinium chelates to such particles, one can synthesize multimodal particles that are useful for MRI techniques. With regard to Au NPs, the highly efficient fluorescence quenching ability of the gold core can be used to build a versatile "off-on" fluorophore-based system that responds to varying levels of cell-based mRNA expression. Such specimens, dubbed "nanoflares," are built with sequences that complement disease-related mRNA (about 18 bases long), such as survivin, and a fluorophore-labeled sequence of "flare" (about 10 bases long) that is hybridized to the particle. In this case, the fluorophore tag is close to the surface of the sample and mainly quenched in its fluorescence. In the cell, the particle nanoflare encounters and binds to its complementary mRNA target, which is longer than the sequence of short flare. This behavior displaces the flare from the surface of the particles and induces an increase in signal an interesting aspect of the nanoflare structure is that the short flare sequence makes the surface strands more rigid and moves the mRNA complement away from the NP layer, resulting in an activated binding site for the mRNA target. For the field of gene regulation, the high cell internalization of SNAs is indeed promising; however, their indiscriminate adoption may present challenges for *in vivo* targeting. In reality, they are suitable for local delivery applications where targeting can be achieved at the genetic level in their current state of development. Unlike chemotherapy, where all cells may be susceptible to drug cytotoxic effects, SNAs target only cancer cell gene expression profiles. However, the nucleic acid shell's chemical tailorability provides an ideal scaffold for chemical change. For example, through modified bases and bioconjugation, one can imagine the covalent attachment of targeting moieties on the shell periphery. In addition, oligonucleotides could be hybridized via targeting "cargo" in a comparatively straightforward fashion. SNAs could be manufactured through a variety of particle sizes, suggesting that they're being tailored to various forms of illness (Leachman et al., 2009; Proksch et al., 2008; Roberts et al., 2007; Zhu et al., 2009).

8.4 CONCLUSION

The nanoparticles, known as SNAs, are compactly packed siRNA around a gold base. SNAs have become a potentially useful tool in biological applications on the basis of their enhanced cellular absorption, stability, biocompatibility, and flexible surface functionality. Originally, a simple concept for the assembly of nanoparticles was developed whereby programmable base-matching communications could be utilized to reversibly shape naturally visible materials from nano-scale segments. Nonetheless, the discovery that the arrangement of oligonucleotides in tightly guided, tightly packed spherical structures results in species able to communicate with biological materials in specific ways offered places for their use in molecular diagnostics, gene regulation, and medicine. The knowledge gained from SNA research as diagnostic and gene-regulating frameworks took the initial study of the whole Genetic code-mediated assembly circle through the understanding of some of the key insights required to crystallize nanoparticles that have arisen as a rich field of study in recent years. As it keeps on expanding across various scientific and technological fields, many scientists around the globe have contributed significantly to the area of SNAs. Nevertheless, much remains to be known about the basic characters of SNAs, their range of usefulness, and the variety of potential conjugate materials. At the molecular level, we do not yet understand their intracellular transport modes, why can tissues and organs penetrate much more effective than other molecular systems, and how they pass inside living systems from cell to cell. Most of the technologies based on them centered on life sciences, but in the fields of electronics, catalysis, and energy harvesting, storage, and conversion, there are major opportunities. It would rely on our capacity to synthesize broader classes of conjugate materials to realize these possibilities. However, although most of the research has centered on SNA-Au NP conjugates, we and others have demonstrated SNAs can be produced from magnetic insulators, semiconductors, and metallic materials, and even pure DNA cores formed using DNA origami methods.

KEYWORDS

- antisense oligonucleotides
- blood-brain barrier
- cetyltrimethylammonium bromide
- deoxyribonucleic acids
- enhanced permeation and retention
- glioblastoma multiforme
- isostructural aluminum diboride

REFERENCES

Banga, R. J., Chernyak, N., Narayan, S. P., Nguyen, S. T., & Mirkin, C. A., (2014). Liposomal spherical nucleic acids. *J. Am. Chem. Soc., 136*(28), 9866–9869.

Barnaby, S. N., Lee, A., & Mirkin, C. A., (2014). Probing the inherent stability of siRNA immobilized on nanoparticle constructs. *Proc. Natl. Acad. Sci. USA, 111*(27), 9739–9744.

Boveri, M., Berezowski, V., Price, A., Slupek, S., Lenfant, A. M., Benaud, C., Hartung, T., et al., (2005). Induction of blood-brain barrier properties in cultured brain capillary endothelial cells: Comparison between primary glial cells and C6 cell line. *Glia., 51*(3), 187–198.

Cerritelli, S. M., & Crouch, R. J., (2009). Ribonuclease H: The enzymes in eukaryotes. *FEBS J., 276*(6), 1494–1505.

Chung, H. J. C., Liangliang, H., Suguna, P. N., Evelyn, A., & Chad, A. M., (2013). *Mechanism for the Endocytosis of Spherical Nucleic Acid Nanoparticle Conjugates*. Pub Med.

Fabian, M. R., Sonenberg, N., & Filipowicz, W., (2010). Regulation of mRNA translation and stability by microRNAs. *Annu. Rev. Biochem., 79*, 351–379.

Giljohann, D. A., et al., (2009). *J. Am. Chem. Society, 131*, 2072–2073.

International Agency for Research on Cancer (IARC), World Health Organization (WHO), (2012). Cancer fact sheets. In: *Globocan 2012: Estimated Cancer Incidence, Mortality, and Prevalence Worldwide in 2012*. International Agency for Research on Cancer (IARC), World Heatlth Organization (WHO), Lyon, France.

Jensen, S. A., Day, E. S., Ko, C. H., Hurley, L. A., Luciano, J. P., Kouri, F. M., Merkel, T. J., et al., (2013). Spherical nucleic acid nanoparticle conjugates as an RNAi-based therapy for glioblastoma, *Sci. Transl. Med., 5*(209).

Jing, Z., Guizhi, Z., Yinhui, L., Chunmei, L., Mingxu, Y., Tao, C., Erqun, S., Ronghua, Y., & Weihong, T., (2013). A spherical nucleic acid platform based on self-assembled DNA biopolymer for high-performance cancer Therapy. *ACS Nano, 7*(8), 6545–6554.

Joshua, I. C., Ke, Z., Dan, Z., Evelyn, A., Andrew, E. P., & Chad, A. M., (2011). Polyvalent nucleic acid nanostructures *J. Am. Chem. Soc., 133*(24), 9254–9257.

Kanasty, R. L., Whitehead, K. A., Vegas, A. J., & Anderson, D. G., (2012). Action and reaction: The biological response to siRNA and its delivery vehicles. *Mol. Ther., 20*(3), 513–524.

Leachman, S. A., Hickerson, R. P., Schwartz, M. E., Bullough, E. E., Hutcherson, S. L., Boucher, K. M., Hansen, C. D., et al., (2009). First-in-human mutation-targeted siRNA Phase Ib trial of an inherited skin disorder. *Mol. Ther., 18*(2), 442–446.

Louis, D. N., Ohgaki, H., Wiestler, O. D., et al., (2007). The 2007 WHO classification of tumors of the central nervous system. *Acta Neuropathologica, 114*(2), 97–109.

Masayoshi, S., Shinya, Y., Ram, K. S., Miguel, C., James, B., Blas, F., David, M. H., et al., (2000). Clearance of Alzheimer's amyloid-β1-40 peptide from brain by LDL receptor-related protein-1 at the blood-brain barrier. *Journal of Clinical Investigation, 106*(12), 1489–1499.

Proksch, E., Brandner, J. M., & Jensen, J. M., (2008). The skin: An indispensable barrier. *Exp Dematol., 17*(12), 1063–1072.

Ravi, L. R., Hyun, B. C., Paulo, J. C. L., Rebecca, W. Y. K., Donovan, A., Jay, N., Muthiah, M., Pieter, R. C., & Brian, A. M. V., (2013). Lipid nanoparticle delivery of siRNA to silence neuronal gene expression in the brain. *Molecular Therapy Nucleic Acids, 2*(12), e136.

Resham, J. B., Natalia, C., Suguna, P. N., SonBinh, T. N., & Chad, A. M., (2014). Liposomal spherical nucleic acids. *J. Am. Chem. Soc., 136*(28), 9866–9869.

Roberts, P. J., & Der, C. J., (2007). Targeting the Raf-MEK-ERK mitogen-activated protein kinase cascade for the treatment of cancer. *Oncogene, 26*(22), 3291–3310.

Sanai, N., & Berger, M. S., (2008). Glioma extent of resection and its impact on patient outcome. *Neurosurgery, 62*, 753–764.

Stegh, A. H., Brennan, C., Mahoney, J. A., Forloney, K. L., Jenq, H. T., Luciano, J. P., Protopopov, A., et al., (2010). Glioma oncoprotein Bcl2L12 inhibits the p53 tumor suppressor. *Genes. Dev., 24*(19), 2194–2204.

Stegh, A. H., Chin, L., Louis, D. N., & DePinho, R. A., (2008). What drives intense apoptosis resistance and propensity for necrosis in glioblastoma? A role for Bcl2L12 as a multifunctional cell death regulator. *Cell Cycle, 7*(18), 2833–2839.

Xiaochen, A. W., Chung, H. J. C., Chuan, Z., Liangliang, H., & Chad, A. M., (2014). Intracellular fate of spherical nucleic acid nanoparticle conjugates. *J. Am. Chem. Soc., 136*(21), 7726–7733.

Young, K. L., Scott, A. W., Hao, L., Mirkin, S. E., Liu, G., & Mirkin, C. A., (2012). Hollow spherical nucleic acids for intracellular gene regulation based upon biocompatible silica shells. *Nano Lett., 12*(7), 3867–3871.

Zhang, H. L., Hurst, S. J., & Mirkin, C. A., (2012). Antibody-linked spherical nucleic acids for cellular targeting. *J. Am. Chem. Soc., 134*(40), 16488–16491.

Zhu, H., Acquaviva, J., Ramachandran, P., Boskovitz, A., Woolfenden, S., Pfannl, R., Bronson, R. T., et al., (2009). Oncogenic EGFR signaling cooperates with loss of tumor suppressor gene functions in gliomagenesis. *Proc. Natl. Acad. Sci. USA, 106*(8), 2712–2716.

CHAPTER 9

Intra-Vital Microscopy: A New Amelioration in Cancer Immunotherapy Monitoring

SANDEEP ARORA, NEELAM SHARMA, and SUKHBIR SINGH

Chitkara College of Pharmacy, Chitkara University, Punjab, India

ABSTRACT

This chapter summarizes progression in intra-vital microscopy (IVM), i.e., high-resolution IVM method, advanced detection methods for simultaneous imaging of multiple cell types and molecules, labeling of drug molecules, and target tissue for IVM imaging, label-free imaging, and fluorescent labeling of drug delivery systems. This chapter also describes the significance of IVM in cancer immunotherapy, which includes investigation of cancer growth and propagation via tumor vasculature imaging, intravital imaging of the tumor-associated immune system, antibody-dependent anticancer activity, visualization of therapeutic delivery at tumor microenvironment, therapeutic delivery in the tumor microenvironment, intra-vital imaging for studying cancer-fibroblast interactions, new tools for living, intra-vital, and in situ imaging in translational cancer research and assessing the efficacy of therapy through IVM.

9.1 INTRODUCTION

Though, absolute surgical removal of primary tumor is proficient remedy for cancer treatment. Unfortunately, metastasis is the cancerous stage at which tumor cells extends to alongside organ to produce secondary tumor (Beerling et al., 2011). *In-vivo* physiology of tumor cells at cellular resolution can be sighted by intra-vital microscopy (IVM). Groom et al. monitored tumor metastasis in the interior embryo using injectable dyes. Green fluorescent protein (GFP) labeled tumor cells were employed to investigate cancerous tissues through confocal scanning microscopy by Farina et al. (1998) and Naumov et al. (1992). Live spatiotemporal dynamics progression of cancer at different levels, i.e., whole-organ, cellular, sub-cellular, and molecular can be directly visualized by intra-vital imaging (Gligorijevic and Condeelis, 2011). IVM has developed as an imperative gadget for investigating the course of action triggering cancer metastasis. Herein, we have summarized the novel advances and applications of IVM in cancer immunotherapy (MacDonald et al., 1992; Chishima et al., 1997).

9.2   CANCER CELLS AND IMMUNE SYSTEM INTERACTIONS

Recent research have demonstrated that immune system can identify and eradicate anomalous cancer cells developing within human body (Zhou, 2013; Narendra et al., 2013; Liu et al., 2012; Rangwala and Tsai, 2011; Hwu, 2010; Hamai et al., 2010; von Boehmer et al., 2012). Consequently, it was established that interaction amongst immune system and cancer is fundamental cause of cancer development. The immune system in cancer patients is not adequately strong to eradicate cancerous cells; signifying suppression of antitumor immune system. Therefore, transplant receiver undergoing continual immune-suppression exhibited considerably larger threat of escalating lung cancer (Dugué et al., 2013) and augmented danger for cervical cancer in women (Feyler et al., 2013). Numerous factors which may produce antitumor immune-suppression include high-avidity antitumor T cells, cellular mediated tumor-induced immune evasion, distorted antigenicity tumor-derived interleukin (IL)-18 induced immune-suppression (Terme et al., 2011, 2012; Cheng et al., 2012). For example, IL-1 up regulated TGF-beta in mesenchymal stem cells induced immune-suppression causing prostate cancer (Egeblad et al., 2008). Therefore, immunological method that eliminate antitumor immune-suppression and augment antitumor immunity possibly will be highly effective in cancer treatment.

9.3   PROGRESSION IN INTRA-VITAL MICROSCOPY (IVM)

9.3.1   HIGH-RESOLUTION INTRA-VITAL MICROSCOPY (IVM) METHOD

Spinning disk confocal microscopy (SDCM), optical frequency domain imaging (OFDI), and multi-photon microscopy (MPM) are examples of high-resolution IVM techniques. Schematic representation of OFDI and their advantages as well as application has been represented in Figures 9.1 and 9.2, respectively.

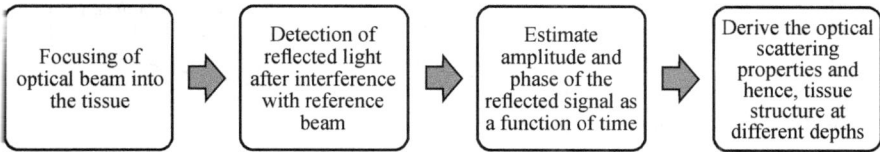

Focusing of optical beam into the tissue	Detection of reflected light after interference with reference beam	Estimate amplitude and phase of the reflected signal as a function of time	Derive the optical scattering properties and hence, tissue structure at different depths

FIGURE 9.1   Schematic representation of OFDI.

Applications	Advantages
• Angiogenesis • Lymph angiogenesis • Tissue viability	• Enabls the imaging of substantial volumes of tissue over prolonged periods without the need for contrast agents.

FIGURE 9.2   Advantages and applications of OFDI.

Tumors which express fluorescent proteins (FPs) are usually detected by SDCM and MPM has been described in Figures 9.3 and 9.4, respectively (Lohela and Werb, 2010; Theer et al., 2003; Campagnola et al., 2002; Helmchen and Denk, 2005; Mohler et al., 2003; Zipfel et al., 2003; Vinegoni et al., 2015). IVM has been preferred technique for intra vital imaging of tumor cell biology due to high-resolution acquisition and deep tissue penetration.

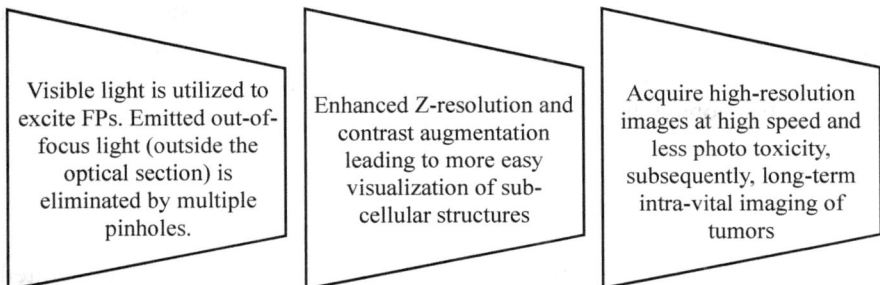

Visible light is utilized to excite FPs. Emitted out-of-focus light (outside the optical section) is eliminated by multiple pinholes.	Enhanced Z-resolution and contrast augmentation leading to more easy visualization of sub-cellular structures	Acquire high-resolution images at high speed and less photo toxicity, subsequently, long-term intra-vital imaging of tumors

FIGURE 9.3   Description of spinning disk confocal microscopy.

Short pulses of infrared (IR) light with a typical wavelength rane of 800-1000 nm penetrate the tissue more than tenfold deeper compared with spinning disk microscopy

IR excitation has capability to create second harmonic generation (SHG) signal extracellular matrix component.

SHG signal does not suffer from photobleaching. SHG microscopy has importance in studying of fibrillar collagen in skin, gut and breast.

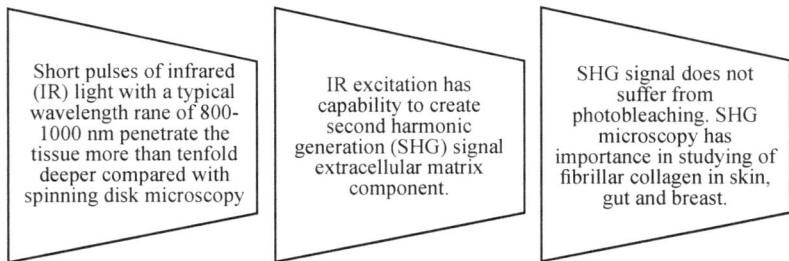

FIGURE 9.4   Description of multi-photon microscopy.

9.3.2   HIGHLY DEVELOPED DETECTION TECHNIQUES FOR INSTANTANEOUS IMAGING OF MULTIPLE CELL TYPES AND MOLECULES

Multi-color IVM exploits colored FPs, e.g., GFP, cyan fluorescent protein (CFP), yellow fluorescent protein (YFP) and red fluorescent protein (RFP) to simultaneously visualize the different types of cell and molecules as well as to study interaction among various cells and molecules in real-time (Helmchen and Denk, 2005; Shimomura et al., 1962; Giepmans et al., 2006; Jalink and van Rheenen, 2009). Foremost drawback of multicolor IVM is overlapping of FPs and dyes excitation and emission spectra which might be differentiated with complicated algorithms (Weigert et al., 2010).

9.3.3   LABELING OF DRUG MOLECULES AND TARGET TISSUE FOR IVM IMAGING

The delivery of diagnostic and therapeutic agents can be envisaged and supervised in live animals through selective labeling of concerned molecules and target tissue at cellular and sub-cellular level which ensures the utmost signal-to-noise ratio. This technique maintains imaging capabilities, trace providence of drug carrier, and its efficacy without troubling ordinary physiological functions within live animals.

9.3.4   LABEL-FREE IMAGING

The label-free technique involves use of cellular/extracellular generated auto-fluorescence and second-harmonic (SHG) signals for multiplexed

IVM imaging. Liver and blood produce auto fluoresce to impart endogenous contrast which could be utilized for recognizing fields of view (FOVs) for comparison of healthy and diseased animal models (Gao et al., 2004; Monici, 2005; Radosevich et al., 2008; Van De Ven et al., 2012). SHG signal has been employed to image collagen and myosin fibers to facilitate differentiation in the microenvironment of tumor diseased and healthy tissue.

9.3.5   FLUORESCENT LABELING OF DRUG DELIVERY SYSTEMS

Fluorescent labeling of drug-loaded particulates facilitates straightforward tracking of drug delivery to target tissues from site-of-injection to targeted organs. Commercially accessible fluorescent molecules have been employed to label silica, iron oxide, liposomal, and polymeric nanoparticles (Kim et al., 2013). For instance, tetramethyl rhodamine-succinyl ester Alexa Fluor™ dye has been successfully utilized to fluorescently label silica nanoparticles derivative with amine functional groups which allowed prolonged IVM imaging of drug delivery systems (Van de Ven et al., 2012). These fluorescent molecules should be reactive to different functional groups and less prone to photo-bleaching. Lipophilic fluorescent dyes facile labeling facilitates the evaluation of vascular flow dynamics in live animals without negotiating the viability of cells. For instance, red blood cells fluorescently labeled with DiD dye was used to indirectly label splenic macrophage and liver cells (Kirui et al., 2014; Zheng et al., 2012).

9.4   SIGNIFICANCE OF IVM IN CANCER IMMUNOTHERAPY

9.4.1   INVESTIGATION OF CANCER GROWTH AND PROPAGATION VIA TUMOR VASCULATURE IMAGING

Cancer cells utilize contiguous stroma to endorse their development and distribution. Tumor vasculature provides required oxygen and nutrients as well as acts as a transporter for circulating cancer cells (Veiseh et al., 2014). Intra-vital imaging tools, i.e., nanoparticles, and FPs have been engaged to understand the relations between cancer and blood vessels along with investigating microvasculature systems in-vivo models (Leong et al., 2014; Minder et al., 2015; Brown et al., 2001; Nobis et al., 2013). Intra-vital imaging of embryonic chicken chorioallantoic membrane (CAM) has been investigated through intravenous injection of agglutinin and fluorescent-tagged cancerous cells for examining molecular scheme implicated in cancerous cells extravasation. Quantum dot (QD) nanoparticles and fluorescent dextrans have been commonly employed to envisage vascular integrity in animate tumor tissues during *in vivo* cancer examination (Gallego-Ortega et al., 2015). Ormandy and colleagues performed intra-vital imaging of QDs in polyoma middle T-model of breast cancer and demonstrated that the primary phase of cancer cells can exploit surrounding vasculature throughout the progression of invasive and metastatic cancer (Cai et al., 2008).

9.4.2   INTRA-VITAL IMAGING OF TUMOR-RELATED IMMUNE SYSTEM

Cancerous cells interconnect with the immune system to assist growth and evade from cell loss (Zal and Chodaczek, 2010; Serrels et al., 2015; Boissonnas et al., 2007; Harney et al., 2015). Intra-vital imaging of immune cells and leaky blood vessels has been utilized for identifying mechanisms of action of drugs. Intra-vital imaging of blood vasculature employing fluorescent dextran and QDs established that Tie2hi-expressing TAMs persuade temporary vascular escape *via* vascular endothelial growth factor A (VEGFA) indicator, consequently assisting cancerous cell extravasation (Zanganeh et al., 2017; Weiner et al., 2012).

9.4.3   ANTIBODY-DEPENDENT ANTICANCER ACTIVITY

Monoclonal antibodies (mAbs) as therapeutic agents have been imperative for cancer therapy (Scott et al., 2012; Gul et al., 2014). Liver imaging through IVM have elucidated the procedure through which mAbs eradicate circulating tumor cells (McDonald et al., 2008). During real-time imaging in murine tumor cell opsonization model, it was investigated that cancerous cells were promptly detected and apprehended through Kupffer cells. Consequently, it was concluded that antibody-dependent phagocytosis (ADPh) *via* macrophages is the foremost mechanism for the elimination of cancerous cells from circulation (Clark et al., 2007; Jain, 2001).

9.4.4   VISUALIZATION OF THERAPEUTIC DELIVERY AT TUMOR MICROENVIRONMENT

Unforeseen developments in IVM imaging have facilitated visualization of therapeutic molecules, cells, and particles through blood vessels and tumor interstitial space (Martinez et al., 2013). IVM imaging has been exploited to design drug carriers that favorably mount up at diseased tissue through enhanced permeability and retention (EPR) effect owing to the tumor microenvironment (Adriani et al., 2012; Decuzzi et al., 2009; Frieboes et al., 2013; Liu, 2009). Various changes in the tumor microenvironment have been depicted in Figure 9.5.

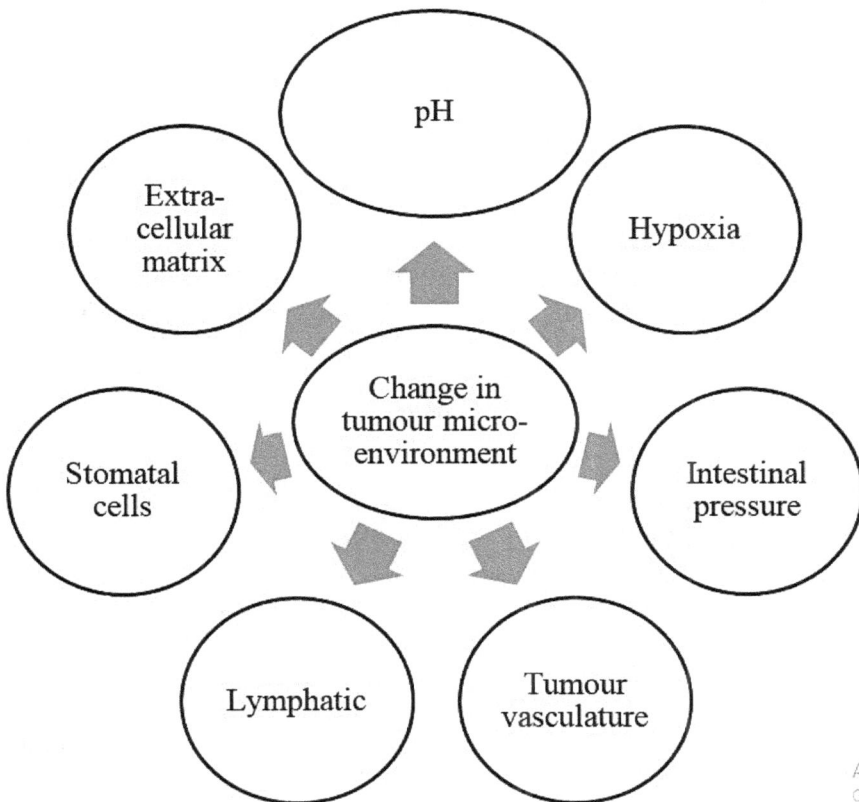

FIGURE 9.5   Changes in the tumor microenvironment.

9.4.5 THERAPEUTIC DELIVERY IN TUMOR MICROENVIRONMENT

IVM investigation of melanoma tumor model discovered that large multi-stage vector (MSV) discoidal particles mount up within tumor microvasculature than smaller counterparts which extravasated out of leaky vascular walls (Kirui et al., 2014). Additional analysis assessed preferential particle accumulation in tumor microenvironment due to surface modifications. The investigation illustrated that arginine-glycine-aspartic acid (RGD) peptide derivatization of MSV particles leads to preferential attachment of particles to $\alpha v\beta 3$ integrins expressed over tumor endothelial walls than uncoated particles (Khawar et al., 2015; Goss and Chambers, 2010).

9.4.6 INTRA-VITAL IMAGING FOR STUDYING CANCER-FIBROBLAST INTERACTIONS

An essential basis of disease setback in tumor dormancy is stromal fibroblasts (Komatsu et al., 2015). Intra-vital imaging has an important role in studying the underline mechanism. Lawson et al. developed a new method for longitudinal imaging of myeloma cells via a dye-dilution system. The technique was successful in labeling and tracking gradually propagating dormant cells and demonstrated that these cells interrelate with host bone cells to pioneer a defensive role for the perseverance of metastasis. Cancer cell-fibroblast interactions facilitate tumor invasion for tumor metastasis.

9.4.7 AN INNOVATIVE APPROACH FOR IN-SITU INTRA-VITAL IMAGING IN TRANSLATIONAL CANCER INVESTIGATION

Fluorescence biosensors are optimistic as a trustworthy gadget to examine method of chemoresistance and drug targeting action. Live imaging of extracellular signal-regulated kinase (Erk), mitogen-activated protein kinase inhibitor (MEKi)-resistant cell lines and S6K fluorescent biosensors have been explored to cross-examine elementary origin of resistance to MEKi in Kras-mutant and Braf-mutant cancer cell lines *in-vitro*. It was illustrated that therapeutic with MEKi, Erk, and PI3K mechanisms could preserve mTORC1 activity and sequentially, promotes cell augmentation, consecutively, causing resistance (Debergh et al., 2010).

9.4.8 EVALUATION OF EFFICIENCY OF TREATMENT THROUGH IVM

IVM can offer exclusive facts on numerous cellular as well as molecular features of drug therapy. Through an investigation of antiangiogenic treatment by means of a dorsal skin chamber, it was examined that antiangiogenic therapy substantially affects characteristics of tumor vessels, i.e., shape irregularities, vessel diameter, and permeability. Moreover, it was revealed that low-molecular-weight heparins (LMWHs) antagonists could bestow survival assistance in cancer patients through decreasing the microvessel density and vascular area fraction.

9.5 CONCLUSIONS AND FUTURE PERSPECTIVES

This chapter described the advantages and significance of IVM in studying the metastatic process and cancer immunotherapy. Progress in IVM includes advanced detection methods for synchronized imaging of multiple cells, high-resolution IVM procedure, drug molecules labeling, and tissue targeting, label-free imaging, and fluorescent labeling of drug delivery systems. Significance of IVM in cancer immunotherapy includes investigation of cancer growth and propagation *via* tumor vasculature imaging, intravital imaging of the tumor-associated immune system, antibody-dependent anticancer activity, visualization of therapeutic delivery at tumor microenvironment, therapeutic delivery in the tumor microenvironment, intra-vital imaging for studying cancer-fibroblast interactions, new tools *in-situ* intra-vital imaging in translational cancer investigation and assessing the efficacy of therapy through IVM.

KEYWORDS

- antibody-dependent phagocytosis
- intra-vital microscopy
- monoclonal antibodies
- multi-photon microscopy
- optical frequency domain imaging
- spinning disk confocal microscopy

REFERENCES

Adriani, G., De Tullio, M. D., Ferrari, M., et al., (2012). The preferential targeting of the diseased microvasculature by disk-like particles. *Biomaterials, 33*(22), 5504–5513.

Amornphimoltham, P., Masedunskas, A., & Weigert, R., (2011). Intravital microscopy as a tool to study drug delivery in preclinical studies. *Advanced Drug Delivery Reviews, 63*(1/2), 119–128.

Beerling, E., Ritsma, L., Vrisekoop, N., Derksen, W. P., & Rheenen, J. V., (2011). Intra-vital microscopy: New insights into metastasis of tumors. *Journal of Cell Science, 124*, 299–310.

Boissonnas, A., Fetler, L., Zeelenberg, I. S., et al., (2007). *In vivo* imaging of cytotoxic T cell infiltration and elimination of a solid tumor. *J. Exp. Med., 204*(2), 345–356.

Brown, E. B., Campbell, R. B., Tsuzuki, Y., et al., (2001). *In vivo* measurement of gene expression, angiogenesis, and physiological function in tumors using multiphoton laser scanning microscopy. *Nat. Med., 7*(7), 864–868.

Cai, W., Gambhir, S. S., & Chen, X., (2008). Molecular imaging of tumor vasculature. *Methods Enzymol., 445*, 141–716.

Campagnola, P. J., Millard, A. C., Terasaki, M., Hoppe, P. E., Malone, C. J., & Mohler, W., (2002). A. Three-dimensional high-resolution second-harmonic generation, imaging of endogenous structural proteins in biological tissues. *Biophys. J., 82*, 493–508.

Chalfie, M., Tu, Y., Euskirchen, G., Ward, W. W., & Prasher, D. C., (1994). Green, fluorescent protein as a marker for gene expression. *Science, 263*, 802–805.

Cheng, J., Li, L., Liu, Y., Wang, Z., Zhu, X., & Bai, X., (2012). Interleukin-1α induces immuno suppression by mesenchymal stem cells promoting the growth of prostate cancer cells. *Molecular Medicine Reports, 6*(5), 955–960.

Chishima, T., Miyagi, Y., Wang, X., Yamaoka, H., Shimada, H., Moossa, A. R., & Hoffman, R. M., (1997). Cancer invasion and micro metastasis visualized in live tissue by green fluorescent protein expression. *Cancer Res., 57*, 2042–2047.

Clark, S. R., Ma, A. C., Tavener, S. A., et al., (2007). Platelet TLR4 activates neutrophil extracellular traps to ensnare bacteria in septic blood. *Nat Med., 13*(4), 463–469.

Claudio, V., Sungon, L., Aaron, D. A., & Ralph, W., (2015). New techniques for motion-artifact-free *in vivo* cardiac microscopy. *Front. Physiol., 6*, 147.

De Visser, K. E., Eichten, A., & Coussens, L. M., (2006). Paradoxical roles of the immune system during cancer development. *Nat Rev Cancer, 6*(1), 24–37.

Debergh, I., Van, D. N., Pattyn, P., Peeters, M., & Ceelen, W. P., (2010). The low-molecular-weight heparin nadroparin, inhibits tumor angiogenesis in a rodent dorsal skin fold chamber model. *Br. J. Cancer, 102*, 837–843.

Decuzzi, P., Pasqualini, R., Arap, W., & Ferrari, M., (2009). Intravascular delivery of particulate systems: Does geometry really matter. *Pharm Res., 26*(1), 235–243.

Dugué, P. A., Rebolj, M., Garred, P., & Lynge, E., (2013). Immunosuppression and risk of cervical cancer. *Expert Review of Anticancer Therapy, 13*(1), 29–42.

Egeblad, M., Ewald, A. J., Askautrud, H. A., Truitt, M. L., Welm, B. E., Bainbridge, E., Peeters, G., et al., (2008). Visualizing stromal cell, dynamics in different tumor microenvironments by spinning disk confocal microscopy. *Dis. Model. Mech., 1*, 155–167.

Farina, K. L., Wyckoff, J. B., Rivera, J., Lee, H., Segall, J. E., Condeelis, J. S., et al., (1998). Cell motility of tumor cells visualized in living intact primary tumors using green fluorescent protein. *Cancer Res., 58*, 2528–2532.

Feyler, S., Selby, P. J., & Cook, G., (2013). Regulating the regulators in cancer-immunosuppression in multiple myeloma (MM). *Blood Reviews, 27*(3), 155–164.

Frieboes, H. B., Wu, M., Lowengrub, J., Decuzzi, P., & Cristini, V., (2013). A computational model for predicting nanoparticle accumulation in tumor vasculature. *PLoS One, 8*(2), e56876.

Gallego-Ortega, D., Ledger, A., Roden, D. L., et al., (2015). ELF5 drives lung metastasis in luminal breast cancer through recruitment of Gr1 + CD11b + myeloid-derived suppressor cells. *PLoS Biol., 13*(12), e1002330.

Gao, S., Lan, X., Liu, Y., Shen, Z., Lu, J., & Ni, X., (2004). Characteristics of blood fluorescence spectra using low-level, 457. 9-nm excitation from Ar+ laser. *Chin Opt Lett., 2*(3), 160–161.

Giepmans, B. N. G., Adams, S. R., Ellisman, M. H., & Tsien, R. Y., (2006). The fluorescent toolbox for assessing protein location and function. *Science, 312*, 217–224.

Gligorijevic, B., & Condeelis, (2011). Stretching the timescale of intra-vital imaging in tumors. *Cell Adhesion and Migration, 3*(4), 313–315.

Goss, P. E., & Chambers, A. F., (2010). Does tumor dormancy offer a therapeutic target? *Nat. Rev. Cancer, 10*(12), 871–877.

Goswitz, C. V., & Peter, S. Z., (2013). Cancer therapy based on a mechanism of action for controlling the immune system and the resulting patent portfolio. *Recent Patents on Endocrine, Metabolic, and Immune. Drug Discovery, 7*(1), 1–10.

Gul, N., Babes, L., Siegmund, K., et al., (2014). Macrophages eliminate circulating tumor cells after monoclonal antibody therapy. *J. Clin. Invest., 124*(2), 812–823.

Hamai, A., Benlalam, H., Meslin, F., Hasmim, M., Carre, T., Akalay, et al., (2010). Immune surveillance of human cancer: If the cytotoxic T-lymphocytes play the music, does the tumoral system call the tune? *Tissue Antigens, 75*(1), 1–8.

Harney, A. S., Arwert, E. N., Entenberg, D., et al., (2015). Real-time imaging reveals local, transient vascular permeability, and tumor cell intravasation stimulated by TIE2hi macrophage-derived VEGFA. *Cancer Discov., 5*(9), 932–943.

Helmchen, F., & Denk, W., (2005). Deep tissue two-photon microscopy. *Nat. Methods, 2*, 932–940.

Hwu, P., (2010). Treating cancer by targeting the immune system. *The New England Journal of Medicine, 8*(363), 779–781.

Jain, R. K., (2001). Delivery of molecular medicine to solid tumors: Lessons from *in vivo* imaging of gene expression and function. *J. Control Release, 74*(1–3), 7–25.

Jalink, K., & Van, R. J., (2009). Filter FRET: Quantitative imaging of sensitized emission. *Laboratory Techniques in Biochemistry and Molecular Biology, 33*, 289–349.

Karreman, M. A., Hyenne, V., Schwab, Y., & Goetz, J. G., (2016). Intravital correlative microscopy: Imaging life at the nanoscale. *Trends in Cell Biology, 26*(11), 848–863.

Khawar, I. A., Kim, J. H., & Kuh, H. J., (2015). Improving drug delivery to solid tumors: Priming the tumor microenvironment. *Journal of Controlled Release, 201*, 78–89.

Kim, P., Ferrari, M., & Yun, S. H., (2013). Real-time intravital microscopy of individual nanoparticle dynamics in liver and tumors of live mice. *Protocol Exchange*.

Kirui, D. K., Mai, J., Palange, A. L., Qin, G., Van, D. V. A. L., Liu, X., et al., (2014). Transient mild hyperthermia induces E-selectin mediated localization of mesoporous silicon vectors in solid tumors. *PloS One, 9*(2), e86489.

Komatsu, N., Fujita, Y., Matsuda, M., et al., (2015). mTORC1 up regulation via ERK-dependent gene expression change confers intrinsic resistance to MEK inhibitors in oncogenic KR as-mutant cancer cells. *Oncogene, 34*(45), 5607–5616.

Leong, H. S., Robertson, A. E., Stoletov, K., et al., (2014). Invadopodia are required for cancer cell extravasation and are a therapeutic target for metastasis. *Cell Rep., 8*(5), 1558–1570.

Liu, S., (2009). Radiolabeled cyclic RGD peptides as integrin αvβ3-targeted radiotracers: Maximizing binding affinity via bivalency. *Bioconjug. Chem., 20*(12), 2199–2213.

Liu, Y., & Zeng, G., (2012). Cancer and innate immune system interactions: Translational potentials for cancer immunotherapy. *Journal of Immunotherapy (Hagerstown, Md.: 1997), 35*(4), 299.

Lohela, M., & Werb, Z., (2010). Intra-vital imaging of stromal cell dynamics in tumors. *Curr. Opin. Genet. Dev., 20*, 72–78.

MacDonald, C., Schmidt, E. E., Morris, V. L., Chambers, A. F., & Groom, A. C., (1992). Intra-vital video microscopy of the chorioallantoic membrane microcirculation: A model system for studying metastasis. *Microvasc. Res., 4*, 185–199.

Martinez, J. O., Boada, C., Yazdi, I. K., et al., (2013). Short and long term, *in vitro* and *in vivo* correlations of cellular and tissue responses to mesoporous silicon nanovectors. *Small, 9*(9/10), 1722–1733.

McDonald, B., McAvoy, E. F., Lam, F., et al., (2008). Interaction of CD44 and hyaluronan is the dominant mechanism for neutrophil sequestration in inflamed liver sinusoids. *J. Exp. Med., 205*(4), 915–927.

Minder, P., Zajac, E., Quigley, J. P., et al., (2015). EGFR regulates the development and microarchitecture of intratumoral angiogenic vasculature capable of sustaining cancer cell intravasation. *Neoplasia, 17*(8), 634–649.

Mohler, W., Millard, A. C., & Campagnola, P. J., (2003). Second-harmonic generation, imaging of endogenous structural proteins. *Methods, 29*, 97–109.

Monici, M., (2005). Cell and tissue auto fluorescence research and diagnostic applications. *Biotechnology Annual Review, 11*, 227–256.

Narendra, B. L., Reddy, K. E., Shantikumar, S., & Ramakrishna, S., (2013). Immune system: A double-edged sword in cancer. *Inflammation Research, 62*(9), 823–834.

Naumov, G. N., Wilson, S. M., MacDonald, I. C., Schmidt, E. E., Morris, V. L., Groom, A. C., et al., (1992). Cellular expression of green fluorescent protein, coupled with high-resolution *in vivo* video microscopy, to monitor steps in tumor metastasis. *J. Cell Sci., 112*, 1835–1842.

Nobis, M., McGhee, E. J., Morton, J. P., et al., (2013). Intra-vital FLIM-FRET imaging reveals dasatinib-induced spatial control of SRC in pancreatic cancer. *Cancer Res., 73*(15), 4674–4686.

Norman, K., (2005). Techniques: Intravital microscopy: A method for investigating disseminated intravascular coagulation. *Trends in Pharmacological Sciences, 26*(6), 327–332.

Radosevich, A. J., Bouchard, M. B., Burgess, S. A., Chen, B. R., & Hillman, E. M. C., (2008). Hyperspectral *in vivo* two-photon microscopy of intrinsic contrast. *Opt. Lett., 33*(18), 2164–2166.

Rangwala, S., & Tsai, K. Y., (2011). Roles of the immune system in skin cancer. *British Journal of Dermatology, 165*(5), 953–965.

Scott, A. M., Wolchok, J. D., & Old, L. J., (2012). Antibody therapy of cancer. *Nat. Rev. Cancer, 12*(4), 278–287.

Serrels, A., Lund, T., Serrels, B., et al., (2015). Nuclear FAK controls chemokine transcription, TREGS, and evasion of antitumor immunity. *Cell, 163*(1), 160–173.

Shimomura, O., Johnson, F. H., & Saiga, Y., (1962). Extraction, purification, and properties of aequorin, a bioluminescent protein from the luminous hydromedusan *Aequorea. J. Cell. Comp. Physiol., 59*, 223–239.

CHAPTER 10

Molecular Imaging: A New Advancement in Cancer Immunotherapy Monitoring

SANDEEP ARORA and NEELAM SHARMA

Chitkara College of Pharmacy, Chitkara University, Punjab, India

ABSTRACT

Molecular imaging is a promptly progressive versatile tool which comprises molecular biology, chemistry, computer, engineering, and medicine. Several imaging modalities for molecular imaging include x-ray computed tomography (CT), optical, radionuclide, ultrasound, magnetic resonance, and multimodality imaging. This chapter summarizes several advantages of molecular imaging, working concepts, and characteristics of molecular imaging technology. Nanoparticle-based novel imaging agent has also been recapitulated. This chapter also outlines the several applications of molecular imaging, which include treatment of cancer patients, cancer surgery, angiogenesis imaging, bone scan, neuroendocrine cancer imaging, and investigate the efficiency of drugs intended for multi-drug resistance.

10.1 INTRODUCTION

Molecular imaging can be defined as "the visualization, characterization, and measurement of biological processes at the molecular and cellular levels in humans and other living systems." The advancement of molecular imaging possibly will generate superlative patient advantage, for instance, prior lesion detection, therapy response supervision, and exclusive cancer remedy. It holds detection technology and contrast agents, reporter probes, and tracers (Cheng et al., 2014). Imaging modalities for molecular imaging have been illustrated in Figure 10.1 (Bulte and Kraitchman, 2004).

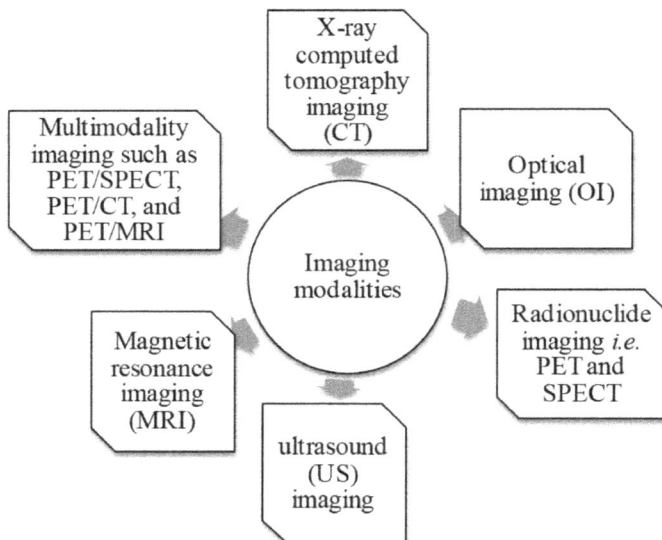

FIGURE 10.1   Imaging modalities for molecular imaging.

During the last three decades, radionuclide imaging, i.e., single-photon emission computed tomography (SPECT) and positron emission tomography (PET) has been significantly utilized (Yuan et al., 2013). Nowadays, it has been pursued by CT, OI, US, and MRI (Xavier et al., 2013; Phelps, 2000; Blake et al., 2003). Multimodality imaging is a combination of imaging technology for providing widespread information for disease diagnosis (Chen and Chen, 2010).

This chapter includes advantages, working concepts, characteristics, nanoparticle-based novel imaging agents and versatile applications of molecular imaging.

10.2   ADVANTAGES OF MOLECULAR IMAGING

Figure 10.2 illustrates the advantages of molecular imaging technology (Xavier et al., 2013; Phelps, 2000; Blake et al., 2003; Chen and Chen, 2010).

10.3   CONCEPT OF MOLECULAR IMAGING WORKING

Figure 10.3 illustrates how does molecular imaging develops disease distribution patterns in the form of pictures.

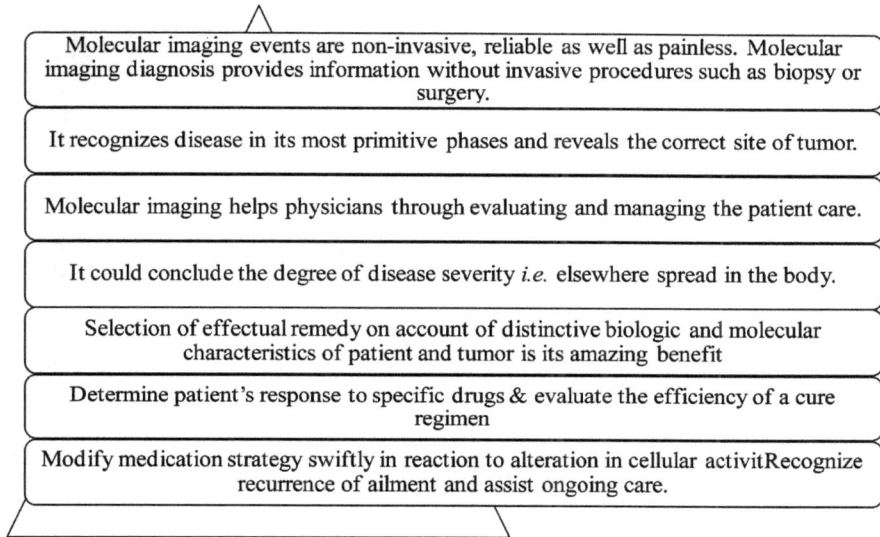

Molecular imaging events are non-invasive, reliable as well as painless. Molecular imaging diagnosis provides information without invasive procedures such as biopsy or surgery.

It recognizes disease in its most primitive phases and reveals the correct site of tumor.

Molecular imaging helps physicians through evaluating and managing the patient care.

It could conclude the degree of disease severity *i.e.* elsewhere spread in the body.

Selection of effectual remedy on account of distinctive biologic and molecular characteristics of patient and tumor is its amazing benefit

Determine patient's response to specific drugs & evaluate the efficiency of a cure regimen

Modify medication strategy swiftly in reaction to alteration in cellular activitRecognize recurrence of ailment and assist ongoing care.

FIGURE 10.2 Advantages of molecular imaging.

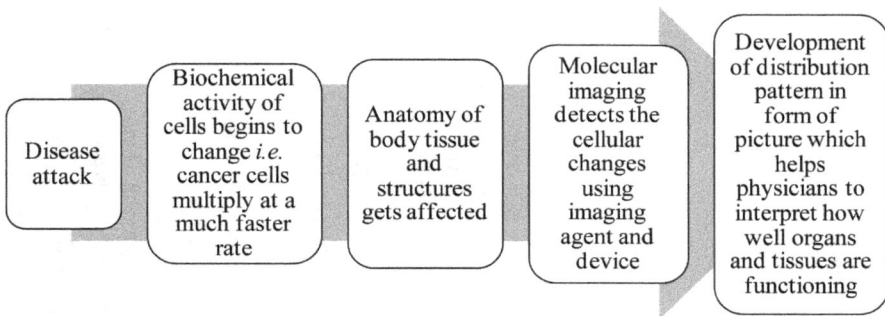

Disease attack

Biochemical activity of cells begins to change *i.e.* cancer cells multiply at a much faster rate

Anatomy of body tissue and structures gets affected

Molecular imaging detects the cellular changes using imaging agent and device

Development of distribution pattern in form of picture which helps physicians to interpret how well organs and tissues are functioning

FIGURE 10.3 How does molecular imaging works?

10.4 CHARACTERISTICS OF MOLECULAR IMAGING TECHNOLOGY

Innovative optical imaging techniques employed fluorescent proteins (FPs) which shifted their light emission nearer to infrared wavelengths which may possibly be straightforwardly detected (Benadiba et al., 2012). Important features of molecular imaging technology are discussed in Table 10.1.

TABLE 10.1 Distinctiveness of Molecular Imaging Technology

Imaging Technology	Characteristics/Principle	Advantages	References
Radionuclide imaging	Functional imaging techniques	Greater sensitivity and quantifiability	Yuan et al. (2013); Zhao (2005); Anderson and Ferdani (2009)
	Includes two technologies, e.g., positron emission tomography and single-photon emission computed tomography	Have significant responsibility in clinical and preclinical investigations	
PET	Functional imaging technique	More sensitive as compared to SPECT.	Xavier et al. (2013); Gore et al. (2011)
	Quantify the signal instigated from release of positrons from radioactive decay of neutron-deficient radioisotopes, e.g., 11C, 15O, 18F, and 131I which are intravenously injected into the body.	Three-dimensional resolution of SPECT is 8–10 mm which is lesser than clinical PET resolution of 5–7 mm.	
	PET radiotracer is 18F-fluorodeoxyglucose (FDG).		
	PET scanner detects photons and generates 3-D images which show FDC distribution in body.		
	Less dense area indicates areas of low metabolic activity (cold spots) and vice-versa.		
	Physicians detects organs and tissues abnormalities through 3-D images	•	
SPECT	Functional imaging technique	More affordable and extensively employed in the clinical routine.	Rapley et al. (2012); Debergh et al. (2014)

Imaging Technology	Characteristics/Principle	Advantages	References
	SPECT directly detects gamma-ray photon discharged through selected radionuclides throughout their decay.	Three-dimensional resolution of micro-organisms by SPECT is superior than PET	Blake et al. (2003); Pan et al. (2009); Li et al. (2010)
Magnetic resonance imaging (MRI)	Anatomic imaging method	Highly versatile imaging modality	
	Molecular MRI needs imaging agent for generating influential signal amplification to enhance its sensitivity.	Provides relatively greater temporal and three-dimensional resolution imaging	
	Imaging agent includes ferromagnetism (positive) and paramagnetic (negative) contrast agents.	Superb tissue penetration	
	Superparamagnetic iron oxide (SPIO), ultra-small superparamagnetic iron oxide (USPIO) and lanthanide chelate (gadolinium) utilized in MRI produces high signal yield.	Employ non-ionizing radiation which are non-invasiveness	
	Employed for soft tissue imaging, e.g., musculoskeletal system, brain, and parenchyma organs.	Synchronized attainment of anatomical structure and physiological activity	
X-ray computed tomography (CT) imaging	Anatomic imaging methods	CT generates a superior resolution of anatomical structure which provides great metabolic information about tumors.	Bzyl et al. (2012); Deshpande et al. (2010); Li et al. (2012); Chen et al. (2010)
	It includes micro-CT (high-resolution small animal CT) as well as organ, tissue to molecular level CT		

TABLE 10.1   *(Continued)*

Imaging Technology	Characteristics/Principle	Advantages	References
.	X-ray CT has comparatively less soft-tissue contrast and cannot differentiate among tissues with a dissimilar constitution; therefore, it requires contrast agents, e.g., polymeric nanoparticle, targeted gold nanoparticle, conjugated 2-deoxy-D-glucose gold nanoparticles.	.	Cai and Chen (2007); Lin et al. (2013)
Optical imaging	Functional imaging system	Since, it is light-based technology and does not involve radiation, hence relatively safer	
	It is founded on proteomics, genomics, and recent optical skills.	Sensitive and low-cost technology	
	Includes bioluminescence imaging (BLI) and fluorescence imaging.	Requires simple detecting devices	
	Has a prime role in examination of tumor incidence, successions, and essential drug progress.	Emitted wavelength cannot penetrate thick tissue layers of human body, therefore, has limited application in human subjects	
	OI is utilized in molecular and cellular imaging and preclinical study.	.	
Ultrasound molecular imaging	Anatomic imaging method	Superior temporal resolution	Cai and Chen (2008); Browning et al. (2013); Abgral et al. (2009); Li et al. (2011)

Imaging Technology	Characteristics/Principle	Advantages	References
	Ultrasound imaging assists particular and perceptive interpretation of molecular targets with the use of ultrasound contrast agent	Quantitative information, instantaneous practice, and non-invasiveness	Evangelista et al. (2014); Ren et al. (2012); Gao et al. (2013); Hackel et al. (2013); Oliveira et al. (2013); Bouchard et al. (2010); Keefe et al. (2010); Hong et al. (2011)
	Can be utilized for diagnostic imaging, therapeutic device and theranostic purposes	Comparatively economical	
		Non-ionizing radiation	
		Specific and sensitive depiction	
Multimodality imaging	Includes PET/SPECT, PET/CT and PET/MRI, OI/US, OI/CT, OI/MRI, and US/MRI	CT, MRI, and the US have small sensitivity while optical and radionuclide imaging have low resolution.	
	Provides enough anatomical and molecular information for clinical diagnosis	The amalgamation of molecular imaging techniques provides synergistic advantages and compensate for the disadvantages.	

10.5   NANOPARTICLE-BASED NOVEL IMAGING AGENT

Molecular imaging extensively utilizes specific and sensitive imaging agents for molecular imaging study (Morawski et al., 2005; Contag and Bachmann, 2002). Targeting molecular imaging agents (TMIA) customarily consisting of signal and targeting components for instance tiny molecule, antibody, aptamer, and peptide have been successfully utilized for diagnosing certain pathological tissues (Bulte and Kraitchman, 2004; Keefe et al., 2010). Multifunctional molecular imaging agents (MMIA) utilizes diverse targeting moieties, different imaging labels, genes, and drugs integrated into nanoparticle to generate multifunctional imaging agents which could be utilized for theranostics appliance and multimodal imaging (Table 10.2) (Hong et al., 2011; Shi et al., 2011).

10.6   APPLICATIONS OF MOLECULAR IMAGING

10.6.1   CANCER PATIENTS

Molecular imaging facilitates physicians to assess the progression of disease more accurately. Novel molecular imaging techniques will envisage the assertiveness of a tumor, predict the upshot of treatment, discover genetic markers of disease and would support physicians in developing additional customized treatment strategy. Hormone analogs have been synthesized for breast and prostate cancer imaging (Mintun et al., 1998). Molecular imaging is a prevailing device for diagnosing the stage of several types of cancers, e.g., prostate, ovarian, lung, breast, and gastrointestinal cancer patients. Physicians utilize PET and PET-CT imaging techniques as presented in Figure 10.4.

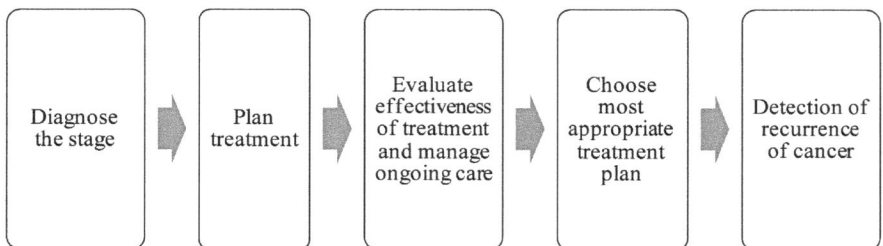

FIGURE 10.4   Application of molecular imaging technology for cancer patients.

TABLE 10.2 Nanoparticle-Based Novel Molecular Imaging Agents

Nanoparticle-Based Novel Imaging Agent	Examples	References
TMIA founded on small molecules of size less than 500 Da	18F-FDG for cancer imaging	Bagalkot et al. (2007); Hwang et al. (2010)
	Gadolinium labeled phosphorothioate-modified human tumor telomerase reverse transcriptase (hTERT) antisense oligonucleotide for targeting hTERT mRNA	
TMIA based on peptide	18F labeled cystine knot peptides for cancer imaging.	Louie (2010); Hall et al. (2012); Madani et al. (2013)
Peptide has improved selectivity and specificity	Polyethylene glycol (PEG) conjugated nanoparticle had five times higher uptake in an urokinase plasminogen activator receptor (uPAR)	.
Have higher stability at atmospheric temperature and less immunogenicity in comparison to antibodies.		
TMIA based on antibodies	Antibody conjugated superparamagnetic iron oxide nanoparticle	John et al. (2012); Ma et al. (2012); Liang et al. (2010)
Binds to targets superior specificity and affinity		
Easy to synthesis		
Utilized for diagnosis and therapy		.
TMIA founded on Aptamer, e.g., single-stranded DNA or RNA oligonucleotides	Activatable Aptamer probe (AAP) for selective binding to membrane proteins of living cancer cells	Yan et al. (2011); Kohl et al. (2005); Rabin et al. (2006); Hyafil et al. (2007); Tardy et al. (2010)

TABLE 10.2 *(Continued)*

Nanoparticle-Based Novel Imaging Agent	Examples	References
Superior affinity with specificity, stable structures, small immunogenicity, simplicity in production	Quantum dot conjugated with prostate-specific membrane antigen RNA aptamer for imaging and curing tumors.	.
Multifunctional molecular imaging agents		
Nanoparticle are fascinating candidates for multimodal imaging probe	Iron oxide nanoparticle augments imaging capacity of ultrasound and MRI	Willmann et al. (2010); Pysz et al. (2010); Fletcher et al. (2008); Juweid and Cheson (2006); Nguyen et al. (2010); van Dam et al. (2011); Wieder and Soloway (1998); Singletary (2002); Meric et al. (2003)
.	Streptavidin nanoparticle-based complexes have been functionalized with biotinylated anti-Her2 Herceptin antibody to detect tumor	
.	Drug-loaded micro bubble functionalized with LyP-1 and breast tumor homing peptide	

10.6.2   CANCER SURGERY

Molecular imaging has great potential to enhance primitive detection and staging of malignancies. The foremost objective of surgical removal of the cancer is to recognize/visualize and eradicate cancerous/diseased tissue to a great extent without causing harm to healthy tissue, nerves, blood vessels, and ureters. Moreover, it provides beneficial intra-operative guidance to the surgeon to make a better outcome (Kaushal et al., 2008; Tran Cao et al., 2012; Nakajima et al., 2011). For blood vessels (Liu and Wang, 2007; Fogelman et al., 2005; Mariani et al., 2001) and ureters (Even-Sapir et al., 2003; Lerman et al., 2007), direct injection of fluorescent probes revealed great assurance for treatment. Fluorescent molecular imaging visualized in a mouse model demonstrated discriminating targeting in nerve tissues within only some hours post-injection (Zhang et al., 2006, 2007). Administration of these probes prior to tumor surgery might significantly support detection and assist in prevention of accidental injury.

10.6.3   ANGIOGENESIS IMAGING

99mTc RGD (Arg-Gly-Asp) peptides have been synthesized for scintigraphy angiogenesis imaging showed great potential for prior breast cancer detection (Jung et al., 2006; Liu et al., 2007).

10.6.4   BONE SCAN

Radiopharmaceuticals based on technetium, for instance, 99mTc-MIBI, 99mTc-MDP and 99mTc (V)-DMSA have been employed to recognize metastases (Jung et al., 2006; Liu et al., 2007).

10.6.5   NEUROENDOCRINE CANCER IMAGING

Neuroendocrine tumors imaging performed by radio-pharmaceuticals is either attributable to the similar molecular structure to hormones which tumors produce or built-in into the different metabolic and cellular progression of tumor cells (Jung et al., 2006; Liu et al., 2007).

10.6.6   TO INVESTIGATE EFFICIENCY OF DRUGS INTENDED FOR MULTI-DRUG RESISTANCE

Lipophilic or cationic radiopharmaceutical agents signal the existence or nonexistence of P-glycoprotein. P-glycoprotein deficit causes translocation of 99mTc-MIBI across the cell membrane and accumulates in the interior of the cell while in the existence of P-glycoprotein, it performs similar to the therapeutic agent and gets pumped out of the cell. Since uptake is little and quantifiable; therefore, radiopharmaceutical can compute the efficiency of drugs intended to care for multi-drug resistance (Jung et al., 2006; Liu et al., 2007).

10.7   CONCLUSION

Molecular imaging technology greatly facilitates the dynamic and quantitative revelation of exclusive biochemical action exclusive of in-vivo distress at cellular as well as molecular level. It ameliorates a comprehensive understanding of the elementary aspect of tumor immunotherapy to provide refined therapeutic strategies. Initial recognition of cancer through imaging technology is possibly the foremost contributor to the decline in mortality for specific cancers. Molecular imaging comprehensively exploits TMIA or MMIA for theragnostic applications and multimodal imaging. Molecular imaging facilitates physicians to assess the progression of the disease more accurately. Novel molecular imaging techniques will envisage the assertiveness of tumors, predict the upshot of treatment, discover genetic markers of disease, and would support physicians in developing an additional customized treatment strategy. Molecular imaging has great potential in the differentiation of diseased tissue and healthy tissue during surgical procedures. It has been extensively utilized for angiogenesis imaging, bone scan, neuroendocrine tumor imaging, and to investigate the efficacy of drugs designed for multi-drug resistance. Novel molecular imaging agents could be developed through a close partnership among academia and information knowledge, biotechnology, and pharmaceutical commerce.

KEYWORDS

- **activatable aptamer probe**
- **molecular imaging**
- **multimodality imaging**

- optical imaging
- radionuclide imaging
- x-ray computed tomography

REFERENCES

Abgral, R., Querellou, S., Potard, G., Le Roux, P. Y., Le Duc-Pennec, A., Marianovski, R., Pradier, O., et al., (2009). Does 18F-FDG PET/ CT improve the detection of post-treatment recurrence of head and neck squamous cell carcinoma in patients negative for disease on clinical follow-up? *J. Nuc. Med., 50*(1), 24–29.

Anderson, C. J., & Ferdani, R., (2009). Copper-64 radiopharmaceuticals for PET imaging of cancer: Advances in preclinical and clinical research. *Cancer Biother. Radiopharm., 24*(4), 379–393.

Bagalkot, V., Zhang, L., Levy-Nissenbaum, E., Jon, S., Kantoff, P. W., Langer, R., & Farokhzad, O. C., (2007). Quantum dot-aptamer conjugates for synchronous cancer imaging, therapy, and sensing of drug delivery based on Bi-fluorescence resonance energy transfer. *Nano Lett., 7*(10), 3065–3070.

Benadiba, M., Luurtsema, G., Wichert-Ana, L., Buchpigel, C. A., & Filho, G. B., (2012). New molecular targets for PET and SPECT imaging in neurodegenerative diseases. *Braz. J. Psychiatry, 34*(2), S125–S148.

Blake, P., Johnson, B., & VanMeter, J. W., (2003). Positron emission tomography (PET) and single photon emission computed tomography (SPECT): Clinical applications. *J. Neuroophthalmol., 23*(1), 34–41.

Bouchard, P. R., Hutabarat, R. M., & Thompson, K. M., (2010). Discovery and development of therapeutic aptamers. *Annu. Rev. Pharmacol. Toxicol., 50*, 237–257.

Browning, Z. S., Wilkes, A. A., Mackenzie, D. S., Patterson, R. M., & Lenox, M. W., (2013). Using PET/CT imaging to characterize 18 F-fluorodeoxyglucose utilization in fish. *J. Fish Dis., 36*(11), 911–919.

Bulte, J. W., & Kraitchman, D. L., (2004). Iron oxide MR contrast agents for molecular and cellular imaging. *NMR Biomed., 17*, 484–499.

Bzyl, J., Lederle, W., Palmowski, M., & Kiessling, F., (2012). Molecular and functional ultrasound imaging of breast tumors. *Eur. J. Radiol., 81*(1), S11–S12.

Cai, W., & Chen, X., (2007). Nanoplatforms for targeted molecular imaging in living subjects. *Small, 3*(11), 1840–1854.

Cai, W., & Chen, X., (2008). Multimodality molecular imaging of tumor angiogenesis. *J. Nuc. Med., 49*(2), 113S–128S.

Chen, K., & Chen, X., (2010). Design and development of molecular imaging probes. *Curr. Topics Med. Chem., 10*(12), 1227–1236.

Chen, Y. Z., Wang, X. Y., Lin, Y., Zhang, J. S., Yang, F., Zhou, L. Q., & Liao, Y. Y., (2014). Advance of molecular imaging technology and targeted imaging agent in imaging and therapy. *Biomed. Res. Int., 2014*, 819324.

Chen, Z. Y., Liang, K., & Qiu, R. X., (2010). Targeted gene delivery in tumor xenografts by the combination of ultrasound-targeted microbubble destruction and polyethylenimine to inhibit surviving gene expression and induce apoptosis. *J. Exp. Clin. Cancer Res.*, *29*(1), 152.

Contag, C. H., & Bachmann, M. H., (2002). Advances *in vivo* bioluminescence imaging of gene expression. *Annu. Rev. Biomed. Eng.*, *4*, 235–260.

Debergh, I., Van, D. N., De Naeyer, D., Smeets, P., Demetter, P., Robert, P., Carme, S., et al., (2014). Molecular imaging of tumor-associated angiogenesis using a novel magnetic resonance imaging contrast agent targeting $\alpha v \beta 3$ integrin. *Ann. Surg. Oncol.*, *21*, 2097–2104.

Deshpande, N., Needles, A., & Willmann, J. K., (2010). Molecular ultrasound imaging: Current status and future directions. *Clin. Radiol.*, *65*(7), 567–581.

Evangelista, L., Cervino, A. R., Chondrogiannis, S., Marzola, M. C., Maffione, A. M., Colletti, P. M., Muzzio, P. C., & Rubello, D., (2014). Comparison between anatomical cross-sectional imaging and 18FFDGPET/ CT in the staging, restaging, treatment response, and long-term surveillance of squamous cell head and neck cancer: A systematic literature overview. *Nuc. Med. Commun.*, *35*(2), 123–134.

Even-Sapir, E., Lerman, H., Lievshitz, G., Khafif, A., Fliss, D. M., Schwartz, A., Gur, E., et al., (2003). Lymphoscintigraphy for sentinel node mapping using a hybrid SPECT/CT system. *J. Nucl. Med.*, *44*(9), 1413–1420.

Fletcher, J. W., Kymes, S. M., Gould, M., Alazraki, N., Coleman, R. E., Lowe, V. J., Marn, C., et al., (2008). A comparison of the diagnostic accuracy of 18F-FDG PET and CT in the characterization of solitary pulmonary nodules. *J. Nucl. Med.*, *49*, 179–185.

Fogelman, I., Cook, G., Israel, O., & Van, D. W. H., (2005). Positron emission tomography and bone metastases. *Semin. Nucl. Med.*, *35*(2), 135–142.

Gao, J., & Zheng, H., (2013). Illuminating the lipidome to advance biomedical research: Peptide-based probes of membrane lipids. *Future Med. Chem.*, *5*(8), 947–959.

Gore, J. C., Manning, H. C., Quarles, C. C., Waddell, K. W., & Yankeelov, T. E., (2011). Magnetic resonance in the era of molecular imaging of cancer. *Magn. Reson. Imaging*, *29*(5), 587–600.

Hackel, B. J., Kimura, R. H., Miao, Z., Liu, H., Sathirachinda, A., Cheng, Z., Chin, F. T., & Gambhir, S. S., (2013). 18F-Fluorobenzoatelabeled cystine knot peptides for PET imaging of integrin $\alpha v \beta 6$. *Nanoscale*, *55*(7), 1101–1105.

Hall, M. A., Kwon, S., Robinson, H., Lachance, P. A., Azhdarinia, A., Ranganathan, R., Price, R. E., et al., (2012). Imaging prostate cancer lymph node metastases with a multimodality contrast agent. *Prostate*, *72*(2), 129–146.

Hansen, L., Unmack, L. E. K., Nielsen, E. H., Iversen, F., Liu, Z., Thomsen, K., Pedersen, M., et al., (2013). Targeting of peptide conjugated magnetic nanoparticles to urokinase plasminogen activator receptor (uPAR) expressing cells. *Nanoscale*, *5*(17), 8192–8201.

Hong, H., Goel, S., Zhang, Y., & Cai, W., (2011). Molecular imaging with nucleic acid aptamers. *Curr. Med. Chem.*, *18*(27), 4195–4205.

Hwang, D. W., Ko, H. Y., Lee, J. H., Kang, H., Ryu, S. H., Song, I. C., Lee, D. S., & Kim, S., (2010). A nucleolin-targeted multimodal nanoparticle imaging probe for tracking cancer cells using an aptamer. *J. Nucl. Med.*, *51*(1), 98–105.

Hyafil, F., Cornily, J. C., Feig, J. E., Gordon, R., Vucic, E., Amirbekian, V., Fisher, E. A., et al., (2007). Noninvasive detection of macrophages using a nanoparticulate contrast agent for computed tomography. *Nat. Med.*, *13*, 636–641.

John, R., Nguyen, F. T., Kolbeck, K. J., Chaney, E. J., Marjanovic, M., Suslick, K. S., & Boppart, S. A., (2012). Targeted multifunctional multimodal protein-shell microspheres as cancer imaging contrast agents. *Mol. Imaging Bio.*, *14*, 17–24.

Jung, K. H., Lee, K. H., Paik, J. Y., Ko, B. H., Bae, J. S., Lee, B. C., Sung, H. J., et al., (2006). Favorable biokinetic and tumor-targeting properties of 99mTc-labeled glucosamine RGD and effect of paclitaxel therapy. *J. Nucl. Med., 47*(12), 2000–2007.

Juweid, M. E., & Cheson, B. D., (2006). Positron-emission tomography and assessment of cancer therapy. *N. Eng. J. Med., 354*, 496–507.

Kaushal, S., McElroy, M. K., Luiken, G. A., Talamini, M. A., Moossa, A. R., Hoffman, R. M., & Bouvet, M., (2008). Fluorophore-conjugated anti-CEA antibody for the intraoperative imaging of pancreatic and colorectal cancer. *J. Gastrointest. Surg., 12*, 1938–1950.

Keefe, A. D., Pai, S., & Ellington, A., (2010). Aptamers as therapeutics. *Annu. Rev. Pharmacol. Toxicol., 9*(7), 537–550.

Kohl, G., (2005). The evolution and state-of-the-art principles of multi slice computed tomography. *Proc. Am. Thorac. Soc., 2*, 470–476.

Lerman, H., Lievshitz, G., Zak, O., Metser, U., Schneebaum, S., & Even-Sapir, E., (2007). Improved sentinel node identification by SPECT/CT in overweight patients with breast cancer. *J. Nucl. Med., 48*(2), 201–206.

Li, B., Abran, M., Matteau-Pelletier, C., Rouleau, L., Lam, T., Sharma, R., Rhéaume, E., et al., (2011). Low-cost three-dimensional imaging system combining fluorescence and ultrasound. *J. Biomed. Opt., 16*(12), 126010.

Li, J., Chaudhary, A., Chmura, S. J., Pelizzari, C., Rajh, T., Wietholt, C., Kurtoglu, M., & Aydogan, B., (2010). A novel functional CT contrast agent for molecular imaging of cancer. *Phys. Med. Biol., 55*(5), 4389–4397.

Li, P., Zheng, Y., Ran, H., Tan, J., Lin, Y., Zhang, Q., Ren, J., & Wang, Z., (2012). Ultrasound triggered drug release from 10-hydroxycamptothecin-loaded phospholipid microbubbles for targeted tumor therapy in mice. *J. Control. Release, 162*(2), 349–354.

Liang, M., Liu, X., Cheng, D., Liu, G., Dou, S., Wang, Y., Rusckowski, M., & Hnatowich, D. J., (2010). Multimodality nuclear and fluorescence tumor imaging in mice using a streptavidin nanoparticle. *Bioconjugate Chem., 21*(7), 1385–1388.

Lin, Y., Chen, Z. Y., & Yang, F., (2013). Ultrasound-based multimodal molecular imaging and functional ultrasound contrast agents. *Curr. Pharm. Des., 19*(18), 3342–3351.

Liu, J., Li, J., Rosol, T. J., Pan, X., & Voorhees, J. L., (2007). Biodegradable nanoparticles for targeted ultrasound imaging of breast cancer cells *in vitro. Phys. Med. Biol., 52*, 4739–4747.

Liu, Y., & Wang, H., (2007). Nanotechnology tackles tumors. *Nat. Nanotechnol., 2*(1), 20–21.

Louie, A., (2010). Multimodality imaging probes: Design and challenges. *Chem. Rev., 110*(5), 3146–3195.

Ma, J., Huang, P., He, M., Pan, L., Zhou, Z., Feng, L., Gao, G., & Cui, D., (2012). Folic acid-conjugated LaF3:Yb, Tm@SiO$_2$ nanoprobes for targeting dual-modality imaging of upconversion luminescence and X-ray computed tomography. *J. Phys. Chem. B, 116*(48), 14062–14070.

Madani, S. Y., Shabani, F., Dwek, M. V., & Seifalian, A. M., (2013). Conjugation of quantum dots on carbon nanotubes for medical diagnosis and treatment. *Int. J. Nanomedicine, 8*, 941–950.

Mariani, G., Moresco, L., Viale, G., Villa, G., Bagnasco, M., Canavese, G., Buscombe, J., et al., (2001). Radio guided sentinel lymph node biopsy in breast cancer surgery. *J. Nucl. Med., 42*, 1198–1215.

Meric, F., Mirza, N. Q., Vlastos, G., Buchholz, T. A., Kuerer, H. M., Babiera, G. V., Singletary, S., et al., (2003). Positive surgical margins and ipsilateral breast tumor recurrence predict disease-specific survival after breast-conserving therapy. *Cancer, 97*, 926–933.

Mintun, M. A., Welch, M. J., Siegel, B. A., Mathias, C. J., Brodack, J. W., McGuire, A. H., & Katzenellenbogen, J. A., (1998). Breast cancer: PET imaging of estrogen receptors. *Radiology, 169,* 45–48.

Morawski, A. M., Lanza, G. A., & Wickline, S. A., (2005). Targeted contrast agents for magnetic resonance imaging and ultrasound. *Curr. Opin. Biotechnol., 16,* 89–92.

Nakajima, T., Mitsunaga, M., Bander, N. H., Heston, W. D., Choyke, P. L., & Kobayashi, H., (2011). Targeted, activatable, *in vivo* fluorescence imaging of prostate-specific membrane antigen (PSMA) positive tumors using the quenched humanized J591 antibody-indocyanine green (ICG) conjugate. *Bioconjug. Chem., 22,* 1700–1705.

Nguyen, Q. T., Olson, E. S., Aguilera, T. A., Jiang, T., Scadeng, M., Ellies, L. G., & Tsien, R. Y., (2010). Surgery with molecular fluorescence imaging using activatable cell-penetrating peptides decreases residual cancer and improves survival. *Proc. Natl. Aca. Sci. U.S.A., 107,* 4317–4322.

Oliveira, S., Heukers, R., Sornkom, J., Kok, R. J., & Van, B. E. H. P. M., (2013). Targeting tumors with nanobodies for cancer imaging and therapy. *J. Control. Release, 172*(3), 607–617.

Pan, D., Williams, T. A., Senpan, A., Allen, J. S., Scott, M. J., Gaffney, P. J., Wickline, S. A., & Lanza, G. M., (2009). Detecting vascular biosignatures with a colloidal, radio-opaque polymeric nanoparticle. *J. Am. Chem. Soc., 131*(42), 5522–15527.

Phelps, M. E., (2000). Positron emission tomography provides molecular imaging of biological processes. *Proc. Nat. Acad. Sci. U.S.A., 97*(16), 9226–9233.

Pysz, M. A., Foygel, K., Rosenberg, J., Gambhir, S. S., Schneider, M., & Willmann, J. K., (2010). Antiangiogenic cancer therapy: Monitoring with molecular US and a clinically translatable contrast agent (BR55). *Radiology, 256,* 519–527.

Rabin, O., Manuel, P. J., Grimm, J., Wojtkiewicz, G., & Weissleder, R., (2006). An X-ray computed tomography imaging agent based on long-circulating bismuth sulphide nanoparticles. *Nat. Mater., 5,* 118–122.

Rapley, P. L., Witiw, C., Rich, K., Niccoli, S., Tassotto, M. L., & Th'ng, J., (2012). *In vitro* molecular magnetic resonance imaging detection and measurement of apoptosis using super paramagnetic iron oxide + antibody as ligands for nucleosomes. *Phys. Med. Bio., 57*(21), 7015–7028.

Ren, B. X., Yang, F., Zhu, G. H., Huang, Z. X., Ai, H., Xia, R., Liu, X. J., et al., (2012). Magnetic resonance tumor targeting imaging using gadolinium labeled human telomerase reverse transcriptase antisense probes. *Cancer Sci., 103*(8), 1434–1439.

Shi, H., He, X., Wang, K., Wu, X., Ye, X., Guo, Q., Tan, W., et al., (2011). Activatable aptamer probe for contrast-enhanced *in vivo* cancer imaging based on cell membrane protein-triggered conformation alteration. *Proc. Nat. Acad. Sci. U.S.A., 108*(10), 3900–3905.

Singletary, S. E., (2002). Surgical margins in patients with early-stage breast cancer treated with breast conservation therapy. *Am. J. Surg., 184,* 383–393.

Tardy, I., Pochon, S., Theraulaz, M., Emmel, P., Passantino, L., Tranquart, F., & Schneider, M., (2010). Ultrasound molecular imaging of VEGFR2 in a rat prostate tumor model using BR55. *Invest. Radiol., 45,* 573–578.

Tran, C. H. S., Kaushal, S., Metildi, C. A., Menen, R. S., Lee, C., Snyder, C. S., Messer, K., et al., (2012). Tumor-specific fluorescence antibody imaging enables accurate staging laparoscopy in an orthotopic model of pancreatic cancer. *Hepatogastroenterology, 59,* 1994–1999.

Van, D. G. M., Themelis, G., Crane, L. M., Harlaar, N. J., Pleijhuis, R. G., Kelder, W., Sarantopoulos, A., et al., (2011). Intraoperative tumor-specific fluorescence imaging in ovarian cancer by folate receptor-alpha targeting: First in-human results. *Nat. Med., 17,* 1315–1319.

Wieder, J. A., & Soloway, M. S., (1998). Incidence, etiology, location, prevention, and treatment of positive surgical margins after radical prostatectomy for prostate cancer. *J. Urol., 160,* 299–315.

Willmann, J. K., Kimura, R. H., Deshpande, N., Lutz, A. M., Cochran, J. R., & Gambhir, S. S., (2010). Targeted contrast-enhanced ultrasound imaging of tumor angiogenesis with contrast micro bubbles conjugated to integrin-binding knottin peptides. *J. Nucl. Med., 51,* 433–440.

Xavier, C., Vaneycken, I., D'huyvetter, M., Heemskerk, J., Keyaerts, M., Vincke, C., Devoogdt, N., et al., (2013). Synthesis, preclinical validation, dosimetry, and toxicity of 68Ga-NOTAAnti-HER2 nanobodies for iPET imaging of HER2 receptor expression in cancer. *J. Nucl. Med., 54*(5), 776–784.

Yan, V. F., Li, X., Jin, Q., Jiang, C., Zhang, Z., Ling, T., Qiu, B., & Zheng, H., (2011). Therapeutic ultrasonic micro bubbles carrying paclitaxel and LyP-1 peptide: Preparation, characterization, and application to ultrasound-assisted chemotherapy in breast cancer cells. *Ultrasound Med. Bio., 37*(5), 768–779.

Yuan, J., Zhang, H., Kaur, H., Oupicky, D., & Peng, F., (2013). Synthesis and characterization of theranostic poly(HPMA)-c(RGDyK)-DOTA-64 cucopolymer targeting tumor angiogenesis: Tumor localization visualized by positron emission tomography. *Mol. Imaging, 12*(3), 203–212.

Zhang, X., & Chen, W., (2007). Differentiation of recurrent astrocytoma from radiation necrosis: A pilot study with 13N-NH3 PET. *J. Neurooncol., 82,* 305–311.

Zhang, X., Changhong, L., Weian, C., & Dong, Z., (2006). PET imaging of cerebral astrocytomas with 13N-ammonia. *J. Neurooncol., 78*(2), 145–151.

Zhao, H., (2005). Emission spectra of bioluminescent reporters and interaction with mammalian tissue determine the sensitivity of detection *in vivo. J. Biomed. Opt., 10*(4), 41210.

CHAPTER 11

Spatiotemporal Genetic Analysis (SAGA) Technique for Cancer Cell Biology Studies

SANDEEP ARORA, SAURABH GUPTA, and NEELAM SHARMA

Chitkara College of Pharmacy, Chitkara University, Punjab, India

ABSTRACT

Spatiotemporal gene expression is the activation of genes during the develop-ment of different tissues of an organism. The patterns of gene activation vary greatly in complexity. Some are simple and stable, like the tubulin pattern that is expressed at all times in life in all cells. One way to identify a specific gene's expression pattern is by putting a reporter gene downstream of its promoter. In this arrangement, only where and when the gene of interest is expressed will the promoter gene cause the reporter gene to be expressed. The reporter gene's expression distribution can be calculated by observing it.

11.1 INTRODUCTION

The stimulation of genes is called spatiotemporal gene expression during the creation of numerous tissues of an organism. The gene activation patterns differ dramatically in intricacy. Some are basic and predictable, like the pattern of tubulin that is expressed in all cells at all times in life. On the other hand, some are highly complex and difficult to predict and model, with speech fluctuating wildly from minute to minute or from cell to cell. Spatiotemporal variability plays a key role in producing the variety of cell types found in developed organisms; since a cell's identity is determined by the set of genes actively expressed within that cell, if gene expression were spatially and temporarily uniform, there could be at most one cell type (Asmussen et al., 1987).

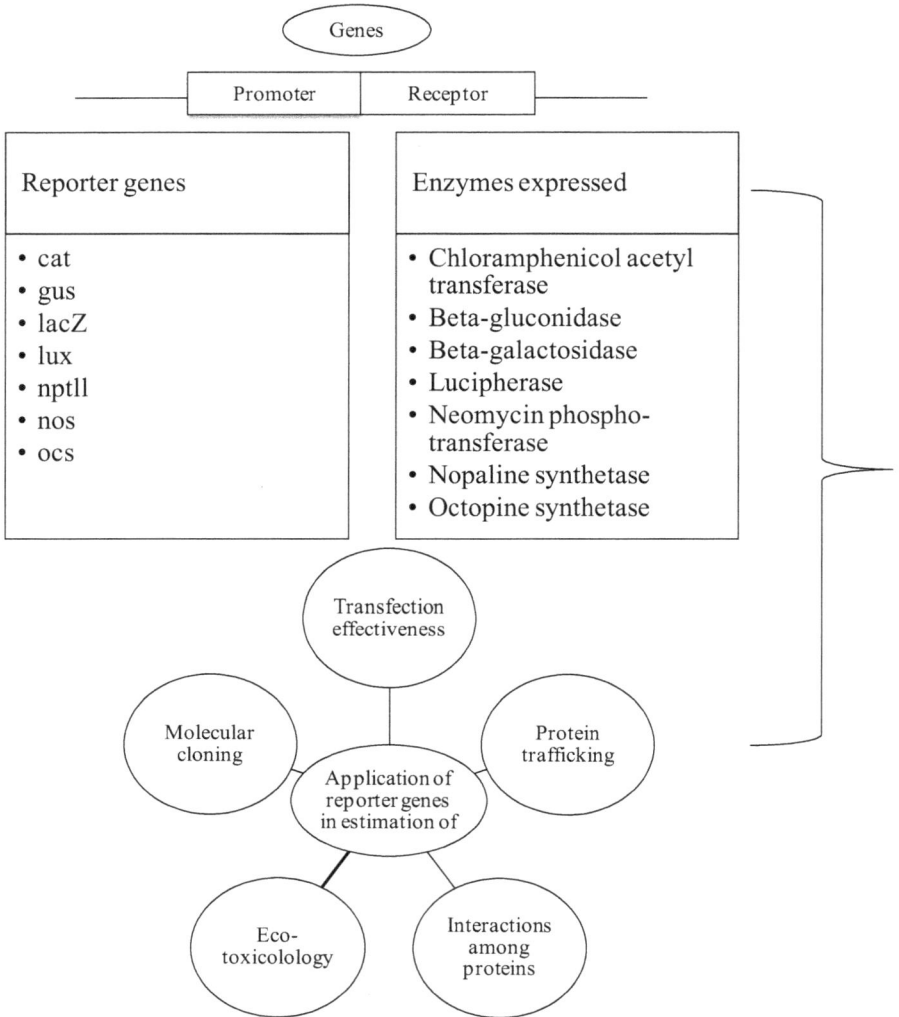

FIGURE 11.1   Graphical representation of reporter genes examples and applications

11.2   IDENTIFYING SPATIOTEMPORAL PATTERNS

To identify a specific gene's expression pattern is by putting a reporter gene downstream of its promoter. The promotor gene can induce the reporter gene to be expressed in this configuration only where and when the gene of interest is expressed. The reporter gene's expression distribution can be calculated by observing it. For example, by activating it with blue light and then using a digital camera to record green fluorescent emissions, the reporter gene can be visualized. If the promoter of the gene of interest is unknown, its spatiotemporal distribution can be defined in several ways. Then a method such as fluorescent labeling can imagine this distribution of this antibody. The benefits of immuno-histochemistry are methodologically feasible and relatively inexpensive. The drawbacks include the antibody's non-specificity contributing to false-positive expression recognition. Poor antibody penetration into the target tissue can result in false-negative outcomes. Also, because immunohistochemistry views the gene-generated protein, where the protein product diffuses between cells or has a relatively short or long half-life compared to the mRNA used to translate the protein, this may result in a skewed understanding of which cells express the mRNA (Blaxter, 2004).

An enhancer-trap screening approach shows the variety of potential patterns of spatiotemporal gene expression in an organism. DNA encoding a reporter gene is randomly inserted into the genome in this technique. The reporter gene will be expressed in different tissues at various developmental stages, depending on the gene promoters proximal to the insertion stage. Although enhancer-trap based patterns of expression do not inherently reflect the actual patterns of specific gene expression, they show the variety of spatiotemporal patterns available for evolution (Blaxter et al., 2005).

11.3   METHODS TO CONTROL SPATIOTEMPORAL GENE EXPRESSION

Many approaches are being sought in various degrees to spatially, tempo-rarily and regulate gene expression. One approach is to use the operon inducer/repressor system that provides temporary gene expression regula-tion. Spatially inkjet printers are being developed to monitor gene expression for printing ligands on gel culture. Other popular method includes the use of light in spatiotemporal fashion to regulate gene expression. Because light can also be easily controlled in space, time, and degree, many methods have been developed and are being studied to regulate gene expression at the level of DNA and RNA. RNA interference (RNAi), for instance, can be controlled using light and gene expression patterning and also been performed in cell monolayer in zebra fish embryos using caged morpholino or peptide nucleic acid (PNA) (Wijlemans et al., 2012) demonstrating spatiotemporal gene expression regulation. Using a transgenic system or caged triplex-forming oligos, light-based control has recently been shown at the DNA level (Floyd et al., 2002; Vincx, 1986).

11.4   EXPLORATION CARRIED OUT IN THE FIELD OF SPATIOTEMPORAL GENETIC ANALYSIS TECHNIQUE IN CANCER CELL BIOLOGY STUDIES

- Christina Curtis and Colin Watts et al. explored that Glioblastoma (GB) is the most common and aggressive primary brain malignancy, with poor prognosis and a lack of effective therapeutic options. Accumulating evidence suggests that intratumor heterogeneity likely is the key to understanding treatment failure. However, the extent of intratumor heterogeneity as a result of tumor evolution is still poorly understood. To address this, they developed a unique surgical multisampling scheme to collect spatially distinct tumor fragments from 11 GB patients. They present an integrated genomic analysis that uncovers extensive intratumor heterogeneity, with most patients displaying different GB subtypes within the same tumor. Moreover, they reconstructed the phylogeny of the fragments for each patient, identifying copy number alterations in EGFR and CDKN2A/B/ p14ARF as early events, and aberrations in PDGFRA and PTEN as later events during cancer progression. They also characterized the clonal organization of each tumor fragment at the single-molecule level, detecting multiple coexisting cell lineages. The results reveal the genome-wide architecture of intratumor variability in GB across multiple spatial scales and patient-specific patterns of cancer evolution, with consequences for treatment design (Sara et al., 2015).
- Roel Deckers et al. demonstrated the use of magnetic resonance temperature imaging (MRI)-guided, high intensity focused ultrasound (HIFU) in combination with a heat-inducible promoter [heat shock protein 70 (HSP70)] for the *in vivo* spatiotemporal control of transgene activation. Local gene activation induced by moderate hyperthermia in a transgenic mouse expressing luciferase under the control of the HSP70 promoter showed a high similarity between the local temperature distribution *in vivo* and the region emitting light. Modulation of gene expression is possible by changing temperature, duration, and location of regional heating. Mild heating protocols (2 min at 43°C) causing no tissue damage were sufficient for significant gene activation. The HSP70 promoter was shown to be induced by the local temperature increase and not by the mechanical effects of ultrasound. Therefore, the combination of MRI-guided HIFU heating and transgenes under control of heat-inducible

HSP promoter provides a direct, noninvasive, spatial control of gene expression via local hyperthermia (Wijlemans et al., 2012).

- Peter Doerner et al. developed a cyclin-GUS reporter to facilitate the spatiotemporal analysis of cell division patterns. The Chimeric reporter protein is turned over every cell cycle and hence its histochemical activity accurately reports individual miotic cells. Using Aribodobsis plants transformed with cyclin-GUS, he visualized patterns of miotic activity in wounded leaves which suggest a role for cell division in structural reinforcement (Carmona et al., 1999).

- Annie Valette et al. discovered that pancreatic ductal adenocarcinoma (PDAC) is one of the most lethal cancers with less than 5% of overall patient survival after 5 years. Local and distant invasion, resistance to chemotherapy and radiotherapy, and lack of early detection are responsible for this poor prognosis. Gemcitabine (2,'2'-difluorode-oxycytidine, a pyrimidine nucleoside analog) chemotherapy is the standard treatment of the patients. The combination of gemcitabine with other chemo- or biotherapies has resulted in a very limited prognostic improvement. Recently, a high throughput RNAi screen identified that checkpoint kinase 1 (CHK1) is a gene conferring resistance to gemcitabine in pancreatic cancer cells (Azorsa et al., 2009). CHK1 is a key component of the cell cycle checkpoints that are activated by genomic and replicative stress (Ma et al., 2010). This checkpoint activation is known to facilitate DNA repair. Consequently, CHK1 may play an important role in the resistance of tumor cells to geno-toxic therapy, raising the possibility that inhibitors of checkpoint kinases may be useful adjuvant agents in chemotherapy of cancer. In the case of pancreatic cancer, *in vitro* and *in vivo* studies have shown that CHK inhibitors enhance the antitumor activity of gemcitabine (Matthews et al., 2007; Parsels et al., 2009). The multicellular tumor spheroid (MCTS) model is generally considered as a better model than two-dimensional cultures to predict the *in vivo* response to drug treatments and it is now widely accepted that MCTS reproduces more accurately the tumor microenvironment than monolayer cell cultures. While growing, spheroids display a gradient of proliferating cells from the outer cell layers with quiescent cells located more centrally. When deprived of oxygen and glucose, central cells die and a necrotic zone is formed. This cell heterogeneity is similar to that found in vascular micro-regions of tumors (Sutherland et al., 1988). It is well established that solid tumor environment induces the level of drug resistance to many chemotherapeutic agents. This phenomenon, called multicellular resistance, emerges as soon as cancer cells have established contacts with surrounding cells or extracellular matrix, i.e., its microenvironment. In MCTS, cancer cells can acquire this multicellular resistance by interacting efficiently in three dimensions with their environment. In order to contribute to the discovery of new anti pancreatic cancer agents or new potent combinations with gemcitabine, the development and the validation of a new spheroid model mimicking the structure and chemo resistance of pancreatic solid tumors compared to conventional 2D cell culture models. The spatio-temporal parameters of the biological response of gemcitabine alone or combined with a CHK1 inhibitor, CHIR-124 (Mellor et al., 2005; Fayad et al., 2009).

- Paul J. Trek et al. determined that human embryonic stem cells (hESCs) express genes in common with PGCs, and that three of these genes, *GDF3, STELLAR,* and *NANOG,* are located on 12p. It was further investigated whether expression of these 12p genes were elevated in seminoma relative to normal testis, and to determine whether elevated expression was unique to seminoma (Vazin et al., 2010).

- Ronald Berezney et al. determined that Fluorescence microscopic analysis of newly; replicated DNA has revealed discrete granular sites of replication (RS). The average size and number of replication sites from early to mid-S-phase suggest that each RS contains numerous replicons clustered together. Researchers are using fluorescence laser scanning confocal microscopy in conjunction with multidimensional image analysis to gain more precise information about RS and, their spatial-temporal dynamics. Using a newly improved imaging segmentation program, researchers report an average of z 1,100 RS after a 5-min pulse labeling of 3T3 mouse fibroblast cells in early S-phase. Pulse chase-pulse double-labeling experiments reveal that RS takes 45 min to complete replication. Appropriate calculations suggest that each RS contains an average of 1 mbp of DNA or 6 average-sized replicons. Double pulse-double chase experiments demonstrate that the DNA sequences replicated at individual RS are precisely maintained temporally and spatially as the cell progresses through the cell cycle and into subsequent generations. By labeling replicated DNA at the G1/Sb orders for two consecutive cell generations, researchers show that the DNA synthesized at early S-phase is replicated at the same time and sites in the next round of replication (Ma et al., 1998).

- Walkley and their colleagues studies generate specific genetic modifications in mice and provides a powerful approach to assess gene function. When genetic modifications have been generated in the germline, the resulting phenotype however often only reflects the first time a gene has an influence on or is necessary for a particular biological process. Therefore, systems allowing conditional genetic modification have been developed (Asmussen et al., 1987); for example, inducible forms of the Cre recombinase from P1 phage have been generated that can catalyze intermolecular recombination between target recognition sequences (*loxP* sites) in response to ligand (Blaxter, 2004; Blaxter et al., 2005; Floyd et al., 2002; Vincx, 1986). It was assessed whether a tamoxifen-inducible form of Cre recombinase (Cre-ERTM) could be used to modify gene activity in the mouse embryo *in utero*. Using the enhancer of the *Wnt1* gene to restrict the expression of Cre-ERTM to the embryonic neural tube, it was found that a single injection of tamoxifen into pregnant mice induced Cre-mediated recombination within the embryonic central nervous system, thereby activating the expression of a reporter gene. Induction was ligand-dependent, rapid, and efficient. The results demonstrate that tamoxifen-inducible recombination can be used to effectively modify gene function in the mouse embryo (Carl et al., 2008).
- Luis F. Parada et al. demonstrated that the mice which are used in laboratory mainly share extensive molecular and physiological similarities to humans and are powerful tool for studying cancer. Unlike invertebrate model systems, tumor development in mice is accompanied by other complex processes such as angiogenesis and metastasis, similar to those in human cancer. More importantly, mouse tumor models provide temporally and genetically controlled systems for studying the tumorigenic process as well as response to treatment. However, initial efforts to create mouse models of glioma using single tumor suppressor knockouts or overexpression of single oncogenes mostly failed. It was subsequently found that, as confirmed by the TCGA project, the core signaling pathways are crucial for gliomas: genetically engineered mice that activate RTK pathways in the brain, along with simultaneous loss of genes involved in cell-cycle control, develop glioma with high penetrance. Also, like human gliomas, additional loss of the tumor suppressor PTEN causes higher-grade malignancy and reduced survival in mouse glioma models (Kwon et al., 2008). Catalyzed by the

profusion of genetic information arising from a number of genome-wide studies that revealed mutations present in human gliomas, as well as advances in molecular biology tools, dozens of genetic mouse glioma models have been generated over the last two decades (Parada et al., 2016).

11.5 CONCLUSION

The awareness of malignant tumors has improved dramatically in recent years, although many concerns and controversies remain. Continuing the integration and verification of spatiotemporal genetic analysis using increasingly sophisticated animal models will further advance our understanding of the cause, development, and treatment of diseases. At the same time, despite the issues highlighted, this methodology not only points to new cancer management approaches that address developmental biology aspects, but also offer insights into tumor maintenance, resistance to treatment, and recurrence. The development of this expertise offers great potential for enhancing and even revolutionizing current diagnosis and treatment for malignant human tumors.

KEYWORDS

- **checkpoint kinase 1**
- **glioblastoma**
- **heat shock protein 70**
- **high intensity focused ultrasound**
- **magnetic resonance imaging**
- **multicellular tumor spheroid**

REFERENCES

Asmussen, M. A., Arnold, J., & Avise, J. C., (1987). Definition and properties of disequilibrium statistics for associations between nuclear and cytoplasmic genotypes. *Genetics, 115*, 755–768.

Azorsa, D. O., Gonzales, I. M., Basu, G. D., Choudhary, A., Arora, S., Bisanz, K. M., Kiefer, J. A., et al., (2009). Synthetic lethal RNAi screening identifies sensitizing targets for gemcitabine therapy in pancreatic cancer. *J. Transl. Med., 7*, 43.

Blaxter, M., (2004). The promise of a DNA taxonomy. *Phil. Trans. Soc. Lond. B, 359*, 669–679.

Blaxter, M., Mann, J., Chapman, T., Thomas, F., Whitton, C., Floyd, R., & Abebe, E., (2005). Defining operational taxonomic units using DNA barcode data. *Phil. Trans. R Soc. B, 360*, 1935–1943.

Carmona, A. C., You, R., Gal, T. H., & Doerner, P., (1999). Spatio-temporal analysis of mitotic activity with a labile cyclin-GUS fusion protein. *The Plant Journal, 20*, 503–510.

Dufau, I., Frongia, C., Sicard, F., Dedieu, L., Cordelier, P., Aussei, F., Ducommun, B., & Valette, A., (2012). Multicellular tumor spheroid model to evaluate Spatio-temporal dynamics effect of chemotherapeutics: Application to the gemcitabine/CHK1 inhibitor combination in pancreatic cancer. *BMC Cancer*, 12–15.

Fayad, W., Brnjic, S., Berglind, D., Blixt, S., Shoshan, M. C., Berndtsson, M., Olofsson, M. H., & Linder, S., (2009). Restriction of cisplatin induction of acute apoptosis to a subpopulation of cells in a three-dimensional carcinoma culture model. *Int. J. Cancer, 125*, 2450–2455.

Floyd, R., Abebe, E., Papert, A., & Blaxter, M., (2002). Molecular barcodes for soil nematode identification. *Mol. Ecol., 11*, 839–850.

Ma, C. X., Janetka, J. W., & Piwnica-Worms, H., (2011). Death by releasing the breaks. CHK1 inhibitors as cancer therapeutics. *Trends Mol. Med., 17*, 88–96.

Ma, H., Samarabandu, J., Rekandu, S., Acharya, D. R., Cheng, P. C., & Ronald, M. C., (1998). Berezney, spatial, and temporal dynamics of DNA replication sites in mammalian cells. *J. Cell Biol., 143*(6), 1415–1425.

Matthews, D. J., Yakes, F. M., Chen, J., Tadano, M., Bornheim, L., Clary, D. O., Tai, A., et al., (2007). Pharmacological abrogation of S-phase checkpoint enhances the antitumor activity of gemcitabine *in vivo. Cell Cycle, 6*, 104–110.

Mellor, H. R., Ferguson, D. J., & Callaghan, R., (2005). A model of quiescent tumor microregions for evaluating multicellular resistance to chemotherapeutic drugs. *Br. J. Cancer, 93*, 302–309.

Parada, L. F., Sheila, R., & Llaguno, A., (2016). Cell of origin of glioma: Biological and clinical implications. *Br. J. Cancer, 115*(12), 1445–1450.

Parsels, L. A., Morgan, M. A., Tanska, D. M., Parsels, J. D., Palmer, B. D., Booth, R. J., Denny, W. A., et al., (2009). Gemcitabine sensitization by checkpoint kinase 1 inhibition correlates with inhibition of a Rad51 DNA damage response in pancreatic cancer cells. *Mol Cancer Ther., 8*, 45–54.

Piccirillo, S. G., Spiteri, I., Sottoriva, A., Touloumis, A., Ber, S., Price, S. J., Heywood, R., et al., (2015). Contributions to drug resistance in glioblastoma derived from malignant cells in the sub-ependymal zone. *Cancer Res., 75*(1), 194–202.

Sutherland, R. M., (1988). Cell and environment interactions in tumor microregions: The multi-cell spheroid model. *Science, 240*, 177–184.

Vazin, T., & Freed, W. J., (2010). Human embryonic stem cells: Derivation, culture, and differentiation: A review. *Restor. Neurol. Neurosci., 28*(4), 589–603.

Vincx, M., (1986). Free-living marine nematodes from the Southern Bight of the North Sea. I. Notes on species of the genera Gonionchus Cobb, 1920, Neochromadora Micoletzky, 1924, and Sabatieria Rouville, 1903. *Hydrobiologia, 140*, 255–286.

Walkley, C. R., Qudsi, R., Sankaran, V. G., Perry, J. A., Gostissa, M., Roth, S. I., Stephen, J., et al., (2008). Conditional mouse osteosarcoma, dependent on p53 loss and potentiated by loss of Rb, mimics the human disease. *Genes Dev., 22*(12), 1662–1676.

Wijlemans, J. W., Bartels, L. W., Deckers, R., Ries, M., Mali, W. P. T. M., Moonen, C. T. W., & Van, D. B. M. A. A. J., (2012). Magnetic resonance-guided high-intensity focused ultrasound (MR-HIFU) ablation of liver tumors. *Cancer Imaging, 12*(2), 387–394.

CHAPTER 12

Plant-Derived Anti-Malarial Compounds and Their Derivatives as Anticancer Agents: Future Perspectives

SANDEEP ARORA,[1] TAPAN BEHL,[1] and SAMIR MEHNDIRATTA[2]

[1]Chitkara College of Pharmacy, Chitkara University, Punjab, India

[2]Taipei Medical University, Taipei, Taiwan

ABSTRACT

Cancer is an occupational lifestyle disease comprising of a group of about 120 different diseases. It affects different parts of the body and is indicated as uncontrolled growth of the cells and invasion to other adjoining tissues thus spreading abnormal cells to healthy tissues, known as metastasis. As a matter of fact, unlike the disease itself, the uncontrolled cell division is the major cause of increased mortality rates among the cancer patients. Currently, there are various chemotherapeutic agents for cancer treatment, both plant derived and synthetic, which also includes target specific/individually designed therapeutic agents.

Prescribed uses of different plant parts like leaves, bark, roots, rhizomes, etc. has been described in ancient texts of Ayurvedic and Chinese medicines for cancer management and cure. These plant products exhibit a broad spectrum of activities which is certainly contributed due to various active ingredients present in them, possessing diverse pharmacological activities. This further support the idea that plant or plant products indicated for one particular disease could be useful in treating other diseases. The traditional medications employed for malaria have been recently investigated for their potential anticancer effects. Malaria has been effectively controlled since ancient times across the globe by herbal medications. The anti-malarial compounds with potent anticancer activities include cinchona alkaloids such as quinine, epiquinne, chloroquine, etc. Apart from Cinchona, other plant constituents used are artemisinin and its derivatives, indole alkaloids, indoloquinolines alkaloid, quassinoids, etc. and can be greatly explored for their potential as anticancer drugs.

12.1   CANCER: FACTS AND FIGURES

Cancer is an occupational lifestyle disease comprising of a group of about 120 different diseases. It affects different parts of the body and is indicated as the uncontrolled growth of the cells and invasion to other adjoining tissues thus spreading abnormal cells to healthy tissues, known as metastasis. As a matter of fact, unlike the disease itself, the uncontrolled cell division is the major cause of increased mortality rates among the cancer patients. Many factors which play a crucial role in the development of these cancers and can be broadly classified as (Torre et al., 2015):

1. **Internal Aspects Promoting Cancer Risks:** Hereditary alterations in the genetic sequence, hormonal involvement, and disturbance in the immune system.
2. **External Aspects Promoting Cancer Risks:** Tobacco or irrelevant dietary consumption and pathogenic intervention.

External parameters can be further categorized based on the type of carcinogen. Such as:

1. **Chemical Carcinogens:** Asbestos, tobacco smoke, contaminants of a potable water (arsenic-As) and food items (aflatoxin).
2. **Physical Agents Producing Cancerous Growth:** Ionizing and ultraviolet radiation.
3. **Biological Carcinogenic Agents:** Some viruses, bacteria, or parasites.

In this multistage process of cancer development, it takes many years (>10) between the vulnerability of the body to external agents and detectable cancer progression where aforesaid factors act together or in sequence. Unlike AIDS, tuberculosis, and malaria, cancer inherits a superior position in producing a greater mortality rate among the population, which constitutes 1 out of every 7 deaths (Torre et al., 2015; Pennathur et al., 2013). According to WHO, in 2012, 8.2 million died from cancer. The global annual occurrence of cancer is about 60% in countries like Africa, Asia, Central, and South America. In the next two decades, WHO estimates an increase of 70% in new cases of cancer with an estimated increase to 22 million annual cases of (WHO, 2015). After the cardiovascular diseases (heart attacks, CHF, arrhythmias, etc.), which poses a greater threat to the lives of the people in developed countries with a high employment rate, cancer occupies the second position. On the other hand, in the developing nations with low employment rate, it occupies the third position after cardiovascular diseases and pathological infections affecting the population primarily (Torre et al., 2015). According to the 2012 data collected by the WHO, men are more susceptible to lung, colorectal, prostate, liver, and stomach cancer whereas women mainly suffer from breast, colorectal, lung, cervix, and stomach cancer. Data published by the American Chemical Society in 2015 shows the top 5 most deadly diseases worldwide, in low-income countries and high-income countries as shown in Table 12.1 (Torre et al., 2015).

TABLE 12.1 Income Levels Affecting the Mortality Rate Globally, 2012 (Thousands)

	Globally			Low and Middle-Income Levels			High-Income Levels		
	Rank	Deaths	%	Rank	Death	%	Rank	Death	%
Cardiovascular diseases	1	17513	31%	1	13075	30%	1	4438	38%
Malignant neoplasm	2	8204	15%	3	5310	12%	2	2894	25%
Infectious/ parasitic diseases	3	6431	12%	2	6128	14%	7	303	3%
Unintentional injuries	4	4040	7%	4	3395	8%	3	645	6%
Respiratory infections	5	3716	7%	5	3212	7%	5	504	4%

The numbers of recognized carcinogens to humans, for example, various new chemical entities, oncoviruses, and other environmental parameters have raised from 50 to 108 within 25 years (1987–2012) due to increase in technology and number of new chemicals and this has also added up to the number of new probably (64) and possibly (271) carcinogens to humans in 2012 (Latosińska and Latosińska, 2013).

Amongst the Asian countries like Japan, India, Taiwan, Singapore, Korea, China, Philippines, etc., Taiwan has the highest prevalence rate for cancer among both the females and males (299 cases per I lakh males) of a particular age. Moreover, Korea and Japan constitute high incidence rates for males; and Singapore and the Philippines for females (Chiang et al., 2010; Chen et al., 2002).

12.1.1   ORIGIN OF CANCER AND CANCER BIOLOGY

Cancer (malignant neoplasm) has been found in dinosaur fossils in Wyoming as well as the ancient mummies preserved in the pyramids, as found in the Great Pyramid of Giza. The remains of a female skull belonging to 1900–1600 B.C. (Bronze Age) comprise of the ancient human specimen with cancerous afflictions. Various cancer cases have been illustrated in the Ramayana (500 B.C.) along with the introduction of arsenic pastes as the first medication to treat the disease progression. Further year-wise developments in understanding cancer and cancer biology are as follows (Table 12.2) (Latosińska and Latosińska, 2013; Chiang et al., 2010; Chen et al., 2002; Vogelstein and Kinzler, 2004).

TABLE 12.2   Year Wise Development of Cancer Biology

Who?	When?	What?
Hippocrates (a Greek physician)	460–370 B.C.	He coined the term cancer (Greek: *carcinos,* meaning venous network around cancer as crab claws), formulated a Humoral theory that illustrates cancer genesis of many types of cancers such as breast, uterus, stomach, etc., and described differences between benign and malignant forms of cancer.
Cornelus Celsus	25 B.C.–50 A.D.	He changed the Greek "carcinos" into the Latin term "cancer" and construed the first surgical aspects of the disease.
Claudius Galen (Roman Empire physician)	129–216 A.D.	He accorded the term "oncos" (Greek word depicting tumor swelling) for cancer.
Antonie van Leeuwenhoek	Late 17th century	Treatment of cancer progression is based on the parameters differentiating a normal cell from a malignant one.
Johannes Peter Muller	1838	He proposed the blastema theory
Karl Thiersch	1860	Cancers metastasis and proliferation by lymph leading to the development of secondary cancer.
Rudolf Virchow	—	Neoplastic cells can be distinguished from the neighboring normal cells from which they mutated.

TABLE 12.2 *(Continued)*

Who?	When?	What?
		Chronic irritation as a factor favoring cancer development
Wilhelm Hofmeister	—	Discovery of chromosome and mitosis
Theodor Boveri	1902	Presence of tumor suppressor genes, oncogenes, and cell-cycle checkpoints.
		The tumor begins with the rapid, uncontrolled proliferation of a single cell that might be due to physical, chemical, and biological aspects.
David Paul von Hansemann	—	Chromosomal theory of cancer
		Formation of tumor due to abnormal number of chromosomes in cells as a result of multipolar mitosis.
Thomas Hunt Morgan	1915	Observed chromosomal changes indicating correctness of Boveri's theory.
G. Steve Martin	1970	Identification of first oncogene (SRC, from sarcoma)
George Knudson	1971	He identified Rb gene (a first tumor suppressor gene) in humans on chromosome 13 (13q14.2).

12.1.2 HALLMARKS OF CANCER

Multistep tumorigenesis elaborates the mutations of normal cells into neoplastic cells as a result of alterations in the genetic sequence of an individual. Douglas Hanahan and Robert A. Weinberg have discussed the eight acquired capabilities of cancer (Table 12.3) (Hanahan and Weinberg, 2000, 2011).

These hallmarks are important for all malignant phenotypes as they are common to all cancer cells and these acquired capabilities are monitored by highly complex protein signaling networks which elaborate that the cell proliferation, motility, and survival regulating cellular signaling pathways in normal cells are altered and form malignant cells. Many possible targets currently under investigation for cancer treatment are signaling proteins that are components of these pathways (Hanahan and Weinberg, 2000, 2011).

Currently, there are various chemotherapeutic agents for cancer treatment, both plant-derived and synthetic, and also include target-specific/individually designed therapeutic agents. Figure 12.1 demonstrates some examples of chemotherapeutic agents.

TABLE 12.3 Hallmarks of Cancer and Their Most Relevant Underlying Causes

Hallmarks of Cancer	Underlying Causes
No need of external stimulus to multiply	Via activation of transforming protein p21
Negligence to growth-inhibiting signals	Retarded action of suppressors of retinoblastoma (retinal cells proliferation)
Concealed apoptosis (programmed cell death)	Production of IGF survival factors
Infinite ability to multiply	Enhanced activity of terminal transferase
Uninterrupted angiogenesis (formation of new vasculature)	Enhanced VEGF inducer activity
Uncontrolled cell division and tissue invasion	Inactivate E-cadherin
Reprogramming energy metabolism	Mutant RAS and upregulated MYC
Evading immune destruction	Secretion of TGF-β or other immuno-suppressors

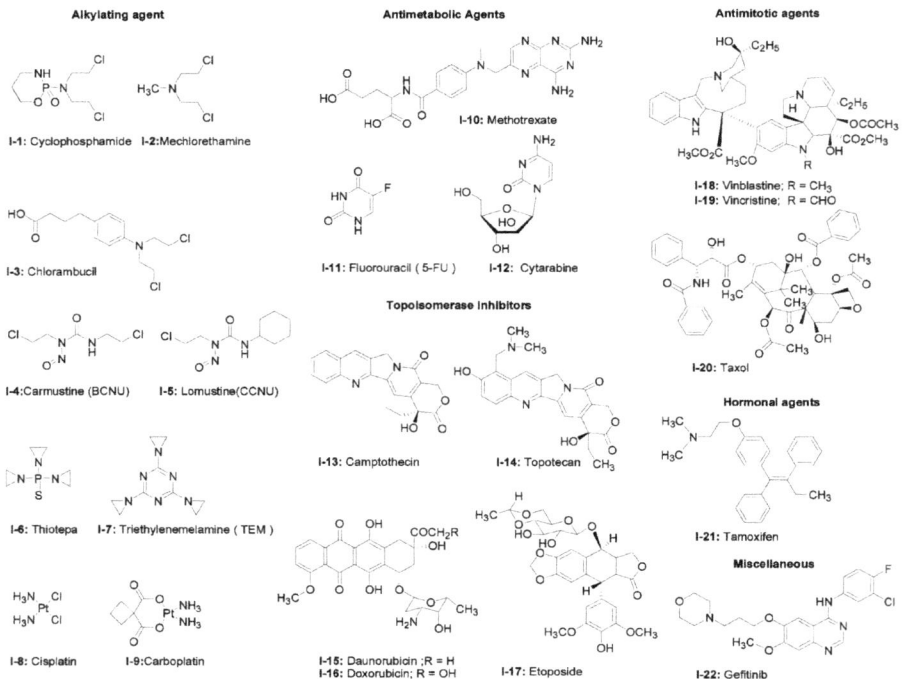

FIGURE 12.1 Chemical structures of various chemotherapeutic agents.

12.2   ANTI-MALARIAL COMPOUNDS WITH POTENT ANTICANCER ACTIVITIES

Treatments using plants and plant products are an important part of human history. Plant-derived natural compounds are the primary source of drugs which contain different secondary metabolites (with differences in structure and biological actions) with potent anticancer actions. Crude plant products have been used for centuries in countries like India, China, Korea, etc., to treat various illnesses. Prescribed uses of different plant parts like leaves, bark, roots, rhizomes, etc., have been described in ancient texts of Ayurvedic and Chinese medicines. Diet rich in natural vegetables and fruits can reduce the risk of various chronic diseases such as heart diseases, diabetes, etc., indicates the importance of these plant products. Moreover, these plant products exhibit a broad spectrum of activities which is certainly contributed due to various active ingredients present in them, possessing diverse pharmacological activities. This further supports the idea that plant or plant products indicated for one particular disease could be useful in treating other diseases. One such observation is; the traditional medications employed for malaria have been recently investigated for their potential anticancer effects. Malaria has been effectively controlled since ancient times across the globe by herbal medications.

12.2.1   CINCHONA ALKALOIDS

Alkaloids are the most significant secondary metabolites that are physiologically active nitrogenous bases rendering potential benefits in malaria, and derived from various bigenetic precursors (Shankar et al., 2012; Saxena et al., 2003; Adebayo and Krettli, 2011). Quinine (1) is the most significant alkaloid employed for cancer therapy and others include quinidine (2), epiquinne (3), cinchonidine (4) and, cinchonine (5) as shown in Figure 12.2, but it was the quinine which drifted the world as an antimalarial (Oliveira et al., 2009; Kaur et al., 2009).

1. **Quinine:** The oldest and most important drug, quinine used first for malaria was the bark extract of *Cinchona* species of South America belonging to family Rubiaceae and was isolated in 1820. Cinchona bark infusion was used to treat malaria since 1632. Recently, potent anticancer potential of quinine has been reported and according to Krishnavedi and Suresh (2015), quinine curbs the replication of cells

and advocates a dose reliant programmed cell death (apoptosis) of the cancerous cell masses (Pranay and Pushpal, 2017; Krishnaveni and Suresh, 2015).

2. **Chloroquine:** It was synthesized in 1940 and has been effectively used in treatment of malaria. Clinical trials have been regulated for the evaluation of chloroquine to potentiate patient response in different anticancer regimens. It inhibits the autophagy (self-eating) of neoplastic cells and sustains the tumor vasculature, thereby following a dual-action mechanism against cancer (Maes et al., 2016). CQ was found to mediate a response of the neoplastic cells to a variety of conventional anticancer medications when used in combinations with them, as per the preclinical studies, thus improving the therapeutic activity. A large number of clinical studies (> 30) are underway to evaluate the action of chloroquine in various forms of cancer. Apart from the cancer cells, chloroquine exercises its effects on the tumor microenvironment as well as it affects the Toll-like receptor 9, p53, and CXCR4-CXCL12 pathway in cancer masses. Moreover, the fibroblasts associated with cancer and the immune system is affected by chloroquine in the stroma of tumor cells (Verbaanderd et al., 2017).

3. **Quinacrine (7):** It is a quinine derivative that has been effectively used in the treatment of breast cancer. It manifests its anticancer actions by significantly suppressing the nuclear factor kappa B, that controls DNA transcription and cytokine production and topoisomerase activity, and activating p53 signaling (Preet et al., 2012).

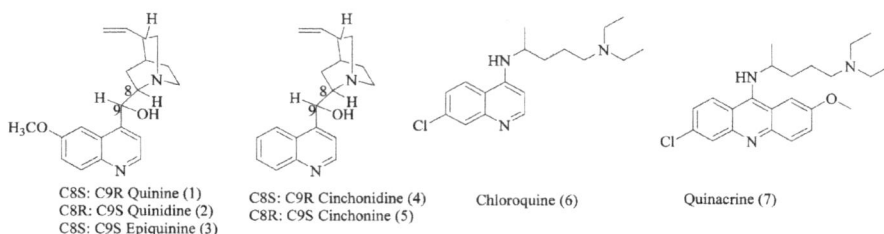

C8S: C9R Quinine (1)
C8R: C9S Quinidine (2)
C8S: C9S Epiquinine (3)

C8S: C9R Cinchonidine (4)
C8R: C9S Cinchonine (5)

Chloroquine (6)

Quinacrine (7)

FIGURE 12.2 Active constituents from Cinchona and their derivatives.

12.2.2 SESQUITERPENES

Apart from Cinchona another plant, called *Artemisia annua* used in China, from the 70s, is an important source of the antimalarial drug-artemisinin.

Artemisinins is a category of antimalarial drugs, comprising of the endo-peroxide group that is essential for its activity and presence of its unique 1,2,4-trioxane ring plays an important role for anti-plasmodial efficacy, and includes artemisinin (**8**), Dihyroxyartemisinin (DHA, **9**), artesunate (**10**), artemether (**11**), and arteether (**12**) (Figure 12.3).

1. **Biological Source:** In 1972, Tu Youyou discovered Qinghaosu (emisinin), an antimalarial constituent from *Artemisia annua*, a Chinese plant and the discovery of this novel sesquiterpene lactone endoperoxide provoked the study of the peroxides occurring in nature, for their anti-schizont activity.

2. **Mode of Action:** The exact mode of action of these drugs is some-what unknown, yet they are believed to act via cytotoxic free radical production by liberating singlet oxygen after being released in the *Plasmodium*. In-vitro studies involving suppression of hypoxanthine labeled with a radioactive atom indicated that artemisinin led to a marked reduction of nucleic acid synthesis. Dihydroartemisinin is more effective (200 times) than artemisinin for the reduction of uptake of 3H-hypoxanthine uptake. For anticancer mechanisms of artemisinins, not much is known. There have been many studies indicating different mechanisms of actions of artemisinin with one possible mechanism could be-inhibition of metastasis-associated angiogenesis (Rücker et al., 1991; Gu et al., 1983; Zhao et al., 1986; Hooft van Huijsduijnen et al., 2013).

Many studies with *in vivo* and *in vitro* conditions constitute more than 188 studies using artemisinin for its role in cancer, aiming at identifying the action mechanism of artemisinin and its synergistic effects with conventional anti-cancer drugs (Zhang et al., 2012; Tin et al., 2012; Wang et al., 2012; Soomro et al., 2011; Gao et al., 2011; Noori and Hassan, 2011; Singh et al., 2011; Weifeng et al., 2011; Zhao et al., 2011; Xu et al., 2011; Crespo-Ortiz and Wei, 2012). However, only a few clinical studies have reported a moderate recovery in advanced cases of NSCLC patients, i.e., patients affected by non-small cell lung cancer (NSCLC) patients. Despite abundant preclinical literature on promising anticancer activity of artemisinin, having excellent, well-established safety profile, there are not many reported cases of off-label use of artemisinin for cancer which could be due to the following reasons:

1. Short half-life;
2. Variability in exposure of drug between patient and over time;

3. Lack of materials suitable for direct therapeutic use (produced according to the requirements of Good Manufacturing Practice) (Hooft van Huijsduijnen et al., 2013).

These problems do not count much while treating malaria patients since its treatment is only a three-day regime; however, it may not lead to appropriate metastasis-associated angiogenesis suppression in cancer patients.

Some reports advocate that artemisinins may suppress the T_{reg} population and promote immune system alteration from T helper type 2 to a T-helper type 1-influenced antineoplastic response (Noori and Hassan, 2011). It can suppress vascular endothelial growth factor along with Ang-1 secretion and interfere with angiogenesis (Chen et al., 2012; Zhou et al., 2007; Wang et al., 2007) and chorioallantois neovascularization. The artemisinin induced programmed cell death in several cancer cell lines is depicted in various writings (Crespo-Ortiz and Wei, 2012) via intrinsic mechanisms (Xu et al., 2011; Zhou et al., 2012; Handrick et al., 2010). These mechanisms include reduced potential across the mitochondrial membrane, cytochrome c release from the mitochondria, activation of protease enzymes (caspases 9 and 3), and involvement of Bak/Bax. The Fe^{2+} mediated activation of artemisinins also appears to play a pivotal role on account of the enhanced iron requirement by neoplastic cells and good cytotoxicity of the mitochondrial heme bound compounds. This further has supported the investigation of the up-regulated transferrin receptor as potential cancer treatment target (Hooft van Huijsduijnen et al., 2013; Kim et al., 2006). Interestingly, this action mechanism varies from those of existing anticancer drugs and thus artemisinins are promising in cancer treatment due to synergistic effects with established treatments (Hooft van Huijsduijnen et al., 2013; Efferth et al., 2007) even more significantly, cancers resisting multiple drugs are responsive to the action of artemisinin (Hooft van Huijsduijnen et al., 2013; Lu et al., 2012).

12.2.3   INDOLOQUINOLINE ALKALOID

Cryptolepine (13), an indoloquinoline alkaloid, is a potent antiplasmodial component, exhibiting effective results recorded *in vitro* conditions against *P. falciparum* resistant and sensitive to chloroquine.

1. **Biological Source:** It is presently obtained from the root extract of *C. sanguinolenta*, along with other alkaloids (Figure 12.4).

2. **Mechanism of Action:** Cryptolepine interacts with deoxyribonucleic acid segments and sustains the covalent complex of topoisomerase II enzyme and deoxyribonucleic acid, thereby inhibiting further DNA synthesis. Studies have revealed the development of charge transfer complex of the nitrogenous bases in DNA (purine and pyrimidine) and cryptolepine, on account of the association between the nitrogen atoms of A-T base pair (adenine-thymine) and cryptolepine (Baba et al., 2014; Kirby et al., 1989) though there are reports indicating the implantation of cryptolepine into DNA segment (Wright et al., 2001 Lisgarten et al., 2002). Experimental investigations proved that cryptolepine has the tendency to suppress the production of β haematin. Haem (hemozoin) is toxic to the parasite but, on conversion to malarial pigment, it can be detoxified and this is identical to β-haematin. It could be concluded that the action pathway of crytolepine varies according to its antimalarial and cytotoxic action.

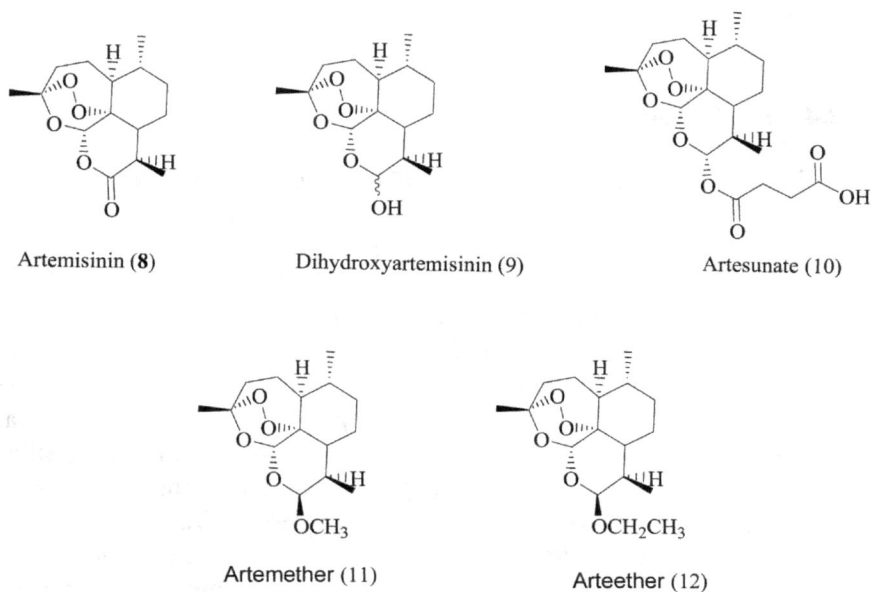

Artemisinin (**8**)   Dihydroxyartemisinin (9)   Artesunate (10)

Artemether (11)   Arteether (12)

FIGURE 12.3   Artemisinin and its derivatives.

Root decoction of this alkaloid is used as an effective cure for malaria in parts of Africa. However, toxic responses have also been observed (Cimanga et al., 1997; Wright, 2005; Wright et al., 2001). Recently, Santosh K. Katiyar et al. have reported (Pal et al., 2017) that the inhibitory action of cryptolepine was linked to the diminished expression of protein-coding genes and loss of potential across the mitochondrial membrane causing disruption of mito-chondrial dynamics. Furthermore, AMPKα1/2-LKB1 (tumor suppressor entity) was activated on account of curtailed ATP levels and mitochondrial masses, associated with rebated mTOR signaling. Mitochondrial biogenesis is significantly retarded due to reduced expression of COX-1 and SDH-A, after administration of cryptolepine.

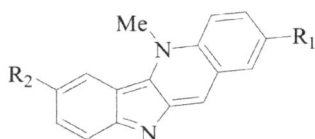

R$_1$=R$_2$=H Cryptolepine (**13**)
R$_1$=R$_2$=Br 2,7-Dibromocryptolepine (**14**)

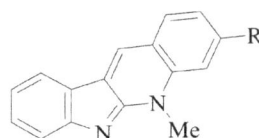

R=H Neocryptolepine (**15**)
R=Br 2-Bromocryptolepine (**16**)

FIGURE 12.4   Various indoloquinoline alkaloids.

12.2.4   INDOLE ALKALOIDS

1. **Biological Source:** Ellipticine (**17**) has been recently isolated from the bark of *Aspidosperma vargasii*. It was initially isolated from evergreen *Ochrosia* species of Australia in 1959.
2. **Chemistry:** The chemical structure of Ellipticine is a planar polycy-clic structure which intercalates with DNA, therefore, manifesting greater binding affinity to DNA (10(6) M(-1)). A unique feature distinguishing ellipticine from other simple intercalators is the presence of protonatable nitrogen of the ring. Under physiological conditions, both monocationic (favoring stabilized binding of ellip-ticine) and uncharged species (lipophilic moiety permeable through membrane barriers) were found to be present. Due to its special pharmacophore, ellipticine exhibit multiple modes of actions such as binding to DNA segment, interactions with membrane barriers (due to lipophilic moiety), oxidative bioactivation, and enzyme function modification (topoisomerase II and telomerase). System-atic structural modification of ellipticine has approved consider-able applications of rational drug design thus masking its toxic side effects (Zhang et al., 2012).

3. **Uses:** Ellipticine has shown exceptional actions in *in vitro* conditions against the K1 strain of *P. falciparum* which exerts significant resistance to the multiple drugs. Ellipticine functions as a synthesis template of Elliptinium acetate (**18**, brand name: Celliptium. R.) which is a clinically used and effectively marketed (France) drug efficient in breast cancer (Figure 12.5) (Garbett and Graves, 2004).

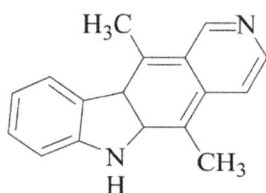

Ellipticine (**17**)   Ellipticinium (**18**)

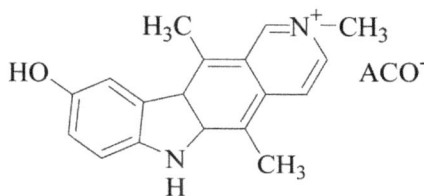

FIGURE 12.5   Indole alkaloids Ellipticine and its derivative.

12.2.5 QUASSINOIDS

The Quassinoids are a class of lactones which are highly oxygenated in nature.

1. **Biological Source:** Two quassinoids are described in this category, i.e., Bruceantin (BCT), and brusatol. BCT was obtained from *Brucea antidysenterica* in Ethiopia.

2. **Chemistry:** Most of the quassinoids constitute a 20 carbon skeleton chain named picrasane (some may also comprise of 18, 19 or 25 carbon atoms), along with different oxygen-containing groups on all the carbon atoms except at carbons C-5, C-9 and the methyl groups at C-4 and C-10. Two quassinoids; more potent BCT (**19**) and brusatol (**20**) Figure 12.6, differ only in the 3,15-ester moiety that accounts for the antimalarial activity. This can be explained by the addition of strong alkyl groups on the 23rd carbon moiety. Researches were conducted for BCT and its role in treating B16 melanoma, colon 38, and P388 leukemia in mice but due to no observed antitumor effect, clinical trials up to phase II were abolished. Recently, the activity of BCT and brusatol has been reinvestigated for the treatment of leukemia. BCT and brusatol treatment caused cell differentiation

via down-regulation of protein-coding gene expression (c-MYC), thus inducing cell differentiation or cell death (Saxena et al., 2003; Kaur et al., 2009; Muhammad and Samoylenko, 2007; Trager and Polonsky, 1981). The animal tumors treated with BCT were marked by a significant elevation in apoptosis (programmed cell death). Treatment of human leukemia cell lines (HL-60 and RPMI 8226) for apoptosis induced by BCT via caspase activation has been studied and established. BCT induced relapse in initial as well as progressive stages of cancer in a study conducted *in vivo* using RPMI 8226 human-SCID xenografts without any significant toxicity. A recent study has explored the cancer stem cell proliferation inhibition potential of BCT mediated by activation of the Notch signaling pathway. NF kappa B activation by brusatol (translocation into nucleus) promotes differentiation of HL-60 cell lines (Issa et al., 2016; Cuendet and Pezzuto, 2004).

3. **Uses:** The quassinoids comprise anti-malarial and anticancer properties, both actions equally significant.

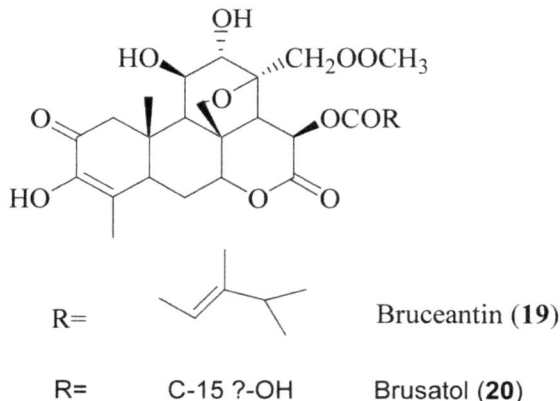

FIGURE 12.6 Quassinoids BCT and brusatol.

These aforesaid examples are only a few out of various available natural antimalarial compounds, which possess potent anticancer activities. Both alkaloidal and non-alkaloidal antimalarials are endowed with cytotoxic activities and chemical architecture of these compounds can be carefully modified to yield synthetics with the desired potential. Plants remain a source of compounds with a wide range of biodiversity and bio-potencies from time immortal. However, the presence of many of these compounds in very low concentrations and usually as a part of complex mixtures in various plant species makes their isolation, purification, and characterization a tedious and highly expensive process. Despite these challenges, plants have given many lead molecules. Now it's onto researchers to explore these bio-diverse molecules, and optimize their activity for human use.

Sesquiterpenes, have shown promising results as anticancer drugs especially artemisinin. With already studied safety profile and FDA approval, it has become leading investigational antimalarial compound with potent anticancer effects. Many other artemisinins have been successfully developed for treatment of malaria such as Artemether, which has already been FDA, approved for the treatment of malaria as an individual drug or in combination with piperaquine and has been shown to be equivalent to artemether/lumefantrine. Another such example is Artesunate which is also FDA approved as a single dose or in a fixed-dose combination with amodiaquine, mefloquine, and pyronaridine. Dihydroartemisinin can also be used as either an individual drug or in association with piperaquine and has shown activity equivalent to artemether/lumefantrine combinations. The key point of these antimalarials is their cytotoxicity which can be carefully monitored and altered to get potent anticancer compounds, e.g., elliptinium acetate from ellipticine. In addition, this inter-related activity creates a huge possibility of finding new lead molecules from cancer/malarial drugs for treatment therapy of malaria/cancer.

KEYWORDS

- **anti-malarial compounds**
- **bruceantin**
- **cinchona alkaloids**
- **dihyroxyartemisinin**
- **indoloquinoline alkaloid**
- **sesquiterpenes**

REFERENCES

Adebayo, J., & Krettli, A., (2011). Potential antimalarials from Nigerian plants: A review. *J. Ethnopharmacol., 133*(2), 289–302.

Baba, G., Adewumi, A., & Jere, S. A., (2014). Toxicity study, phytochemical characterization and anti-parasitic efficacy of aqueous and ethanolic extracts of *Sclerocarya birrea* against *Plasmodium berghei* and salmonella typhi. *Br. J. Pharmacol. Toxicol.*, *5*(2), 59–67.

Chen, C. J., You, S. L., Lin, L. H., Hsu, W. L., & Yang, Y. W., (2002). Cancer epidemiology and control in Taiwan: A brief review. *Japanese Journal of Clinical Oncology*, *32*(1), S66–S81.

Chen, X., Lin, H., Wen, J., Rong, Q., Xu, W., et al., (2012). Dihydroartemisinin suppresses cell proliferation, invasion, and angiogenesis in human glioma U87 cells. *African J. Pharmacy and Pharmacol.*, *6*, 2433–2440.

Chiang, C. J., Chen, Y. C., Chen, C. J., You, S. L., & Lai, M. S., (2010). Taiwan cancer registry task, F. cancer trends in Taiwan. *Jpn. J. Clin. Oncol.*, *40*, 897–904.

Cimanga, K., De Bruyne, T., Pieters, L., Vlietinck, A. J., & Turger, C. A., (1997). *In vitro* and *in vivo* antiplasmodial activity of cryptolepine and related alkaloids from *Cryptolepis sanguinolenta*. *J. Nat. Prod.*, *60*(7), 688–691.

Crespo-Ortiz, M. P., & Wei, M. Q., (2012). Antitumor activity of artemisinin and its derivatives: From a well-known antimalarial agent to a potential anticancer drug. *J. Biomed. Biotechnol.*, 247597.

Cuendet, M., & Pezzuto, J. M., (2004). Antitumor activity of bruceantin: An old drug with new promise. *J. Nat. Prod.*, *67*(2), 269–272.

Efferth, T., Giaisi, M., Merling, A., Krammer, P. H., & Li-Weber, M., (2007). Artesunate induces ROS-mediated apoptosis in doxorubicin-resistant T leukemia cells. *PLoS One, 2*, e693.

Gao, N., Budhraja, A., Cheng, S., Liu, E. H., Huang, C., et al., (2011). Interruption of the MEK/ERK signaling cascade promotes dihydroartemisinin-induced apoptosis *in vitro* and *in vivo*. *Apoptosis, 16*, 511–523.

Garbett, N. C., & Graves, D. E., (2004). Extending nature's leads: The anticancer agent ellipticine. *Curr. Med. Chem. Anticancer Agents, 4*(2), 149–172.

Genome, E. H., (1990–2003). Available from: http://www.ornl.gov/sci/techresources/Human_Genome/project/hgp.shtml (accessed on 23 July 2020).

Gu, H., Warhurst, D., & Peters, W., (1983). Rapid action of Qinghaosu and related drugs on incorporation of [3 H] isoleucine by Plasmodium falciparum *in vitro*. *Biochem. Pharmacol., 32*(17), 2463–2466.

Hanahan, D., & Weinberg, R. A., (2000). The hallmarks of cancer. *Cell, 100*, 57–70.

Hanahan, D., & Weinberg, R. A., (2011). Hallmarks of cancer: The next generation. *Cell, 144*, 646–674.

Handrick, R., Ontikatze, T., Bauer, K. D., Freier, F., & Rubel, A., (2010). Dihydroartemisinin induces apoptosis by a Bak-dependent intrinsic pathway. *Mol Cancer Ther., 9*, 2497–2510.

Hooft, V. H. R., Guy, R. K., Chibale, K., Haynes, R. K., Peitz, I., Kelter, G., Phillips, M. A., et al., (2013). Anticancer properties of distinct antimalarial drug classes. *PLoS One, 8*(12), e82962.

Issa, M. E., Berndt, S., Carpentier, G., Pezzuto, J. M., & Cuendet, M., (2016). Bruceantin inhibits multiple myeloma cancer stem cell proliferation. *Cancer Biol. Ther., 17*(9), 966–975.

Kaur, K., Jain, M., Kaur, T., & Jain, R., (2009). Antimalarials from nature. *Bioorg. Med. Chem., 17*(9), 3229–3256.

Kim, S. J., Kim, M. S., Lee, J. W., Lee, C. H., & Yoo, H., (2006). Dihydroartemisinin enhances radio sensitivity of human glioma cells *in vitro*. *J. Cancer Res. Clin Oncol., 132*, 129–135.

Kirby, G. C., O'Neill, M. J., Phillipson, J. D., & Warhurst, D. C., (1989). *In vitro* studies on the mode of action of quassinoids with activity against chloroquine-resistant *Plasmodium falciparum. Biochem. Pharmacol., 38*(24), 4367–4374.

Krishnaveni, M., & Suresh, K., (2015). Induction of apoptosis by quinine in human laryngeal carcinoma cell line (KB). *Int. J. Curr. Res. Aca. Rev., 3*(3), 169–178.

Latosińska, J. N., & Latosińska, M., (2013). Anticancer drug discovery—from serendipity to rational design. In: *Drug Discovery.* Intech Open.

Lisgarten, J. N., Coll, M., Portugal, J., Wright, C. W., & Aymami, J., (2002). The antimalarial and cytotoxic drug cryptolepine intercalates into DNA at cytosine-cytosine sites. *Nat. Struct. Mol. Biol., 9*(1), 57–60.

Lu, J. J., Chen, S. M., Ding, J., & Meng, L. H., (2012). Characterization of dihydroartemisinin-resistant colon carcinoma HCT116/R cell line. *Mol Cell Biochem., 360*, 329–337.

Maes, H., Kuchnio, A., Carmeliet, P., & Agostinis, P., (2016). Chloroquine anticancer activity is mediated by autophagy-independent effects on the tumor vasculature. *Mol Cell Oncol., 3*(1), e970097.

Muhammad, I., & Samoylenko, V., (2007). Antimalarial quassinoids: Past, present, and future. *Expert Opinion on Drug Discovery, 2*(8), 1065–1084.

Noori, S., & Hassan, Z. M., (2011). Dihydroartemisinin shift the immune response towards Th1, inhibit the tumor growth *in vitro* and *in vivo. Cell Immunol., 271*, 67–72.

Oliveira, A. B., Dolabela, M. F., Braga, F. C., Jácome, R. L., Varotti, F. P., & Póvoa, M. M., (2009). Plant-derived antimalarial agents: New leads and efficient phythomedicines. Part I. Alkaloids. *Anais da Academia Brasileira De Ciencias, 81*(4), 715–740.

Pal, H. C., Prasad, R., & Katiyar, S. K., (2017). Cryptolepine inhibits melanoma cell growth through coordinated changes in mitochondrial biogenesis, dynamics, and metabolic tumor suppressor AMPKα1/2-LKB1. *Sci. Rep., 7*(1), 1498.

Pennathur, A., Gibson, M. K., Jobe, B. A., & Luketich, J. D., (2013). Esophageal carcinoma. *Lancet, 381*, 400–412.

Pranay, G., & Pushpal, D., (2017). Spectrum of biological properties of cinchona alkaloids: A brief review. *J. of Pharmacog. Phytochem., 6*(4), 162–166.

Preet, R., Mohapatra, P., Mohanty, S., Sahu, S. K., Choudhuri, T., Wyatt, M. D., & Kundu, C. N., (2012). Quinacrine has anticancer activity in breast cancer cells through inhibition of topoisomerase activity. *Int. J. Cancer, 130*(7), 1660–1670.

Rücker, G., Walter, R., Manns, D., & Mayer, R., (1991). Antimalarial activity of some natural peroxides. *Planta Med., 57*(3), 295.

Saxena, S., Pant, N., Jain, D., & Bhakuni, R., (2003). Antimalarial agents from plant sources. *Curr. Sci., 85*(9), 1314–1329.

Shankar, R., Deb, S., & Sharma, B., (2012). Antimalarial plants of northeast India: An overview. *J. Ayurveda Integr. Med., 3*(1), 10.

Singh, N. P., Lai, H. C., Park, J. S., Gerhardt, T. E., Kim, B. J., et al., (2011). Effects of artemisinin dimers on rat breast cancer cells *in vitro* and *in vivo. Anticancer Res., 31*, 4111–4114.

Soomro, S., Langenberg, T., Mahringer, A., Konkimalla, V. B., Horwedel, C., et al., (2011). Design of novel artemisinin-like derivatives with cytotoxic and antiangiogenic properties. *J. Cell Mol. Med., 15*, 1122–1135.

Tin, A. S., Sundar, S. N., Tran, K. Q., Park, A. H., Poindexter, M., et al., (2012). Antiproliferative effects of artemisinin on human breast cancer cells requires the downregulated expression of the E2F1 transcription factor and loss of E2F1-target cell cycle genes. *Anticancer Drugs, 23*, 370–379.

Torre, L., Siegel, R., & Jemal, A., (2015). Global cancer facts and figures. *Atlanta: American Cancer Society, 2.*

Trager, W., & Polonsky, J., (1981). Antimalarial activity of quassinoids against chloroquine-resistant *Plasmodium falciparum in vitro. Ame. J. Ttrop. Med. Hyg., 30*(3), 531–537.

Verbaanderd, C., Maes, H., Schaaf, M. B., Sukhatme, V. P., Pantziarka, P., Sukhatme, V., & Bouche, G., (2017). Repurposing drugs in oncology (ReDO)—chloroquine and hydroxychloroquine as anticancer agents. *E Cancer Medical Science, 11*, 781.

Vogelstein, B., & Kinzler, K. W., (2004). Cancer genes and the pathways they control. *Nature Medicine, 10*, 789–799.

Wang, J., Guo, Y., Zhang, B. C., Chen, Z. T., & Gao, J. F., (2007). Induction of apoptosis and inhibition of cell migration and tube-like formation by dihydroartemisinin in murine lymphatic endothelial cells. *Pharmacology, 80*, 207–218.

Wang, Z., Yu, Y., Ma, J., Zhang, H., Zhang, H., et al., (2012). LyP-1 modification to enhance delivery of artemisinin or fluorescent probe loaded polymeric micelles to highly metastatic tumor and its lymphatics. *Mol. Pharm., 9*, 2646–2657.

Weifeng, T., Feng, S., Xiangji, L., Changqing, S., Zhiquan, Q., et al., (2011). Artemisinin inhibits *in vitro* and *in vivo* invasion and metastasis of human hepato cellular carcinoma cells. *Phytomedicine, 18*, 158–162.

WHO, (2015). http://www.who.int/mediacentre/factsheets/fs297/en/ (accessed on 23 July 2020).

Wright, C. W., (2005). Plant-derived antimalarial agents: New leads and challenges. *Phytochem. Rev., 4*(1), 55–61.

Wright, C. W., Addae-Kyereme, J., Breen, A. G., Brown, J. E., Cox, M. F., Croft, S. L., Gökçek, Y., et al., (2001). Synthesis and evaluation of cryptolepine analogues for their potential as new antimalarial agents. *J. Med. Chem., 44*(19), 3187–3194.

Xu, Q., Li, Z. X., Peng, H. Q., Sun, Z. W., Cheng, R. L., et al., (2011). Artesunate inhibits growth and induces apoptosis in human osteosarcoma HOS cell line *in vitro* and *in vivo. J. Zhejiang Univ. Sci. B., 12*, 247–255.

Zhang, C. Z., Pan, Y., Cao, Y., Lai, P. B., Liu, L., et al., (2012). Histone deacetylase inhibitors facilitate dihydroartemisinin-induced apoptosis in liver cancer *in vitro* and *in vivo. PLoS One, 7*, e39870.

Zhang, C. Z., Zhang, H., Yun, J., Chen, G. G., & Lai, P. B., (2012). Dihydroartemisinin exhibits antitumor activity toward hepatocellular carcinoma *in vitro* and *in vivo. Biochem Pharmacol., 83*, 1278–1289.

Zhao, Y., Hanton, W. K., & Lee, K. H., (1986). Antimalarial agents, 2. Artesunate, an inhibitor of cytochrome oxidase activity in plasmodium Berghei. *J. Nat. Prod., 49*(1), 139–142.

Zhao, Y., Jiang, W., Li, B., Yao, Q., Dong, J., et al., (2011). Artesunate enhances radiosensitivity of human non-small cell lung cancer A549 cells via increasing NO production to induce cell cycle arrest at G2/M phase. *Int. Immunopharmacol., 11*, 2039–2046.

Zhou, C., Pan, W., Wang, X. P., & Chen, T. S., (2012). Artesunate induces apoptosis via a Bak-mediated caspase-independent intrinsic pathway in human lung adenocarcinoma cells. *J. Cell Physiol., 227*, 3778–3786.

Zhou, H. J., Wang, W. Q., Wu, G. D., Lee, J., & Li, A., (2007). Artesunate inhibits angiogenesis and down regulates vascular endothelial growth factor expression in chronic myeloid leukemia K562 cells. *Vascul. Pharmacol., 47*, 131–138.

CHAPTER 13

Epigenetic Control of the Immune System and its Applications in Metastatic Diseases

SANDEEP ARORA, SUKHBIR SINGH, NEELAM SHARMA,
TAPAN BEHL, and NIDHI GARG

Chitkara College of Pharmacy, Chitkara University, Punjab, India

ABSTRACT

Immunity is termed as an organism's capability to fight against numerous foreign agents that can harm the human system. Epigenetics can be defined as the changes in the gene activity without any alteration in the DNA sequence. Epigenetics exerts its own effects, including uniqueness (as the epigenetic of each individual is different in terms of distinctive features; making each single individual unique), regulates turning off and on genes. Epigenetics is responsible for controlling genes as well as it also regulates chemical alterations in genes, thereby exerting their job in regulating immunity and thus helps in fighting with diseases like cancer and Alzheimer's disease. It also helps in the differentiation of helper T cells, helps in the activation of Ifng and Il4 genes, which are responsible for transcription of cytokine gene along with induction of lineage deciding activators T-bet and GATA-3, which are essential for their role in immunity.

13.1 INTRODUCTION

Immunity can be defined as the ability of an organism to act against various foreign agents (bacteria, viruses, pathogens, tiny droplets, pollens, etc.) and stopping them from entering or harm the human system. The special cells, proteins, tissues, and organs concerned in defense mechanisms comprise the system. Cells are the basic operating units of each individual. The chemical

DNA (DNA) contains all the essential data for the correct operating of the cell. An individual's DNA consists of 3 billion bases of nucleotides. The DNA contains adenine (A), cytosine (C), guanine (G), and thymine (T). The sequence within which bases are organized regulates our life directions. A fraction of distinction within the sequence of DNA makes every person differ from each other.

The term EPIGENETICS signify the changes in gene activity while not bringing any alterations to the DNA sequence. An alternative method, it may be aforementioned that phenotypical changes come, whereas no impact is seen on the genotype. The surroundings, lifestyle, increasing age, the sickness someone is tormented by, etc., conjointly bring epigenetic changes. The 'turning off' or 'turning on' mechanism of a varied set of genes or epigenetic silencing renders individuality to the cells, tissues, and organs of the human system that's why although all the cells have the same DNA however some are liver cells, others are pancreatic cells or heart cells, etc. The classic example to depict gene silencing is genetic twins though they're born through the same maternity however varies phenotypically. There are three kinds of the mechanism during a cell concerned with silencing genes and produce phenotypical changes (Egger et al., 2004; Simmons, 2008).

13.1.1 DNA METHYLATION

The chemical action that facilitates the addition of the methyl group to DNA continuously occurs in CpG sites. CpG sites are high in C nucleotide present adjacent to guanine via phosphate linkage (Egger et al., 2004; Jones and Baylin, 2002; Robertson, 2002). This addition of methyl teams at the CpG station brings changes to the looks and functioning of DNA. In some sequences, a development referred to as 'imprinting' happens to differentiate the gene copy rooted from and from mother, respectively (Simmons, 2008).

13.1.2 HISTONE MODIFICATION

Histones are the proteins present in a very condensed kind to make chromatin granule. The DNA strands wind around the histone polymer. DNA transcription can solely turn up once chromatin granule is not in compact or condensed kind. Acetylation and methylation bring changes to the histone compound. There happens either addition of acetyl radical to lysine present on histone. In active chromatin, granule acetylation appears, whereas, in heterochromatin, deacetylation occurs. But methylation is related to each dynamic and dormant areas/locales of chromatin granule. e.g., lysine (K9) on histone (H3) once undergoes methylation leads to DNA silencing throughout heterochromatin. This leads to an inactivating X chromosome of females, therefore depicting an epigenetic modification. On the contrary, lysine (K4) on the same histone (H3) once undergoes methylation leads to gene activation (active gene) (Egger et al., 2004; Simmons, 2008).

13.1.3   RNA ASSOCIATED SILENCING

At the point when RNA is inside the antisense transcripts, RNA interference (RNAi), it closes down the genes. Either ribonucleic acid (RNA) causes the formation of heterochromatin or leads to triggering modification of histones and methylation of DNA, which can result in gene expression (Egger et al., 2004; Simmons, 2008) (Figure 13.1).

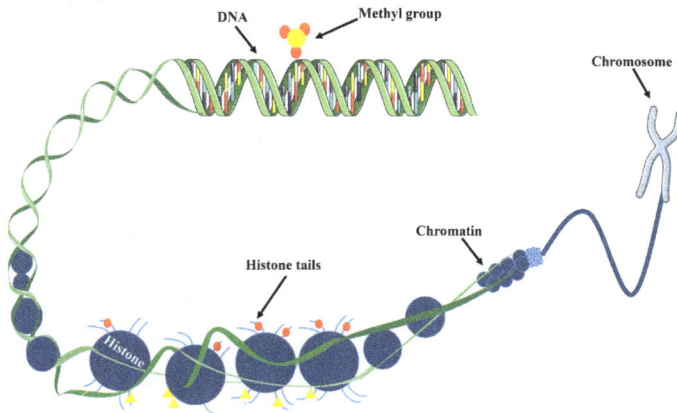

FIGURE 13.1   Depiction of chromatin composition which becomes available to the epigenetic marks comprising of histones and DNA

13.2   HISTORY

The term 'epigenesis' was coined way earlier, and then the word 'epigenetic' evolved. Around 1650, the medical practitioner and physiologist William Harvey gave the term 'epigenesis' to unravel the mechanism by which an inseminated zygote develops into a complex organism. Conrad Waddington in 1942 brought the term 'epigenetics' draws its roots from the earlier nomenclature 'epigenesis.' He speculated a couple of biological systems during which "concatenations of

processes are joined along in a network so that a disturbance at an early stage
could step by step cause additional and additional comprehensive abnormali-
ties in many various organs and tissues" (Waddington, 1942, p. 10). In 1958,
microbiologist Nanney planned two cellular management systems, "library of
specificities" that control template replicating mechanisms and "auxiliatory
mechanisms" that control gene expression. In 1961, Jacob and Monod gave the
operon model of gene regulation (Figure 13.2).

13.3   EPIGENETICS AND CANCER

In 1983, cancer was connected to epigenetics by creating it as the primary
malady to be related to epigenetics. It had been found that once the pathologic tissue from the patients laid low with the large intestine, cancer was
extracted, and it demonstrated fewer DNA methylation compared to non-
sick or ordinary tissue of the patient (Feinberg and Vogelstein, 1983). The
genes that are methylated are ordinarily turned off; therefore, there happens
abnormally high gene activation because of the debit of DNA methylation
and alteration in the arrangement of chromatin granule. In distinction, a great
amount of methylation can reverse the operating of tumor suppressor genes.

CpG sites are the foremost favorable spots for DNA methylation;
however, there are spots in DNA close to the promoter region that is freed
from methylation despite the abundance of CpG sites present there. In
cancer, cells CpG sites get extensively methylated, resulting in the silencing
of genes. This is often a hot example of epigenetics that happens in the earlier
development of tumors or cancer (Oscar Palmer Robertson, 2002).

13.4   EPIGENETICS CORRELATION WITH MENTAL RETARDATION

Fragile X is a condition bringing about extreme cerebral impairment, differed
verbal advancement, and "autistic-like" conduct. It notably has an effect on
males as a result of only 1 X chromosome, so one fragile X can show a larger
and severe impact. The condition is termed fragile X syndrome because the
part of the chromosome that has gene abnormality seems to like hanging
by a thread and might be simply broken. The FMR1 gene gets affected
during this syndrome. The population without this condition has six to fifty
repeats of CGG trinucleotide in the FMR1 gene; however, once the repeats
transcend 200, showing full mutation, the symptoms of the syndrome arise.

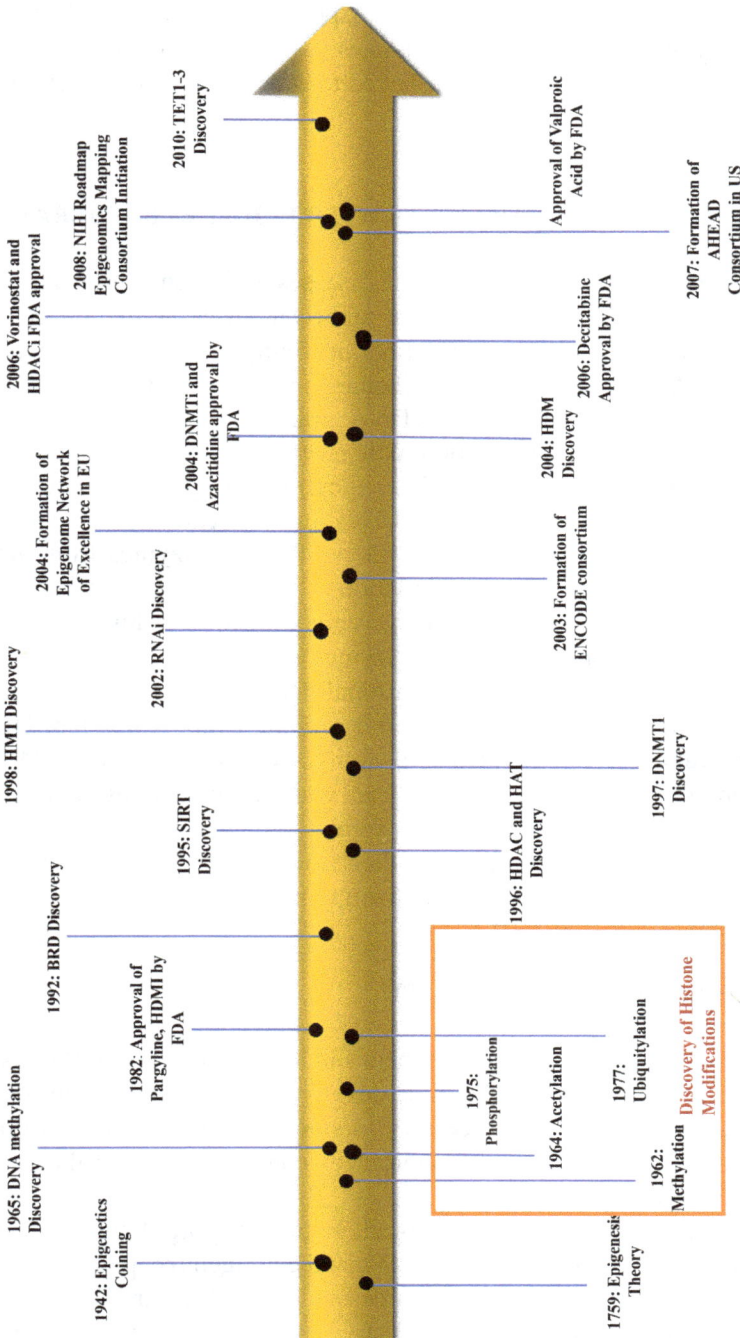

FIGURE 13.2 Timeline of Milestones in the History of Epigenetics

These extensive CGG repeats end up in CpG at the site of the FMR1 gene to get methylated. This methylation makes the gene off and stops FMR1 to manufacture an important protein referred to as fragile X mental retardation protein.

13.5   ENCOUNTERING AILMENTS WITH EPIGENETIC THERAPY

Epigenetic has its say in a plethora of diseases and even in our existence. This epigenetics may be used to fight numerous diseases like cancer. The epigenetic treatment aims at targeting or fixing DNA methylation and histone acetylation. The epigenetic changes may be targeted as a result of these changes is reversible, whereas DNA mutations cannot.

Inhibition of DNA methylation will reactivate suppressed genes. For instance, 5-azacytidine and 5-aza-2'-deoxycytidine (Egger et al., 2004), they act like C nucleotides and fuse themselves into replicating DNA. Once the drug gets incorporated into DNA, it blocks DNMT enzymes from acting, resulting in inhibition of DNA methylation.

Drugs intended for histone alterations are alluded to as histone deacetylase (HDAC) antagonist. They are enzymes responsible for the expulsion of the acetyl group from the lysine terminal that gathers chromatin granule. HDAC inhibitors block this method and activate gene expression. HDAC inhibitors are phenyl butyric acid and valproic acid (Egger et al., 2004).

Epigenetic medical aid ought to be used with caution as a result of epigenetic processes, and changes are widely spread. If epigenetic treatments don't seem to be specific to irregular cells, then it would result in the stimulation of gene expression in cells rendering them mutated.

13.6   EPIGENETICS IN IMMUNITY

The development of lymphocytes happens in bone marrow once B cells and T cells are concerned. When WBC is developing, they set up their antigen receptor genes. This can be necessary to shield the body against a microorganism that contains antigenic substances complementary to the antigen receptor (Steven et al., 2005).

The sequence of development in T-cell includes the pro-T cells once enter the thymus; they do not express CD8. When the antigen receptors present on one chain happens, large proliferation ensues and ends up in the expression of each CD4 and CD8 cells. At this time, the antigen receptors present on the opposite chain reorganize themselves. Further, CD4 and CD8 cells called the two lineage markers to endure down-regulation during a non-mitotic conversion. The genetic silencing of the CD4 gene leads to the maturation of CD8+ cells from CD4+CD8+ cells. The CD4+ and CD8+ thymocytes move towards the peripheral lymphoid organs, and proliferation and differentiation of naïve CD4+ T cells happen in response to pathogens. When the developing B and T lymphocytes exist in bone marrow and thymus, respectively, they get mature and prepared for action. Until the time the cell does have any encounter with the antigen, it is a naïve cell anyway; once it comes in contact with the antigen, it experiences partition. Its daughters will be comparably attributable to explicit acquired recombination anyway can differ with respect to gene controllers of the immune response. This kind of process is eluded as proliferation or differentiation (Steven et al., 2005).

The involvement of epigenetic in helper T cell differentiation: In progenitor naïve cells, Ifng and Il4 genes are present in a restrictive fashion. Once they are activated by the antigens, an occasional level transcription of the cytokine gene and gene induction of lineage deciding activators T-bet and GATA-3 occur. TH1 cells end up in silencing of the GATA-3 gene, whereas TH2 cells silence the T-bet gene (Zheng et al., 1997). The forfeiture of CpG methylation within the Ifng and Il4 gene ends up in the development of TH1 and TH2 cells. This ends up in heritable remodeling of cytokine that does not need T-BET and GATA-3 (Steven et al., 2005).

A few details concerning epigenetics are summarized below:

- *Epigenetics controls genes:* Nature—epigenetics is a branch that defines a cell's specialization, i.e., deciding the skin cells, blood cells, hair cells, etc., actively or dormantly as the fetus turns into a baby. Along with this, the environment plays a major role in turning on and off the genes.
- *Epigenetics is everywhere:* All the activities including maturing of an individual can be the purpose behind chemical alterations in the genes which will additionally kill those genes on or after some time. Furthermore, in different sicknesses, a few genes will assume the contrary job than their typical job like in Cancer and Alzheimer's disease.
- *Epigenetics makes us unique:* The uniqueness of each person is a gift from epigenetics, like different tastes, distinctive features, even the act of being social. The diverse combo of genes that are turned on or off is the thing that makes every one of us interesting.

13.7   EFFECT OF LIFESTYLE ON EPIGENETICS AND HEALTH OF AN INDIVIDUAL

- Our epigenetics can be modified by our decisions about our lifestyle and by the influence of the environment, even though our epigenetics are stable throughout our life especially during our adulthood. It is mostly observed that these effects, i.e., the epigenetic effects occur during the complete lifespan of the individual rather than the time that the individual has spent in the womb. Numerous samples related to epigenetics show that how this modification can alter the streak on prime of DNA and do its job in pivotal health outcomes.
- The environment is an incredible impact on epigenetic labels and malady susceptibility. According to research, air pollution could change methyl tags on DNA and result in brain-related disorders. Strangely, Vitamin B has the capacity to battle these harmful epigenetic impacts of air pollution.
- It has additionally been discovered that a diet that has elevated measures of lipids and satisfactory proteins promotes an epigenetic compound created by the organism.

KEYWORDS

- adenine
- cytosine
- epigenetics
- guanine
- histone deacetylase
- thymine

REFERENCES

Avni, O., Lee, D., Macian, F., Szabo, S. J., Glimcher, L. H., & Rao, A., (2002). T(H) cell differentiation is accompanied by dynamic changes in histone acetylation of cytokine genes. *Nat. Immunol., 3*, 643–651.

Egger, G., et al., (2004). Epigenetics in human disease and prospects for epigenetic therapy. *Nature, 429*, 457–463. doi: 10.1038/nature02625.

Feinberg, A. P., & Vogelstein, B., (1983). Hypomethylation distinguishes genes of some human cancers from their normal counterparts. *Nature, 301*, 89–92. doi: 10.1038/301089a0.

Fields, P. E., Kim, S. T., & Flavell, R. A., (2002). Cutting edge: Changes in histone acetylation at the IL-4 and IFN-gamma loci accompany Th1/Th2 differentiation. *J. Immunol., 169*, 647–650.

Grogan, J. L., Mohrs, M., Harmon, B., Lacy, D. A., Sedat, J. W., & Locksley, R. M., (2001). Early transcription and silencing of cytokine genes underlie polarization of T helper cell subsets. *Immunity, 14*, 205–215.

Grogan, J. L., Wang, Z. E., Stanley, S., Harmon, B., Loots, G. G., Rubin, E. M., & Locksley, R. M., (2003). Basal chromatin modification at the *IL-4* gene in helper T cells. *J. Immunol., 171*, 6672–6679.

Jacob, F., & Monod, J., (1961). Genetic regulatory mechanisms in the synthesis of proteins. *J. Mol. Biol., 3*, 318–356.

Jones, P. A., & Baylin, S. B., (2002). The fundamental role of epigenetic events in cancer. *Nature Reviews Genetics, 3*, 415–428. doi: 10.1038/nrg816.

Kaati, G., et al., (2002). Cardiovascular and diabetes mortality determined by nutrition during parents' and grandparents' slow growth period. *European Journal of Human Genetics, 10*, 682–688.

Lee, D. U., & Rao, A., (2004). Molecular analysis of a locus control region in the T helper 2 cytokine gene cluster: A target for STAT6 but not GATA3. *Proc. Natl. Acad. Sci. USA, 101*, 16010–16015 (Epubl. 2004 Oct. 16026).

Nanney, D. L., (1958). Epigenetic control systems. *PNAS, 44*, 712–717.

Penagarikano, O., et al., (2007). The pathophysiology of fragile X syndrome. *Annual Review of Genomics and Human Genetics, 8*, 109–129. doi: 10.1146/annurev.genom.8.080706.092249.

Robertson, K. D., (2002). DNA methylation and chromatin: Unraveling the tangled web. *Oncogene, 21*, 5361–5379. doi: 10.1038/sj.onc.1205609.

Shnyreva, M., Weaver, W. M., Blanchette, M., Taylor, S. L., Tompa, M., Fitzpatrick, D. R., & Wilson, C. B., (2004). Evolutionarily conserved sequence elements that positively regulate IFN-gamma expression in T cells. *Proc. Natl Acad. Sci. USA, 101*, 12622–12627 (Epubl. 2004 Aug. 12610).

Simmons, D., (2008). Epigenetic influence and disease. *Nature Education, 1*(1), 6.

Steven, L. R., (2005). Epigenetic control in immune response. *Human Molecular Genetics, 14*(1), R41–R46.

Waddington, C. H., (1942). *The Epigenotype* (Vol. 1, pp. 18–20). Endeavor.

Waddington, C. H., (1957). *The Strategy of the Genes: A Discussion of Some Aspects of Theoretical Biology*. Ruskin House/George Allen and Unwin Ltd., London.

Zheng, W., & Flavell, R. A., (1997). The transcription factor GATA-3 is necessary and sufficient for Th2 cytokine gene expression in CD4 T cells. *Cell, 89*, 587–596.

CHAPTER 14

Immune Checkpoint Inhibitors

SANDEEP ARORA, SAURABH GUPTA, and NIDHI GARG

Chitkara College of Pharmacy, Chitkara University, Punjab, India

ABSTRACT

Immune checkpoint blockade has emerged as one of the most promising therapeutic options for patients in the history of cancer treatment. In the context of cancer, where negative T-cell regulatory pathways are often over-active, immune checkpoint blockade has proven to be an effective strategy for enhancing the effector activity and clinical impact of antitumor T-cells. In recent years, checkpoint inhibitors targeting CTLA-4, PD-1, and PD-L1 have yielded unprecedented and durable responses in a significant percentage of cancer patients, leading to U.S. FDA approval of six checkpoint inhibitors for numerous cancer indications. In this review, we highlight the role and clinical success of immune checkpoint inhibitors and discuss current challenges and future strategies that must be considered going forward to maximize the efficacy of immune checkpoint blockade therapy for cancer.

14.1 INTRODUCTION

Our immune system embraces a distinctive ability to distinguish normal body cells from foreign cells and substances; attacking and engulfing the latter to provide immunity. Certain molecules called 'checkpoints' are present on immune cells which on activation or inactivation initiate an immune response and produce immunoprotective effects. The checkpoints shield cancer cells from the attack of immune cells (Pardoll, 2012). A new promising therapy for treating cancer includes the discovery of new drug compounds that effectively target these checkpoints and cause the destruction of cancer cells.

The cells of our immune system mainly T-lymphocytes on activation of certain proteins prevent engulfing of cancer cells. This mechanism is blocked by the action of an immune checkpoint inhibitor which keeps a check on the immune system and cancer cells. The blocking of these expressed proteins releases 'brakes' on immune cells which aid in better killing of cancer cells. The following proteins namely CTLA-4/B7-1/B7-2 and PD-1/PD-L1 are present as checkpoints on cancer or immune cells. Various inhibitors of immune checkpoint proteins are used as a therapy in the treatment of cancer by blocking proteins which prevent cancer cells from attack of immune cells thereby enhancing their destruction (Marin-Acevedo et al., 2018). Drugs used in cancer act through various mechanisms and fail to fit into a specific treatment type as they are categorized into a number of different groups. Checkpoint inhibitors generally aim for treatments specific to target proteins and can also act as a monoclonal antibody (Mab) (Wei et al., 2012).

14.2   HOW DO CHECKPOINT INHIBITORS FUNCTION?

The immune system of our body protects us from exposure to various diseases by destroying foreign antigens including bacteria and viruses. T-cells are the principal immune cells that preserve immunity. There are specific proteins expressed on them which initiate an immune response with the release of other proteins called checkpoints for slowing immune reactions. Highly reactive T-cells if not checked for their activity start targeting healthy cells and tissues. Therefore, checkpoints assist inactivation of T-cells (Sharma and Allison, 2015).

Cancer cells synthesize high levels of proteins which suppress the activity of T-cells, and prevents them from being attacked hence dodge the immune system. This prevents destruction of cancer cells as T-cells fail to recognize and kill cancer cells (Figure 14.1a).

Checkpoint inhibitors are the drugs that block checkpoint proteins (Figure 14.1b). They stimulate the immune system and prevent its suppression due to expression of proteins on the cancer cells and T-cells causing engulfing of cancer cells (Dunn et al., 2004).

14.3   HISTORY OF INHIBITORS OF IMMUNE CHECKPOINT

Our immune system performs a crucial role in control and progression of neoplasm. Immunotherapy was invented to help patients with cancer in which

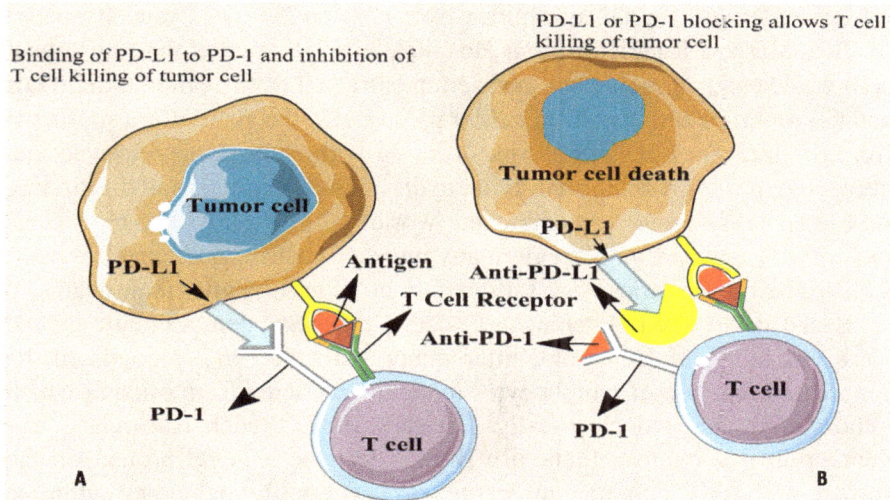

FIGURE 14.1 (A) PD-1 protein present on the T- lymphocytes and PD-L1 protein present on the cancer cells help to maintain the immune system of the body. The attachment of the PD-1 protein to the PD-L1 protein protects the tumor cells from the attack by the T-cells. (B) The tumor cells can be killed by the T-cells with the inhibition of the immune checkpoints (anti- PD-L1 or anti- PD-1) by hindering the binding between the immune checkpoints.

tumors could not be removed surgically. William B Coley from New York technically laid the roots of immunotherapy in 1891. Streptococcus bacteria and beef broth were mixed and injected to an Italian cancer patient in his arm who suffered from an inoperable neck tumor. At first, the 40-year-old man got extremely sick and developed fever with vomiting and chills but one month later, it was observed that his tumor had shrunk considerably. William Coley replicated this process on thousands of other cancer patients but the FDA stopped him. These were the first roots of immunotherapy (Park et al., 2018).

Coley's principles in 1890 were stated to be precise after the use of bacteria was justified in 1976 for evaluating the efficiency in the treatment of superficial cancer of bladder persuaded by the bacterium Bacillus Calmette-Guérin (BCG). A research by Old in 1959 served as the foundation for this clinical trial which showed BCG to possess an antitumor effect by using mouse as animal model. Old also carried out extensive research on other CI-related topics besides his work on BCG, and after many attempts successfully discovered tumor necrosis factor (TNF) in the year 1975. Coley and Old are referred as the "Father of Immunotherapy" owing to the exceptional discoveries they made and also lifelong dedication they had in this field, and perhaps are the pair with best-shared titles (Coley, 1991).

Ernest Freund and Gisa Kaminer, two Austrian Jewish physicians, based in Vienna at the Rudolf-Stiftung Hospital, in 1910 spotted that the cancer cells could easily dissolve in blood serum extracted from healthy individuals and not in serum obtained from cancer patients. By the year 1924 a substance from the intestines of the patients suffering with cancer was retrieved that decreased the ability of normal serum to dissolve cancer cells and this finding was later broadcasted throughout the world. In 1938, both the physicians took off to London after Nazi Germany invaded Austria (Zhou and Levitsky, 2012). Their discoveries were forgotten in no time soon after their deaths.

Based in the Fred Hutchinson Cancer Center-Sweden, a couple named Karl and Ingegerd Hellstrom, after many years in 1966, recognized the suppressed reaction of lymphocytes in serum extracted from mice in which tumors were induced chemically. Later in 1987, French researchers and their group led by Jean-Francoise Brunet detected a novel protein on the surface of T-cells. This new molecule was successfully named as cytotoxic T-lymphocyte-associated antigen 4 (CTLA-4) and its role remained unidentified for many years (Drake et al., 2014). Two teams working independently from each other in 1995 solved the mysterious role of CTLA-4. One team from the University of California in Berkeley led by James Allison while the other team from the University of California, San Francisco, guided by Jeffrey Bluestone, demonstrated that the activity of T-cells could be inhibited by CTLA-4 (Zou and Chen, 2008). The first person to comprehend the role of this mechanism in the treatment of cancer was Allison, and he later developed a monoclonal antibody (Mab) for blocking CTLA-4.

Allison's patent was finally licensed by the year 1999 to a small company of biotechnology in Princeton named Medarex which was founded in 1987. Alan Korman and Nils Lonberg were the two key scientists in the company who grasped the potential of Allison's work and initiated this patent. The first clinical trial of Medarex with human Mab that binds to CTLA-4 was launched in 2000 (Schwartz, 1992). This paved the way for treatment of metastatic melanoma by approving ipilimumab in 2011 by FDA. Ipilimumab hence became the first checkpoint inhibitor to make its way to the market.

Another checkpoint inhibitor developed by Medarex named nivolumab was approved by FDA three years later. Nivolumab was founded after the discovery of CTLA-4 related other proteins which are present on T-cells and inhibit their activity. In 1992, Tasuko Honjo with his colleagues at Kyoto University first spotted this protein and named it as PD-1 (Rudd et al., 2009). The function of the protein PD-1 continued to be mysterious till it was witnessed to suppress immune responses after elimination of disease in late 1990s. The capability of cancer cells to duck attack by immune cells by hijacking protein PD-1 was further demonstrated by Gordon Freeman at the Dana-Farber Institute along with his colleagues (Parry et al., 2005). It is estimated that more than 1000 immune checkpoints will be running underway for clinical trials by 2015. The trials do not refrain at exploring new pathways for immune checkpoints but also run to discover various immune checkpoint inhibitor combinations besides chemotherapy, radiations, and targeted therapies (Table 14.1) (Qureshi et al., 2011).

TABLE 14.1   Major events in the development of immune checkpoint inhibitors

Year of event	Event	Scientist
1910	Witnessed the destruction of cancer cells in blood serum obtained from cancer victimized individuals	Freund and Kaminer, 1910
1924	A substance from the intestine of cancer patients was retrieved that possessed the ability to decrease dissolution of cancer cells obtained from normal serum	Freund and Kaminer, 1924
1969	Observed blocked reaction of lymphocytes due to presence of chemically induced tumours in the serum of mice	Nelson et.al., 1980
1971	They suggested that immune system fail to detect cancer cells as the latter are masked by binding of antibodies	Sjögren et al., 1971
1992	Discovery of PD-1 (programmed cell death protein 1)	Tasuku Honjo
1995	Inhibition of T cells activity by CTLA-4 was demonstrated by two independent teams	Jeffrey Bluestone and James Alison
2005	A humanized antibody to PD-1 protein was developed for treating cancer by	Ono and Medarex Pharmaceuticals and entered research alliance
2006	The anti-CTLA-4 treatment was observed to be enhanced by inducible co-stimulator (ICOS) protein for inducing cancer cell destruction	Paulson, Tom. Seattle PI, Feb. 23, 2006
2008	The first ever antibody against PD-1 protein for treatment of cancer entered phase 1 clinical trial	
2011	Ipilimumab, Yervoy®, the first drug that inhibited the immune checkpoint by targeting CTLA4 was approved by FDA	
2014	An immune checkpoint inhibitor for treatment of melanoma called nivolumab (Opdivo®) that acted by targeting PD-1 protein was approved by FDA. US FDA approved the first ever immune checkpoint inhibitor drug that targeted PD-1 protein	

TABLE 14.1   *(Continued)*

Year of event	Event	Scientist
2015	An enhanced sensitivity to anti–CTLA-4 therapy was demonstrated through experiments in tumour cells of azacytidine treated mice	
	Experiments on mice demonstrated the response of CTLA-4 checkpoint inhibitor mediated immunotherapy on tumours and it was observed to improve due to modified gut microbiome	
2017	Diseased individuals with superior range of bacteria in the gut are reported by researchers to acquire better response to immunotherapy for cancer	
	An accelerated approval by FDA granted to avelumab, a PD-L1 checkpoint inhibitor for treatment of an unusual type of cancer of the skin named Merkel cell carcinoma in patients 12 years and older in age	
	NHS patients with advanced lung cancer were exposed to treatment with Nivolumab (Opdivo®)	
	A quicker relapse and shorter survival time was observed in cancer patients who routinely administered antibiotics before and after treatment by inhibition of PD-1 checkpoint	
	Experiments on mice depicted diminished tumour growth on administration of faecal transplants obtained from patients who responded positively to cancer immunotherapy	
2018	Nobel Prize in Physiology or Medicine was awarded to for their discovery of immune checkpoint inhibitors in treatment of cancer	James Allison and Tasuku Honjo

14.4   IMPORTANCE OF IMMUNE CELL INHIBITORS

- Drugs inhibiting immune checkpoints have come out to be a major breakthrough in treatment of cancer.
- The long-lasting action of checkpoint inhibitor drugs and the durability in responses achieved is the most impressive thing about them. Patients who are originally given a survival period of a week survive for years following treatment therapy (Wing et al., 2008).
- Individuals suffering with lung cancer and melanoma have been proven to be most helpful from immune checkpoint drug inhibitors.
- The diseases that were believed to be fatal at some point of time have successfully been transformed into a chronic condition with the aid of these drugs.
- The drugs are highly recommended for the treatment of urothelial cancer, head, and neck cancer, carcinoma of renal cells, ovarian cancer, non-small cell lung cancer (NSCLC), and various lymphomas and types of melanomas (Topalian et al., 2015).

14.5   MAIN IMMUNE CHECKPOINTS

14.5.1   PD-1 AND PDL-1

Inhibition of immune checkpoints is rising as a front-line treatment for various cancer types. A new novel approach emerged for treatment of cancers includes inhibition of PD-1 protein and PD-L1 protein molecules imparted on the exterior of immune cells (Tumeh et al., 2014). The inhibitors of proteins PD-1 and PD-L1 produce their effects by refraining the binding of receptor programmed cell death protein 1 (PD-1) to its ligand programmed death-ligand 1 (PD-L1) protein. To prevent autoimmune diseases and limit the killing of bystander host cells, this surface protein interacts and suppresses our immune system on exposure to infections (Sunshine and Taube, 2015). The checkpoints on immune cells are highly functional during pregnancy besides conditions of tissue allograft and in certain types of cancer.

The inhibitors of checkpoints that block PD-1 proteins are nivolumab (Opdivo) and pembrolizumab (Keytruda). The therapeutic uses of Nivolumab and pembrolizumab include management of:

- Melanoma skin cancer;
- Hodgkin lymphoma;
- Non-small cell lung cancer; and
- Cancer of the urinary tract (urothelial cancer).

14.5.1.1   MOLECULAR MECHANISM OF ACTION OF PD-1

Maintenance of tolerance in the periphery and responses to T-cells in a precise physiological range are the primary biological functions of PD-1. The regulatory system of PD-1/PD-L1 is persuaded by immune responses forming a negative feedback loop that will attenuate native responses of T-cells in order to minimize tissue damage. PD-1 expresses itself on T-cell activation by interacting with PD-L1 and PD-L2 which further stimulate the regulation of T-cells. The ligands localized in non-lymphoid tissues on expression through PD-1 cells attenuate activation of T-cells in the periphery. Inflammatory cytokines like IFNγ induce manifestation of PD-L1 and PD-L2 protein, the latter being expressed to a lesser extent (Iwai et al., 2002). The PD-L1 stimulated regulation of T-cell activity arises as a retort to T-cell effector and cytolytic function [e.g., CD8 cytotoxic T-lymphocyte and helper 1 (Th1) CD4 T-cells] in a tempting manner. PD-1 transmits a negative costimulatory signal on direct contact with PD-L2 and PD-L1 through tyrosine phosphatase SHP2 mechanism, thereby attenuating activation of T-cells. The TCR signaling is directly depreciated on SHP2 recruitment after proximal signaling elements are dephosphorylated. A dichotomy is reflected by regulatory modes employed by PD-1 protein and CTLA4 association through this mechanism. PD-1 in contrast to regulation mediated by CTLA4 manages signaling of TCR as indicated by data reports to attenuate activity of T-cells (Mahoney et al., 2015). Recent evidences, however, claim CD28 to be the principal target responsible for attenuating signaling of T-cells via induction of PD-1 proteins. A reconstitution model comprising a cell-free membrane was utilized in the studies conducted for scrutinization of functional relationships for the period of activation of T-cells and it was revealed that it's not TCR but PD-1 that is responsible for preferential dephosphorylation of CD28 on recruitment of SHP2. Therefore, similar molecular mechanism is involved in attenuation of CD28-mediated costimulation (signal 2) via CTLA-4 and PD-1 proteins. Thus, CTLA-4 and PD-1 mediated regulation can represent a point of functional convergence on modulating signaling of C28. SHP2 through recent findings has been indicated to be non-essential for responses inducing exhaustion of T-cells or anti-PD-1 protein therapy *in vivo*. A functional redundancy is hence highlighted in signaling pathways of PD-1 protein (Alsaab et al., 2017). It moreover becomes vital to demarcate the instantaneous signaling events that are downstream of PD-1 and CTLA4 to differentiate shared and marked molecular mechanisms involved in regulatory pathways of T-cells (Figure 14.2) (Chauvin et al., 2015; Walunas et al., 1994; Parry et al., 2005).

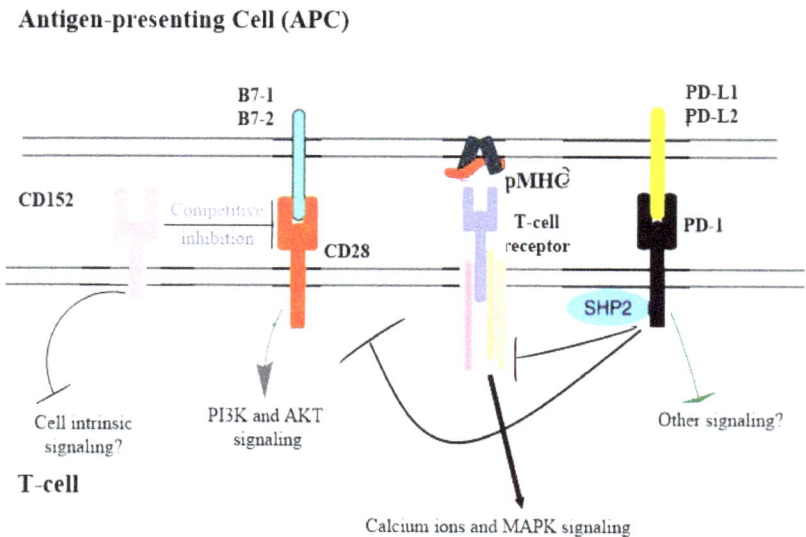

FIGURE 14.2   Decreased activation of T-cell via the molecular mechanisms (PD-1 and CTLA-4).

14.5.2 CTLA4

Another protein receptor named cytotoxic T-lymphocyte-associated protein 4 or CTLA-4, also called CD152 or cluster of differentiation 152, operates as an immune checkpoint inhibitor to diminish immune reactions. This protein is highly expressed in regulatory T-cells and upregulate on activation only in conventional T-cells—a phenomenon comprising of utmost importance in cancers (Chemnitz et al., 2004). On binding to the surface of antigen-presenting cells, CD80 or CD86 acts as an "off" switch (Grohmann et al., 2002).

14.5.2.1 MOLECULAR MECHANISM OF ACTION OF CTLA4

The expression and function of CTLA-4 are fundamentally correlated with activation of T-cells. On interaction with T-cell receptors (TCR), CTLA-4 is immediately upregulated (signal 1) and expresses on 2 to 3 days of activation. CTLA-4 is more attracted towards the ligands for B7 including B7-1 (CD80) and B7-2 (CD86) and competes with CD28, a costimulatory molecule for the ligand sites thus reducing TCR signaling (Krummel and Allison, 1996). CD28 through B7 ligands imparts positive costimulatory signals and weaken T-cell activation by competitively inhibiting both molecules of CTLA-4. A rapid binding kinetics is displayed by CD28 and CTLA-4 with B7-1 with differences in binding strengths that allow competitive inhibition by CTLA-4 swiftly (Grohmann et al., 2002). On activation of T-cells, the expression of CTLA-4 is highly upregulated causing trafficking of CTLA-4 stored in intracellular vesicles to the immunologic synapse. The amount of CTLA-4 that is recruited to immunologic synapse is in direct correlation with TCR signal strength. CTLA-4 is stabilized by binding with B7 ligand on reaching the immunologic synapse which causes its accumulation and allows it to compete with CD28 effectively (Buchbinder and Desai, 2016). This mechanism debilitates the CD28 associated positive costimulation through CTLA-4 and limits PI3K and AKT mediated signaling of CD28. This concludes a vigorous rise in amplitude of receptor signal regulation of T-cells besides their activity. The negative costimulation of CTLA-4 protein is associated with the expression of B7 ligand and positive costimulation by CD28 which is responsible for the regulation of activity of T-cells at their priming sites, e.g., secondary lymphoid organs. The activation of T-cells is also attenuated by CTLA4 in the peripheral tissues besides the above core function as the ligands of B7 are constitutively expressed by antigen-presenting cells to altering degrees but can also be articulated by activation of T-cells (Demaria et al., 2005).

Opdivo (nivolumab), Yervoy (ipilimumab), Keytruda (pembrolizumab), Bavencio (avelumab), and Tecentriq (atezolizumab) are some of the inhibitors of immune checkpoints which are approved for their use in treatment of cancers by the U.S. Food and Drug Administration (FDA).

14.6   CHECKPOINT INHIBITORS

14.6.1   *IPILIMUMAB*

- The trade name of Ipilimumab is Yervoy.
- Ipilimumab is a Mab which by targeting a protein receptor CTLA-4 activates immune system of the body which was initially downregulated (Hodi et al., 2010).
- The cancer cells are successfully recognized and destroyed by Cytotoxic T-lymphocytes (CTLs) but some inhibitory mechanisms interrupt this destruction pathway which can be overcome by treatment with ipilimumab and aid in restoring functions of CTL (Wolchok et al., 2013).
- The U.S. FDA approved ipilimumab in 2011 for treatment of melanoma, a type of skin cancer. It is being explored for treatment of non-small cell lung carcinoma (NSCLC), bladder cancer, small cell lung cancer (SCLC) and metastatic hormone-refractory prostate cancer and is under clinical trials (Figure 14.3) (Weber et al., 2012).

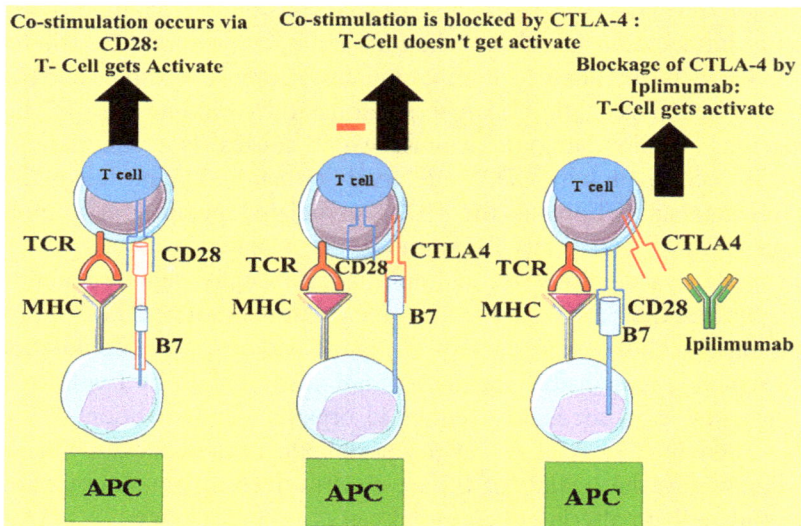

FIGURE 14.3   The depiction of T-cell receptor MHC in antigen presenting cell (APC).

CTLA-4 is an inhibitory receptor and also an alternative ligand for B7 which limits activation of T-cells as they are least expressed on the T-cell surfaces.

- **Step 1:** The costimulation via ligation of B7/CD28 causes activation of T-cells.
- **Step 2:** After 48–72 hours of B7/CD28-induced, activation of T-cells CTLA4 becomes upregulated.

CTLA competes for binding to B7 with CD28 as it has a higher affinity for B7 than the former (Wolchok et al., 2017). The T-cell responses are downregulated on ligation of CTLA4 to activated T-cells producing brakes on their activation.

14.6.2 PEMBROLIZUMAB

- Keytruda is the trade name of pembrolizumab.
- Pembrolizumab is a humanized antibody mainly used in the treatment of cancers (Robert et al., 2015).
- It belongs to an IgG4 isotype antibody that allows the immune system to attack cancer cells by blocking their protective mechanisms.
- The PD-1 receptor of lymphocytes is the most targeted (Garon et al., 2015).
- It was initially approved for its use in the treatment of metastatic melanoma by FDA. It was in 2017 when FDA approved its use in treatment of any metastatic solid tumors with genetic anomalies making it the first cancer drug to be approved that treats tumors rooted with genetics than type of tumor or its site (Bellmunt et al., 2017).

14.6.3 NIVOLUMAB

- Nivolumab, or trade named Opdivo is also a medication used in the treatment of cancer.
- Nivolumab is an IgG4 anti-PD-1 humanized Mab (Robert et al., 2015).
- Drug of choice for treatment of inoperable or metastatic melanoma in adjunction with ipilimumab and is used as a second-line treatment for carcinoma of renal cells.
- Nivolumab blocks signaling molecules that shield cancer cells from being attacked by immune cells and act as a checkpoint inhibitor thereby clearing the cancer cells (Motzer et al., 2015).

14.6.4   ATEZOLIZUMAB

- Atezolizumab is a completely humanized, engineered Mab effective against programmed cell death ligand (PD-L1) protein belonging to IgG1 isotype and is popular under the trade name Tecentriq (Rosenberg et al., 2016).
- Atezolizumab was acknowledged with an accelerated approval in May 2016 by FDA for its effective treatment in locally advanced or metastatic urothelial carcinoma after a disappointing treatment with chemotherapy based on cisplatin, however, the confirmatory trial failed to achieve its principal endpoint of overall survival.
- This drug was approved for its therapeutic use in metastatic non-small cell lung cancer (NSCLS) later in October 2016 by FDA in patients with progressed disease following or while treatment with platinum-containing chemotherapy (Fehrenbacher et al., 2016).

14.7   HOW TO MANAGE IMMUNE-RELATED TOXICITY?

The commonly occurring side effects are enlisted in subsections.

14.7.1   GASTROINTESTINAL DIARRHEA/COLITIS

- For the management of mild symptoms, budesonide is administered daily with a dose of 9 mg.
- For managing moderate symptoms immunotherapy must be delayed with administration of oral dose of 0.5–1 mg/kg/day of methylprednisolone which is equivalent to its IV strength. Gastrointestinal doctors should be consulted with colonoscopy and taper over at least 4 weeks if symptoms improve to Grade 1 or less.
- For the management of severe symptoms, the immunotherapy must be discontinued. Methylprednisolone is administered IV in a dose of 1–2 mg/kg/day. Steroids are tapered for a minimum of 4 weeks if symptoms improve to Grade 1 or less, and if the symptoms do not improve within 48–72 hours, second line immunosuppression should be considered (Villadolid and Amin, 2015).

14.7.2   PNEUMONITIS

- On exposure to mild symptoms, immunotherapy is delayed initially with proper monitoring of symptoms. The chest radiographs should be repeated every 2–4 weeks.

- The immunotherapy should be delayed in case of moderate symptoms with proper monitoring of symptoms. Hospitalization should be considered if symptoms worsen. The chest of the patient should be re-imaged every 1–3 days with consultancy and bronchoscopy. Methylprednisolone IV or oral dose equivalent to 1–2 mg/kg/day should be administered. Steroids are tapered for a minimum of 4 weeks on the improvement of symptoms (Brahmer et al., 2018).
- The severe symptoms are prevented by discontinuing immunotherapy and administration of 2–4 mg/kg/day of methylprednisolone IV. Steroids are tapered for a minimum of 6 weeks if symptoms improve. When no improvement in symptoms is observed, second-line immunosuppression should be considered (Eigentler et al., 2016).

14.7.3   HEPATITIS

- When mild symptoms of hepatitis are observed, the I-O therapy should be continued and repeat LFTs in 1 week.
- To overcome moderate symptoms, the I-O therapy is delayed with LFTs which are repeated after 3–5 days. 0.5–1 mg/kg/day of methylprednisolone is administered. When symptoms improve to milder states, steroids are tapered for a minimum of 4 weeks.
- In cases with severe symptoms of hepatitis, the therapy is discontinued with an increased LFT monitoring frequency for 1–2 days. A dose of 12 mg/kg/day of methylprednisolone is administered IV. A GI specialist should be consulted if no improvement is observed within 48–72 h with consideration of second-line immunosuppression (Kumar et al., 2017).

14.7.4   DERMATOLOGICAL TOXICITIES

- The mild dermatological toxicities can be treated by continuing immunotherapy with the application of low potency topical steroids and antihistaminics. In cases with moderate symptoms 0.5–1 mg/kg/day of methylprednisolone with equivalent oral dose is administered despite optimal topical management. When symptoms begin to resolve steroids are tapered over for at least 4 weeks and dermatological evaluations are carried along with skin biopsy.

- Patients facing severe symptoms are advised to discontinue immunotherapy. A dose of 1–2 mg/kg/day of methylprednisolone is administered IV or to its equivalent oral dose. If symptoms resolve or become milder, steroids are tapered for a minimum of 4 weeks with consideration of skin biopsy (Postow et al., 2018).

14.8   NEW GUIDELINES FOR CHECKPOINT INHIBITORS THAT AIM AT RECOGNIZING AND MANAGING SIDE EFFECTS ASSOCIATED WITH THEM AND HELP DOCTORS

According to the guidelines patients with cancer exposed to:

- Milder grade 1 toxicity, except hematological and neurological complications must continue treatment.
- Moderate grade 2 toxicities must exclude the use of checkpoint inhibitors on a temporary basis until milder symptoms and better laboratory reports are not observed. Till then, corticosteroids can be used as a substitute therapy.
- Severe grade 3 toxic conditions must administer high dose corticosteroids for a minimum of six weeks with exceedingly high caution before resuming the therapy as indicated by the physician in case he decides to execute the same therapy again.
- In extreme grade 4 toxic conditions, the use of checkpoint inhibitors must be stopped immediately (Brahmer et al., 2018; Friedman et al., 2016).

14.9   RECENTLY APPROVED IMMUNE CHECKPOINT INHIBITORS IN DRUG DISCOVERY

- A new immunotherapeutic drug named cemiplimab-rwlc under brand name Libtayo has been approved by U.S. FDA for treatment of patients with a type of skin cancer named cutaneous squamous cell carcinoma.
- Cemiplimab-rwlc is highly useful for patients with metastatic cutaneous squamous cell carcinoma or locally advanced cutaneous squamous cell carcinoma that cannot be treated with curative surgery or curative radiation.

- A new molecular therapeutic target has been approved recently by the U.S. FDA named talazoparib (Talzenna) for treatment of patients diagnosed with breast cancer with positive tests for a cancer-associated BRCA1 or BRCA2 (BRCA1/2) mutation.
- Talazoparib is highly intended for patients diagnosed with metastatic or locally advanced HER2-negative breast cancer and also those inherited with BRCA1/2 mutation. Besides approving talazoparib for this therapeutic application, the FDA also approved a genetic test—the BRAC Analysis CDx test to detect patients who have inherited BRCA1/2 mutation and patients with positive breast cancer (La-Beck et al., 2015; Dine et al., 2017; Franklin et al., 2017; Hazarika et al., 2004).

14.10   CONCLUSION

- Immunotherapy undoubtedly exhibits promising antitumor effects in NSCLC but also accompanies exclusive side effects depending upon the mechanism of action of the immune system.
- An appropriate selection of patients (biomarker) is the key for developing a single agent in combination with other therapies.
- The inhibitors of immune checkpoints have emerged as an advanced therapy for treatment of patients suffering with solid tumors, and show positive results on further clinical testing, thus creating hope for patients affected with the disease.

KEYWORDS

- **bacillus Calmette-Guérin**
- **cytotoxic T-lymphocytes**
- **lymphocyte activation gene 3**
- **monoclonal antibody**
- **non-small cell lung cancer**
- **small cell lung cancer**
- **T-cell receptors**

REFERENCES

Alsaab, H. O., Sau, S., Alzhrani, R., Tatiparti, K., Bhise, K., Kashaw, S. K., & Iyer, A. K., (2017). PD-1 and PD-L1 checkpoint signaling inhibition for cancer immunotherapy: Mechanism, combinations, and clinical outcome. *Frontiers in Pharmacology, 8*, 561.

Bellmunt, J., De Wit, R., Vaughn, D. J., Fradet, Y., Lee, J. L., Fong, et al., (2017). Pembrolizumab as second-line therapy for advanced urothelial carcinoma. *New England Journal of Medicine, 376*(11), 1015–1026.

Brahmer, J. R., Lacchetti, C., Schneider, B. J., Atkins, M. B., Brassil, K. J., Caterino, J. M., et al., (2018). Management of immune-related adverse events in patients treated with immune checkpoint inhibitor therapy: American Society of Clinical Oncology Clinical Practice Guideline. *Journal of Clinical Oncology, 36*(17), 1714–1768.

Buchbinder, E. I., & Desai, A., (2016). CTLA-4 and PD-1 pathways: Similarities, differences, and implications of their inhibition. *American Journal of Clinical Oncology, 39*(1), 98.

Coley, W. B., (1991). The classic: The treatment of malignant tumors by repeated inoculations of erysipelas with a report of ten original cases. *Clinical Orthopaedics and Related Research®, 262*, 3–11.

Demaria, S., Kawashima, N., Yang, A. M., Devitt, M. L., Babb, J. S., Allison, J. P., & Formenti, S. C., (2005). Immune-mediated inhibition of metastases after treatment with local radiation and CTLA-4 blockade in a mouse model of breast cancer. *Clinical Cancer Research, 11*(2), 728–734.

Dine, J., Gordon, R., Shames, Y., Kasler, M. K., & Barton-Burke, M., (2017). Immune checkpoint inhibitors: An innovation in immunotherapy for the treatment and management of patients with cancer. *Asia-Pacific Journal of Oncology Nursing, 4*(2), 127.

Drake, C. G., Lipson, E. J., & Brahmer, J. R., (2014). Breathing new life into immunotherapy: Review of melanoma, lung, and kidney cancer. *Nature Reviews Clinical Oncology, 11*(1), 24.

Dunn, G. P., Old, L. J., & Schreiber, R. D., (2004). The three Es of cancer immuno editing. *Annu. Rev. Immunol., 22*, 329–360.

Eigentler, T. K., Hassel, J. C., Berking, C., Aberle, J., Bachmann, O., Grünwald, V., et al., (2016). Diagnosis, monitoring, and management of immune-related adverse drug reactions of anti-PD-1 antibody therapy. *Cancer Treatment Reviews, 45*, 7–18.

Fehrenbacher, L., Spira, A., Ballinger, M., Kowanetz, M., Vansteenkiste, J., Mazieres, J., et al., (2016). Atezolizumab versus docetaxel for patients with previously treated non-small-cell lung cancer (POPLAR): A multicentre, open-label, phase 2 randomized controlled trial. *The Lancet, 387*(10030), 1837–1846.

Franklin, C., Livingstone, E., Roesch, A., Schilling, B., & Schadendorf, D., (2017). Immunotherapy in melanoma: Recent advances and future directions. *European Journal of Surgical Oncology (EJSO), 43*(3), 604–611.

Friedman, C. F., Proverbs-Singh, T. A., & Postow, M. A., (2016). Treatment of the immune-related adverse effects of immune checkpoint inhibitors: A review. *JAMA Oncology, 2*(10), 1346–1353.

Garon, E. B., Rizvi, N. A., Hui, R., Leighl, N., Balmanoukian, A. S., Eder, J. P., et al., (2015). Pembrolizumab for the treatment of non-small-cell lung cancer. *New England Journal of Medicine, 372*(21), 2018–2028.

Grohmann, U., Orabona, C., Fallarino, F., Vacca, C., Calcinaro, F., Falorni, A., et al., (2002). CTLA-4-Ig regulates tryptophan catabolism *in vivo. Nature Immunology, 3*(11), 1097.

Hazarika, M., White, R. M., Johnson, J. R., & Pazdur, R., (2004). FDA drug approval summaries: Pemetrexed (Alimta®). *The Oncologist, 9*(5), 482–488.

Hodi, F. S., O'day, S. J., McDermott, D. F., Weber, R. W., Sosman, J. A., Haanen, J., et al., (2010). Improved survival with ipilimumab in patients with metastatic melanoma. *New England Journal of Medicine, 363*(8), 711–723.

Iwai, Y., Ishida, M., Tanaka, Y., Okazaki, T., Honjo, T., & Minato, N., (2002). Involvement of PD-L1 on tumor cells in the escape from host immune system and tumor immunotherapy by PD-L1 blockade. *Proceedings of the National Academy of Sciences, 99*(19), 12293–12297.

Krummel, M. F., & Allison, J. P., (1996). CTLA-4 engagement inhibits IL-2 accumulation and cell cycle progression upon activation of resting T-cells. *Journal of Experimental Medicine, 183*(6), 2533–2540.

Kumar, V., Chaudhary, N., Garg, M., Floudas, C. S., Soni, P., & Chandra, A. B., (2017). Current diagnosis and management of immune-related adverse events (irAEs) induced by immune checkpoint inhibitor therapy. *Frontiers in Pharmacology, 8*, 49.

La-Beck, N. M., Jean, G. W., Huynh, C., Alzghari, S. K., & Lowe, D. B., (2015). Immune checkpoint inhibitors: New insights and current place in cancer therapy. *Pharmacotherapy: The Journal of Human Pharmacology and Drug Therapy, 35*(10), 963–976.

Mahoney, K. M., Freeman, G. J., & McDermott, D. F., (2015). The next immune-checkpoint inhibitors: PD-1/PD-L1 blockade in melanoma. *Clinical Therapeutics, 37*(4), 764–782.

Marin-Acevedo, J. A., Dholaria, B., Soyano, A. E., Knutson, K. L., Chumsri, S., & Lou, Y., (2018). Next generation of immune checkpoint therapy in cancer: New developments and challenges. *Journal of Hematology and Oncology, 11*(1), 39.

Motzer, R. J., Escudier, B., McDermott, D. F., George, S., Hammers, H. J., Srinivas, S., et al., (2015). Nivolumab versus everolimus in advanced renal-cell carcinoma. *New England Journal of Medicine, 373*(19), 1803–1813.

Pardoll, D. M., (2012). The blockade of immune checkpoints in cancer immunotherapy. *Nature Reviews Cancer, 12*(4), 252.

Park, Y. J., Kuen, D. S., & Chung, Y., (2018). Future prospects of immune checkpoint blockade in cancer: From response prediction to overcoming resistance. *Experimental and Molecular Medicine, 50*(8), 109.

Parry, R. V., Chemnitz, J. M., Frauwirth, K. A., Lanfranco, A. R., Braunstein, I., Kobayashi, et al., (2005). CTLA-4 and PD-1 receptors inhibit T-cell activation by distinct mechanisms. *Molecular and Cellular Biology, 25*(21), 9543–9553.

Postow, M. A., Sidlow, R., & Hellmann, M. D., (2018). Immune-related adverse events associated with immune checkpoint blockade. *New England Journal of Medicine, 378*(2), 158–168.

Qureshi, O. S., Zheng, Y., Nakamura, K., Attridge, K., Manzotti, C., Schmidt, E., et al., (2011). Trans-endocytosis of CD80 and CD86: A molecular basis for the cell-extrinsic function of CTLA-4. *Science, 332*(6029), 600–603.

Robert, C., Long, G. V., Brady, B., Dutriaux, C., Maio, M., Mortier, L., et al., (2015). Nivolumab in previously untreated melanoma without BRAF mutation. *New England Journal of Medicine, 372*(4), 320–330.

Robert, C., Schachter, J., Long, G. V., Arance, A., Grob, J. J., Mortier, L., et al., (2015). Pembrolizumab versus ipilimumab in advanced melanoma. *New England Journal of Medicine, 372*(26), 2521–2532.

Rosenberg, J. E., Hoffman-Censits, J., Powles, T., Van, D. H. M. S., Balar, A. V., Necchi, A., et al., (2016). Atezolizumab in patients with locally advanced and metastatic urothelial carcinoma who have progressed following treatment with platinum-based chemotherapy: A single-arm, multicentre, phase 2 trial. *The Lancet*, *387*(10031), 1909–1920.

Rudd, C. E., Taylor, A., & Schneider, H., (2009). CD28 and CTLA-4 co-receptor expression and signal transduction. *Immunological Reviews*, *229*(1), 12–26.

Schwartz, R. H., (1992). Costimulation of T-lymphocytes: The role of CD28, CTLA-4, and B7/BB1 in interleukin-2 production and immunotherapy. *Cell*, *71*(7), 1065–1068.

Sharma, P., & Allison, J. P., (2015). The future of immune checkpoint therapy. *Science*, *348*(6230), 56–61.

Sunshine, J., & Taube, J. M., (2015). Pd-1/Pd-L1 Inhibitors. *Current Opinion in Pharmacology*, *23*, 32–38.

Topalian, S. L., Drake, C. G., & Pardoll, D. M., (2015). Immune checkpoint blockade: A common denominator approach to cancer therapy. *Cancer Cell*, *27*(4), 450–461.

Tumeh, P. C., Harview, C. L., Yearley, J. H., Shintaku, I. P., Taylor, E. J., Robert, L., et al., (2014). PD-1 blockade induces responses by inhibiting adaptive immune resistance. *Nature*, *515*(7528), 568.

Villadolid, J., & Amin, A., (2015). Immune checkpoint inhibitors in clinical practice: Update on management of immune-related toxicities. *Translational Lung Cancer Research*, *4*(5), 560.

Weber, J. S., Kähler, K. C., & Hauschild, A., (2012). Management of immune-related adverse events and kinetics of response with ipilimumab. *Journal of Clinical Oncology*, *30*(21), 2691–2697.

Wei, S. C., Duffy, C. R., & Allison, J. P., (2018). Fundamental mechanisms of immune checkpoint blockade therapy. *Cancer Discovery*, *8*(9), 1069–1086.

Wing, K., Onishi, Y., Prieto-Martin, P., Yamaguchi, T., Miyara, M., Fehervari, Z., et al., (2008). CTLA-4 control over Foxp3+ regulatory T-cell function. *Science*, *322*(5899), 271–275.

Wolchok, J. D., Chiarion-Sileni, V., Gonzalez, R., Rutkowski, P., Grob, J. J., Cowey, C. L., et al., (2017). Overall survival with combined nivolumab and ipilimumab in advanced melanoma. *New England Journal of Medicine*, *377*(14), 1345–1356.

Wolchok, J. D., Kluger, H., Callahan, M. K., Postow, M. A., Rizvi, N. A., Lesokhin, A. M., et al., (2013). Nivolumab plus ipilimumab in advanced melanoma. *New England Journal of Medicine*, *369*(2), 122–133.

Zhou, G., & Levitsky, H., (2012). Towards curative cancer immunotherapy: Overcoming post-therapy tumor escape. *Clinical and Developmental Immunology*.

Zou, W., & Chen, L., (2008). Inhibitory B7-family molecules in the tumor microenvironment. *Nature Reviews Immunology*, *8*(6), 467.

CHAPTER 15

Tyrosine Kinase Inhibitors in Lymphocytic Leukemia

SANDEEP ARORA, TAPAN BEHL, SUKHBIR SINGH,
NEELAM SHARMA, and NIDHI GARG

Chitkara College of Pharmacy, Chitkara University, Punjab, India

ABSTRACT

Chronic lymphocytic leukemia is cancer affecting lymphocytes (white blood corpuscles), initially leading to the formation of the tumor inside the bone marrow and its further proliferation to organs, including the spleen, liver, lymph node. It can be detected clinically through physical examination, flow cytometry, gene test, and cytogenetic test. Enzyme tyrosine kinase (TK) is found in humans, and acts as vital mediators during the process of signaling, further responsible for cell metabolism, proliferation, apoptosis, and differentiation. TK acts as a major category of enzymes, which are responsible for catalyzing the phosphorylation of specific tyrosine residues in the target protein, acquiring the aid of ATP. Numerous steps of neoplastic progression followed by its development is controlled by tyrosine kinase. Thus, dysregulated proliferation and development results in apoptotic sensitivity and exert their role in tumor and cancerous conditions. Epigenetic and genetic changes are observed in cancerous cells where dysregulated tyrosine pathways are observed (amplified autocrine expression, stimulation, and functioning). Tyrosine kinase can be responsible for causing lymphocytic leukemia, and the management of the same can be done via the introduction of efficacious TK inhibitors (including duvelisib, venetolax, and idealisib).

15.1 INTRODUCTION

Bruton's tyrosine kinase (BTK) consists of 659 amino acid, belonging to Tec family of kinases that serves as the second leading class of cytoplasmic protein tyrosine kinase next to SRC family kinases (SGKs). It comprises of the five major mammalian members including bone marrow kinase that is present on the X-chromosome, resting lymphocyte kinase, IL-2 inducible T-cell kinase, and Tec. Chronic lymphocytic leukemia (CLL) is caused due to BTK. It is defined as the type of cancer in blood cells that develops in lymphocytes and various other B-cell lymphomas (Kolibaba and Druker, 1997). Thus, the development as well as the introduction of BTK inhibitors in clinical practice marks a crucial advancement in the management of chronic leukemia of lymph that is lymphocytic leukemia and other B-cell lymphomas viz., idelalisib, duvelisib, and venetoclax. Another drug named as zanubrutinib showed promising results in phase I clinical trials for both front-line and relapsed/refractory mantle cell lymphoma (MCL), refractory lymphocytic leukemia, or small lymphocytic lymphoma and refractory follicular lymphoma with 92% of on the whole response rate and presenting a higher selectivity as well as low toxicity in comparison to other BTK inhibitors (Clark et al., 1988).

15.2   LEUKEMIA

Leukemia is a term used for cancerous stage which initially commences in the blood cells or bone marrow and later on develops into leukemia cell which do not mature and also divide faster than the normal rate. This increases their number more than the normal cells. Eventually, they move from the bone marrow and spread in the bloodstream. This ultimately leads to massive growth in the total count of white blood cells (WBCs) present in the blood. Later it may spread to the various body parts including the vital organs, causing a disturbance in their functioning. Based on the nature of cancer, leukemia is mainly of four different types on classifying whether they are chronic or acute and lymphocytic or myeloid: acute myeloid leukemia, acute lymphocytic leukemia, chronic myeloid leukemia, CLL (Rosenberg and Witte, 1988).

15.3   CHRONIC LYMPHOCYTIC LEUKEMIA (CLL)

It is leukemia that most commonly affects adults. It affects white blood corpuscles (lymphocytes) formed inside the bone marrow and proliferate to other organs including the liver, spleen, lymph node, etc. CLL are of two types: CLL that proliferates at a very slow rate and thus involves a long time treatment and the other is a faster-growing CLL causing the severe condition and needs immediate treatment (Daley et al., 1990). For diagnosing the type of CLL, there are lab tests for checking proteins known as CD38 and ZAP-70. Leukemia tends to proliferate slowly with better long-term outcomes when the amounts of these respective proteins are low. The most widespread leukemia prevalent in the west of the United States is CLL. The diagnosed average age of a patient suffering from CLL is 72 years, and 2/3 among the diagnosed cases is aged 65 and older (Kelliher et al., 1990). The age-related occurrence of CLL is approximately 3.9/100,000 people, increasing to 22.3/100,000 among greater than 65-year-olds and an estimated under-reporting of 10 to 30% of cases.

15.3.1   NATURAL HISTORY OF CLL

The historical records of CLL began in 1845, but were first known in 1749 when the initial white cells, "the globulialbicanates," were marked by Joseph Lieutaud. The basic etiologies as well as the treatment involved were encouraged because of the various advancements. Rai discussed three topics on the history of CLL: (1) the acknowledgment of CLL to act as a clinical entity, 1845–1924; (2) preliminary clinical investigations, 1924–1973; and (3) 1973–2002 marked as the modern era (Lugo et al., 1990).

15.3.2   RISK FACTORS FOR CLL

On an average, about 9 out of 10 people suffering from CLL are over 50 years of age. Some studies revealed that an exposure to Agent Orange which is a herbicide that was exploited at the time of the Vietnam War increases the risk of CLL. This can also be due to a family history in which the first-degree relatives that include mainly the parents, siblings, or children of people affected with CLL to be more prone for this cancer involving twice the risk factor and this disease is to some extent more common in males as compared to women though the reason is yet unknown. Cases of CLL are more commonly found in Europe and North America than in Asia (Lugo et al., 1990).

15.3.3   CLINICAL PRESENTATION OF CLL

Many people with CLL rarely show any symptoms on being first diagnosed. It is commonly found from the blood test reports (Buchdunger et al., 1995). A person is having CLL if he shows the following signs and symptoms, if he feels weak or tired, experienced sudden weight loss, chills, fever, night sweats, and observes lumps under the skin that depicts swollen lymph nodes and if a person feels pain or "fullness" sense in the belly which is probably due to an enlarged liver or spleen. Following diagnostic tests are done for detecting CLL: they include physical examination, medical history, blood tests-peripheral blood smear complete blood count (CBC), flow cytometry (for detection of Biopsy of lymph node and imaging tests CT scan, MRI, and Ultrasound (Buchdunger et al., 1996).

15.4   ROLE OF TYROSINE KINASE AND BTK IN THE DEVELOPMENT OF CLL

Enzyme tyrosine kinase is found in humans and is responsible for transferring a phosphate group from Adenosine Tri Phosphate to a protein in a cell. These act as vital mediators in the process of signal transduction that further leads to cell proliferation, metabolism, differentiation, and apoptosis. For example, EGFR, PDGFR, FGFR, SRC, ABL, Janus kinase, and FAK. Tyrosine kinases form a major category of enzymes, that are required for catalyzing the phosphorylation of specific tyrosine residues in target protein acquiring the aid of ATP (Zimmermann et al., 1996). This covalent post-translational modification plays a vital role in the maintenance of homeostasis along with the normal cellular communication. Various steps of neoplastic progression and its development are implicated by tyrosine kinases. Signaling of these kinases usually, cause deregulated proliferation, prevention, and also contributes towards apoptotic stimuli sensitivity. Tyrosine kinase signaling pathways are frequently epigenetically or genetically changed in cancerous cells so as to pass on a selective advantage to the cancer cells (Druker et al., 1996). Thus, it won't be any more surprising to acknowledge that increased signaling arising from tyrosine kinase bestows a leading oncoprotein status to these enzymes, those results in signaling network malfunction. The finding of SRC oncogene acquiring transforming activity of non-receptor tyrosine kinase in addition to the discovery of primary receptor tyrosine kinase, known to be EGFR marked the significance and the role played by tyrosine kinase in cancer. Thus, the process of identification and development of therapeutic agents for disease states related with tyrosine kinases activation because of increased autocrine stimulation, stimulation, and expression is very relevant (Carroll et al., 1997). This leads to an abnormal downstream oncogenic signaling that have proved to be effective targets for cancer therapy (Figure 15.1).

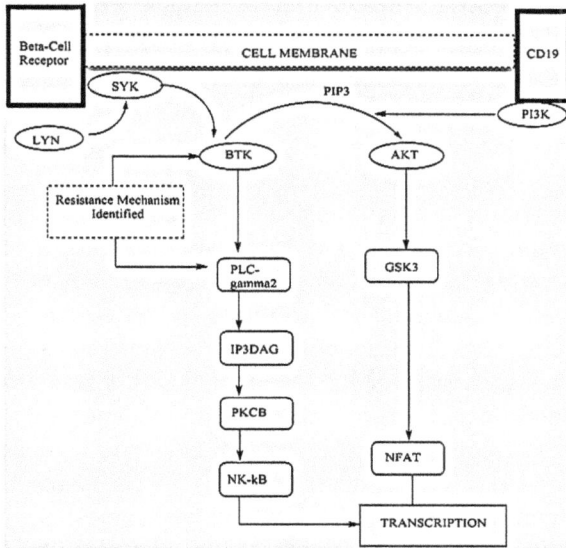

FIGURE 15.1   Outline representing BTK and PI3K signaling in CLL B cell (Awan and Byrd, 2014)

15.5   MECHANISM OF ACTION OF TYROSINE KINASE

Tyrosine phosphorylation is a well-known post-translational alteration which is necessary for metazoans intra- and intercellular communications. The enzyme protein tyrosine kinase is involved in catalyzing/transferring of phosphoryl into tyrosine residues residing within protein substrates with the help of ATP that acts as a phosphate donor. In the human genome, these are comprised of proteins that are of 58 receptor types (RTKs) along with 32 non-receptor types (Deininger et al., 1997). The RTK family comprises of fibroblast growth factor receptors, epidermal growth factor receptors (EGFRs), platelet-derived growth factor receptors, vascular endothelial growth factor receptors, ephrin receptors, hepatocyte growth factors also known as scatter factor receptor and the insulin receptors. These RTKs are vital machineries of cellular signaling pathways which are found to be highly active for the time period of adult homeostasis as well as embryonic development. RTKs are used during the onset and succession of many types of cancers because of their growth factor receptor activity by receptor overexpression or by receptor gain of function mutations (le Coutre et al., 1999). The utmost level of preservation between RTKs is displayed by an ATP binding intracellular catalytic domain which plays the role of catalyzing receptor auto-phosphorylation. The ATP binding site provides an essential site required for binding of specific cytoplasmic signaling proteins that contains protein tyrosine binding (PTB) domains and Src homology-2 (SH2). Moreover, the same proteins further employ supplementary effector molecules that consist of PTB, SH3, SH2, and the Pleckstrin homology (PH) domain that causes assembling of these signaling complexes over the activated membrane receptors and successive activation of intracellular biochemical signals (Beran et al., 1998). These activities define the role of biological response to signals and resulting in repression or activation of various subsets of genes. Throughout these processes, migration of receptors inside the plasma membrane occurs and their internalization takes place via the clathrin-coated invagination, that ultimately isolate in order to form an endocytic vesicle. Degradation of lysosomal enzyme may take place during the process of fusion of the endocytic vesicle with the lysosomes. The endocytic vesicles tend to fuse with the available lysosomes. During this, fused receptor and ligand can cause degradation to take place by the lysosomal enzymes. In some of the cases, re-cyclization of receptor and dissociation of ligand-receptor complex takes during receptor internalization that causes a termination of signaling reaction (Figure 15.2) (Oda et al., 1994; Druker et al., 1999).

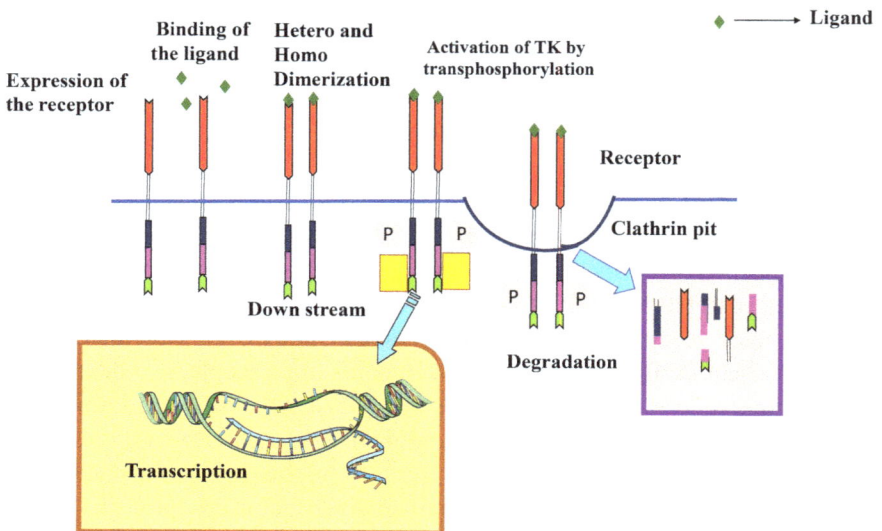

FIGURE 15.2   Mechanism of action of enzyme, tyrosine kinase by activation and degradation.

15.6 ONCOGENIC ACTIVATION OF TYROSINE KINASE

Tyrosine kinase can attain transforming functions by several mechanisms, but ultimately leads to the activation of normally controlled pathways that cause activation of secondary messengers and also the other signaling proteins available. This further provides to hinder various regulatory functions taking place in cellular responses such as cellular growth, division, and cell death. The several processes include:

15.6.1 ACTIVATION BY MUTATION

Certain mutations in the extracellular province such as EGFRv III mutant lacking amino acid 6–273 that promotes constitutive activity of receptor tyrosine kinase that results into proliferation of the cell, causing a dearth of ligands in the glioblastomas, lung carcinoma and ovarian carcinomas (Toledo et al., 1999). Cervical and human bladder carcinomas are associated with the somatic mutations in the EGFR 2 and 3. Cut-off points all through atypical chromosomal translocation also serve as a vital source of mutation. Mutations can also occur in the transmembrane domain (TMD) (such as lung cancer cells show driver mutations) and juxtamembrane domain (JMD) (such as KIT V560G and PDGFRA V561D mutation in GIST) of RTKs (Figure 15.3).

15.6.2 HUMAN LEUKEMIA AND BCR-ABL

CML stands for chronic myelodysplastic hematopoietic stem cell disorder syndrome that takes place because of the reciprocal translocation involving chromosome 9 and chromosome 22. The fusion protein can be seen in three forms based on site including the breakpoint on BCR and this shows a dysregulated PTK activity in comparison to a normal ABL (Traxler et al., 1997). The initial exon of c-ABL that is a 210 KDa mutant protein gets replaced by the BCR sequences fabricated by fusion genes. It encodes either 902 or 927 amino acid. An additional BCR-ABL fused protein is diagnosed in 10% adults. The individuals whom are having 185 KDa and include the commencement of the BCR sequence leading to exon 1 fused to exon 2–11 of c-ABL. This tyrosine kinase activity present in BCR-ABL chimeric gene product is many times higher as when compared with standard counterpart and it associates with phenotype of disease (Zhu et al., 1999). As a result of which, unnecessary tyrosine

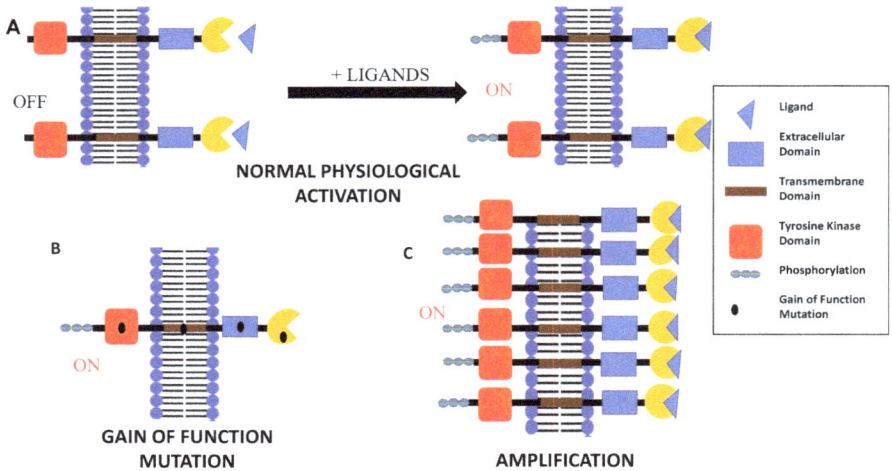

FIGURE 15.3 Activity of Tyrosine Kinase (a) Representation of the physiological activation; (b) Representation of the activation of altered genes due to gain of function mutation (c) Representation of activation of altered genes due to amplification

related phosphorylation of intracellular proteins like BCR-ABL takes place. Though it is not necessary that all the interaction of BCR-ABL with various additional proteins are phosphotyrosine dependent type, but the mutational analysis clearly clarifies that for malignant transformation, the PTK activity is a basic requirement and that any downstream effector is unable to complement it (Faderl et al., 1999). In disparity to it, currently, it is yet unclear that BCR-ABL activates which of the signaling pathways (i.e., phosphatidylinositol 3′-kinase, RAS, and JAK-STAT, i.e., Janus-activated kinase-signal transducers and activators of transcription pathway) is crucial for transformation.

15.6.3   *HUMAN LEUKEMIA AND TEL-ABL*

Unlike ABL-BCR and TEL-ABL, the phosphorylation is constitutive in tyrosine kinase because of the reciprocal translocation in the case of ALL and in patients suffering from CML by a complex karyotype. In frame fusion of an alleged fusion factor TEL along with exon-2 belonging to ABL proto-oncogene, results in formation of fusion protein as a product having increased activity of tyrosine kinase (Kantarjian et al., 1991; Buchdunger et al., 1996). Various other important translocations involve production of TEL-PDGF receptor with the contribution of CMML.

TEL consists of specific helix-loop and helix shape which is known for persuading kinase activation as well as to cause homo-dimerization of the TEL-ABL and TEL-PDGFRβ fusion proteins. Following this, constitutive activation of NPM-ALK fusion products takes place in anaplastic large cell lymphoma.

15.6.4   AUTOCRINE-PARACRINE LOOPS

A vital method for the constitutive tyrosine kinase activation especially of receptor tyrosine kinases (RTKs) is mainly by the activation of Autocrine-paracrine. Stimulation of this activation loop leads to an abnormal or overexpression of tyrosine kinas receptor, this occurs in incidence of its related ligand or in case when an overexpression of the ligand takes place in existence of its related receptor. Activation of autocrine-paracrine loops has a vital role in broad range of human cancers. Various examples include IGF, PDGFR, and EGFR receptors (Trotti et al., 2000).

15.7   TYROSINE KINASES AS POTENT TARGETS FOR ANTICANCER AGENTS

Tyrosine kinase shows an immense function in molecular pathogenesis of cancer as these kinases have been proven to be potential targets of anticancer drugs and so are dispensed in the market. Successive reports of the human genome project provided with more possibilities of drug discovery by an increase in number and complexity of the tyrosine kinases (Spencer et al., 1995). Recent discovery in molecular pathophysiology of cancer explains the presence of tyrosine kinases downstream or upstream of epidemiologically related tumor suppressor or oncogenes, particularly the RTKs.

15.7.1   TARGETING SITES

By 1980, clear confirmations of presence of low molecular weight tyrosine kinase inhibitors acting against tyrosine kinases are competent of inquisiting with the protein substrate or ligand binding which is usually very difficult. Though this bisubstrate inhibitor approach is of little progress but is quite promising and various efforts of generating allosteric inhibitors have also lacked behind in proving ATP competitive inhibitors be a potent target choice (Thiesing et al., 2000).

15.7.2   THE ATP BINDING SITE

Adenosine triphosphate binding takes place in a deep cleft shaped present between the two lobes of tyrosine kinase domain making its architecture highly conserved in the region that is proximal to ATP binding site and provides variety for designing of a new drug possessing prospective of application in drug discovery (Mahon et al., 2000).

15.7.3   KEY FEATURES OF ATP BINDING SITE

The interaction between the N-1 and N-6 amino group present in the adenine ring leads to the formation of the hydrogen bond in this adenine region. These hydrogen bonds are used by many potential inhibitors. Sugar region consisting of a hydrophilic region, except EGFR. Hydrophobic pocket plays a major role in selectivity of inhibitor though not much used. Hydrophobic channels are variously modified for inhibitory specifications. For this inhibitor specificity, a phosphate-binding region gets improved (Mahon et al., 2000) (Figure 15.4).

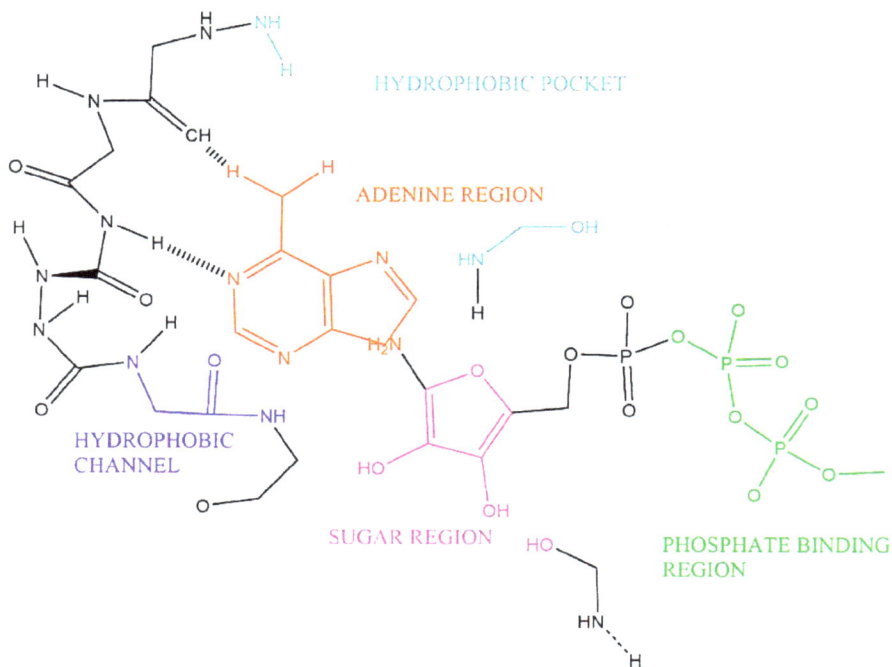

FIGURE 15.4   Structure of tyrosine kinase showing exposed ATP-binding sites.

15.7.4 SMALL MOLECULE INHIBITOR

By the 1980s, it was found that EGF-dependent cell proliferation could be blocked by the molecular weight EGFR inhibitors. Within a short phase of time, various reports regarding the effectiveness of tyrosine kinase inhibitors acting as promising key in anticancer development and advanced research in this regard made clear the targets of neglected kinases against biases (Weisberg and Griffin, 2000). Most tyrosine kinase inhibitors formed are ATP mimics that are converted by the addition of nitrogen of benzene malononitrile into the second ring. Minimum two aromatic rings are present in compounds that are ATP mimics. The ATP binding site serves as an easy target because of a minor difference in the kinase domain that results in hydrophobic interactions as well as hydrogen bonding leading to a change in affinity.

Kinases inhibitors are one of the alternative options for patients suffering from CLL and also can also transform the treatment pattern for the disease effectively (le Coutre et al., 2000). Earlier some of the BTK inhibitors like ibrutinib, (imbruvica) and P13 K (phosphatidylinositol-4,5-bisphosphate 3-kinase) Inhibitors like idelalisib, duvelisib showed a positive clinical impact and promising efficiency and now several drugs are also under investigation. One of those drugs is zanubrutinib, a small molecule and an inhibitor of BTK evaluated in late phase three clinical trials conducting at 150 centers in the US, China, Europe, Australia, and New Zealand for both front-line and relapsed or refractory lymphocytic leukemia, relapsed MCL, and relapsed follicular cancer.

15.8 CONCLUSIONS

The specific role of tyrosine kinase to regulate cellular differentiation, as well as growth takes an important part in human neoplastic diseases (Gorre et al., 2001). The intrinsic role of tyrosine kinase inhibitors in clinical application is well represented by remarkable illustrations like Imbruvica, Ibrutinib as well as P13 K (phosphatidylinositol-4,5-bisphosphate 3-kinase). Inhibitors include idelalisib and duvelisib. Several small-molecule inhibitors are undertaken human trials to act as a channel in drug discovery and the specific actions of such drugs are limited to CLL along with other comorbid conditions. The spontaneous selection of epidemiologically applicable tyrosine kinase targets and other sites such as p13 k coupled to the effective finding of lead requires an intense involvement throughout cancer genome-based molecular therapeutics (Hofmann et al., 2002). All these efforts paved a silver lining in cancer therapeutics. In the present time scenario, tyrosine kinase inhibitors serve as primary/principal therapy because of an apparent theory for its usage, appropriate preclinical data, and established use in a set of patients. Kinase inhibitors are effective for previously untreated patients and for relapsed conditions of CLL including patients with high risks. In the recent research of CLL, zanubrutinib is being compared with a standard of care immune-chemotherapy regimen, AbbVie/Johnson and Johnson's imbruvica (ibrutinib), and it has a 92% overall response rate. It is shown that zanubrutinib has higher selectivity against BTK than ibrutinib and is also associated with less toxicity.

KEYWORDS

- Bruton's tyrosine kinase
- chronic lymphocytic leukemia
- fluorescent in situ hybridization
- juxtamembrane domain
- mantle cell lymphoma
- pleckstrin homology
- protein tyrosine binding
- receptor tyrosine kinases

REFERENCES

Awan, F. T., & Byrd, J. C., (2014). New strategies in chronic lymphocytic leukemia: Shifting treatment paradigms. *Clin. Cancer Res., 20*(23), 5869–5874.

Beran, M., Cao, X., Estrov, Z., Jeha, S., Jin, G., O'Brien, S., Talpaz, M., et al., (1998). Selective inhibition of cell proliferation and BCRABL phosphorylation in acute lymphoblastic leukemia cells expressing Mr 190,000 BCR-ABL protein by a tyrosine kinase inhibitor (CGP57148). *Clin. Cancer Res., 4*, 1661–1672.

Buchdunger, E., Zimmermann, J., Mett, H., Meyer, T., Müller, M., Regenass, U., & Lydon, N. B., (1995). Selective inhibition of the platelet-derived growth factor signal transduction pathway by a protein-tyrosine kinase inhibitor of the 2-phenylaminopyrimidine class. *Proc. Natl. Acad. Sci. U.S.A., 92*, 2558–2562.

Buchdunger, E., Zimmermann, J., Mett, H., Meyer, T., Müller, M., Druker, B. J., & Lydon, N. B., (1996). Inhibition of the Abl protein-tyrosine kinase *in vitro* and *in vivo* by a 2-phenylaminopyrimidine derivative. *Cancer Res., 56,* 100–104.

Carroll, M., Ohno-Jones, S., Tamura, S., Buchdunger, E., Zimmermann, J., Lydon, N. B., Gilliland, D. G., & Druker, B. J., (1997). CGP 57148, a tyrosine kinase inhibitor, inhibits the growth of cells expressing BCR-ABL, TEL-ABL, and TEL-PDGFR fusion proteins. *Blood, 90,* 4947–4952.

Clark, S. S., McLaughlin, J., Timmons, M., Pendergast, A. M., Ben-Neriah, Y., Dow, L. W., Crist, W., et al., (1988). Expression of a distinctive BCR-ABL oncogene in Ph1-positive acute lymphocytic leukemia (ALL). *Science, 239,* 775–777.

Daley, G. Q., Van, E. R. A., & Baltimore, D., (1990). Induction of chronic myelogenous leukemia in mice by the P210bcr/abl gene of the Philadelphia chromosome. *Science, 247,* 824–830.

Deininger, M. W., Goldman, J. M., Lydon, N., & Melo, J. V., (1997). The tyrosine kinase inhibitor CGP57148B selectively inhibits the growth of BCR-ABL-positive cells. *Blood, 90,* 3691–3698.

Druker, B. J., Bauer, G., Rice, C. R., Rothschild, J. C., Carbonaro, D. A., Valdez, P., Hao, Q. I., et al., (1999). Clinical efficacy and safety of an Abl specific tyrosine kinase inhibitor as targeted therapy for chronic myelogenous leukemia. *Blood, 94,* 368–371.

Druker, B. J., Tamura, S., Buchdunger, E., Ohno, S., Segal, G. M., Fanning, S., Zimmermann, J., & Lydon, N. B., (1996). Effects of a selective inhibitor of the ABL tyrosine kinase on the growth of BCR-ABL positive cells. *Nat. Med., 2,* 561–566.

Faderl, S., Talpaz, M., Estrov, Z., O'Brien, S., Kurzrock, R., & Kantarjian, H. M., (1999). The biology of chronic myeloid leukemia. *N. Engl. J. Med., 341,* 164–172.

Gorre, M. E., Mohammed, M., Ellwood, K., Hsu, N., Paquette, R., Rao, P. N., & Sawyers, C. L., (2001). Clinical resistance to STI-571 cancer therapy caused by BCR-ABL gene mutation or amplification. *Science, 293,* 876–880.

Hofmann, W. K., Jones, L. C., Lemp, N. A., De Vos, S., Gschaidmeier, H., Hoelzer, D., Ottmann, O. G., & Koeffler, H. P., (2002). Ph(+) acute lymphoblastic leukemia resistant to the tyrosine kinase inhibitor STI571 has a unique BCR-ABL gene mutation. *Blood, 99,* 1860–1862.

Kantarjian, H. M., Talpaz, M., Keating, M. J., Estey, E. H., O'Brien, S., Beran, M., McCredie, K. B., et al., (1991). Intensive chemotherapy induction followed by interferon-alpha maintenance in patients with Philadelphia chromosome-positive chronic myelogenous leukemia. *Cancer, 68,* 1201–1207.

Kelliher, M. A., McLaughlin, J., Witte, O. N., & Rosenberg, N., (1990). Induction of a chronic myelogenous leukemia-like syndrome in mice with v-abl and BCR/ABL. *Proc. Natl. Acad. Sci. U.S.A., 87,* 6649–6653.

Kolibaba, K. S., & Druker, B. J., (1997). Protein tyrosine kinases and cancer. *Biochim. Biophys. Acta., 1333,* F217–F248.

Le Coutre, P., Mologni, L., Cleris, L., Marchesi, E., Buchdunger, E., Giardini, R., Formelli, F., & Gambacorti-Passerini, C., (1999). *In vivo* eradication of human BCR/ABL-positive leukemia cells with an ABL kinase inhibitor. *J. Natl. Cancer Inst., 91,* 163–168.

Le Coutre, P., Tassi, E., Varella-Garcia, M., Barni, R., Mologni, L., Cabrita, G., Marchesi, E., et al., (2000). Induction of resistance to the Abelson inhibitor STI571 in human leukemic cells through gene amplification. *Blood, 95,* 1758–1766.

Lugo, T. G., Pendergast, A. M., Muller, A. J., & Witte, O. N., (1990). Tyrosine kinase activity and transformation potency of BCR-ABL oncogene products. *Science, 247*, 1079–1082.

Mahon, F. X., Deininger, M. W. N., Schultheis, B., Chabrol, J., Reiffers, J., Goldman, J. M., & Melo, J. V., (2000). Selection and characterization of BCR-ABL positive cell lines with differential sensitivity to the tyrosine kinase inhibitor STI571: Diverse mechanisms of resistance. *Blood, 96*, 1070–1079.

Oda, T., Heaney, C., Hagopian, J. R., Okuda, K., Griffin, J. D., & Druker, B. J., (1994). CRKL is the major tyrosine-phosphorylated protein in neutrophils from patients with chronic myelogenous leukemia. *J. Biol. Chem., 269*, 22925–22928.

Rosenberg, N., & Witte, O. N., (1988). The viral and cellular forms of the Abelson (abl) oncogene. *Adv. Virus Res., 35*, 39–81.

Spencer, A., O'Brien, S. G., & Goldman, J. M., (1995). Options for therapy in chronic myeloid leukaemia. *Br. J. Haematol., 91*, 2–7.

Thiesing, J. T., Ohno-Jones, S., Kolibaba, K. S., & Druker, B. J., (2000). Efficacy of STI571, an abl tyrosine kinase inhibitor, in conjunction with other antileukemic agents against BCR-ABL-positive cells. *Blood, 96*, 3195–3199.

Toledo, L. M., Lydon, N. B., & Elbaum, D., (1999). The structure-based design of ATP-site directed protein kinase inhibitors. *Curr. Med. Chem., 6*, 775–805.

Traxler, P., Bold, G., Frei, J., Lang, M., Lydon, N., Mett, H., Buchdunger, E., et al., (1997). Use of a pharmacophore model for the design of EGF-R tyrosine kinase inhibitors: 4-(phenylamino)pyrazolo[3,4-d]pyrimidines. *J. Med. Chem., 40*, 3601–3616.

Trotti, A., Byhardt, R., Stetz, J., Gwede, C., Corn, B., Fu, K., Gunderson, L., et al., (2000). Common toxicity criteria: Version 2.0. an improved reference for grading the acute effects of cancer treatment: Impact on radiotherapy. *Int. J. Radiat. Oncol. Biol. Phys., 47*(1), 13–47.

Weisberg, E., & Griffin, J. D., (2000). Mechanism of resistance to the ABL tyrosine kinase inhibitor STI571 in BCR/ABL-transformed hematopoietic cell lines. *Blood, 95*, 3498–3505.

Zhu, X., Kim, J. L., Newcomb, J. R., Rose, P. E., Stover, D. R., Toledo, L. M., Zhao, H., & Morgenstern, K. A., (1999). Structural analysis of the lymphocyte-specific kinase Lck in complex with nonselective and Src family selective kinase inhibitors. *Structure, 7*, 651–661.

Zimmermann, J., Caravatti, G., Mett, H., Meyer, T., Müller, M., Lydon, N. B., & Fabbro, D., (1996). Phenylamino-pyrimidine (PAP) derivatives: A new class of potent and selective inhibitors of protein kinase C (PKC). *Arch. Pharm. (Weinheim), 329*, 371–376.

CHAPTER 16

Cyclooxygenase-1 (COX-1) Inhibitors in the Management of Neoplastic Disorders

SANDEEP ARORA, SAURABH GUPTA, and SUMAN BAISHNAB

Chitkara College of Pharmacy, Chitkara University, Punjab, India

ABSTRACT

Cyclooxygenase (COX) majorly acts as a substrate or precursor for numerous molecules, including prostacyclin, prostaglandin, and thromboxane. COX exists in its two major isoforms termed as COX-1 and COX-2; both of them catalyze arachidonic acid into prostaglandin via bis-deoxygenation. Cancer is associated with chronic inflammation and leukocyte infiltration, which is a marked feature of neoplastic disorders. Arachidonic acid regulates the process of homeostatic inside tissues and cells. Along with this, prostaglandins and thromboxane (also termed as prostanoids) exert their role in neoplastic disorders via PGE2 and PGF2a. Elevated levels of PGE2 are associated with carcinomas. Prostaglandins like PGD2 exert their role in colon cancer; TXA2 is associated with the pathophysiology of colon cancer, lung cancer, and multiple myeloma. Along with this, they can be responsible for genetic as well as epigenetic changes that can induce an inflammatory reaction. Thus, the antagonism of COX can be a target for the management of neoplastic disorders. COX inhibitors can be targeted by selectively COX-1, COX-2 inhibitors, or nonselective inhibitors that exert their action in inhibiting COX and thus can be used for managing such disorders.

16.1 CYCLOOXYGENASE

Cyclooxygenase (COX) acts as a precursor for various molecules, including prostaglandins (PGs), prostacyclin, and thromboxane, and is a rate-limiting enzyme responsible for transition of arachidonic acid (AA) into PG H2 (Ohike et al., 2005).

The most meticulously researched and understood mammalian oxygen-ases are cyclooxygenase isoforms (COX-1 and COX-2). The enzyme possesses two distinct yet connected active sites, which enable it to catalyze AA to PG G_2 and PGH_2 via bis-deoxygenation.

16.2   COX-1 AND COX-2: STRUCTURAL AND FUNCTIONAL DIFFERENCES

16.2.1   STRUCTURAL DIFFERENCES (RESEARCH GATE, 2005)

COX-1 is generally spread and expressed in tissues. Ptgs-1 (prostaglandin-endoperoxide synthase 1) gene is associated with COX-1 and codes for a comparatively stable mRNA. In contrast, Ptgs-2 (prostaglandin-endoperoxide synthase 2), gene associated with COX-2 is an instant, early gene which is activated by inflammatory and proliferative stimuli replacing COX-2 mRNA with the 3″ untranslated area producing unstable sequences (Smith et al., 2000; Rouzer et al., 2003).

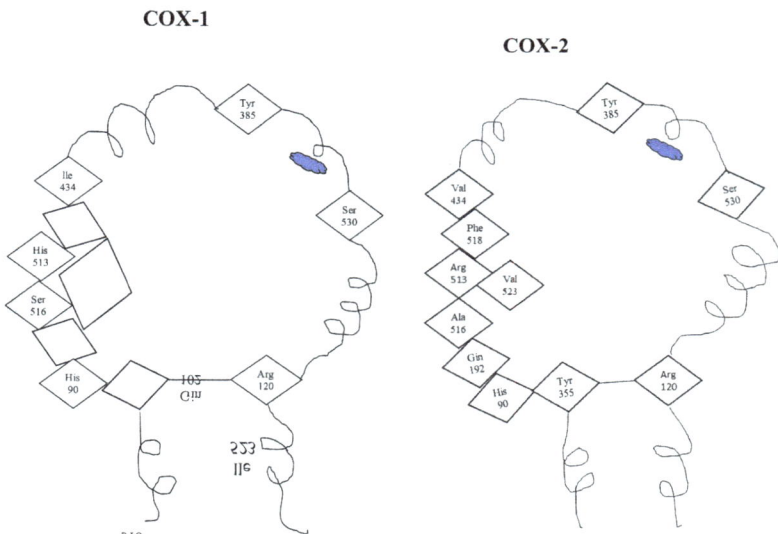

16.2.2   CYCLOOXYGENASE-1 AND CYCLOOXYGENASE-2: DIFFERENTIAL EXPRESSION

According to a study that was performed by autopsy of 20 healthy subjects (human) showed uniform articulation of cyclooxygenase-1 injury multiple tissues, with the majority of the protein situated in the blood vessels, delicate muscle cells, interstitial cells, tract platelets, and mesothelial cells. In spite of the fact that the COX-2 protein is extremely variable, it is found in practically all tissues of parenchymal cells (Zidar et al., 2008). The cerebrum, kidney, and female conceptive framework shows constitutive COX-2 articulation which were later demonstrated for account the enlistment of COX-1 during the inflammatory and cellular differentiation of lipopolysaccharide (LPS) (McAdam et al., 2000; Lipsky et al., 2000; Langenbach et al., 1999; Wallace et al., 1998; Gudis et al., 2005).

16.2.3   CYCLOOXYGENASE-1 AND CYCLOOXYGENASE-2: DIFFERENTIAL FUNCTIONS

The distinctive genetic expression explains variations between the COX isoforms, indicating the absence of any significant phenotype which can substitute the COX-2 gene with COX-1. However, better expression of the Cyclooxygenase-1 in place of Cyclooxygenase-2 in mice partly fills the PGI_2formation deficiency and does not completely reduce reproductive or renal function defects linked to the removal of COX-2 (Yu et al., 2007). These findings show obviously that Cyclooxygenase-1 and Cyclooxygenase-2 at protein level cannot be interchanged functionally.

It could be explained that COX-2 needs less hydroperoxide levels for the activation than COX-1 does (Kulmacz et al., 2005). While that distinction generally does not impact kinetic parameters measured *in vitro*, it translates into a COX-2 capacity to operate at reduced AA levels than COX-1 within the reduction setting of the intact cell (Yu et al., 2007; Smith et al., 2001; Morita et al., 2002).

16.3   INVOLVEMENT OF CYCLOOXYGENASE-1 (COX-1) IN CANCER

The characteristic feature of cancer development is chronic inflammation (Hanahan et al., 2011; Ben-Neriah et al., 2011) as a German pathologist in the year 1863 found that few neoplastic disorders were related to Leukocyte infiltration (Balkwill et al., 2001).

Chronic inflammation that is associated with events like persistent infections, exposure to irritants (prolonged), any damage caused by the immune system can be the cause of cancer.

Genetic and epigenetic changes can induce a chronic inflammatory reaction. These modifications can also lead to modifications in the homeostasis of the tissue. The inflammatory cells and mediators that are irrespective of the nature of the process could be identified in the majority of the tumor tissues. They help in determining a microenvironment that promotes tumors by acting on both the cells, i.e., tumor and stromal cells (Coussens et al., 2013).

The metabolites of AA play an important part in the homeostasis of cells and tissues (Dennis et al., 2015). The prostanoids (prostaglandins and thromboxane) are the result of a series of actions of Cyclooxygenase-1 or Cyclooxygenase-2 and particular synthases. These components show an effect on the surface of the cell through GPCR (G Protein-Coupled Receptor) in an autocrine and/or paracrine manner (Hirata et al., 2011).

The role of PGs in neoplastic disorders was first observed in esophageal carcinoma cell of humans, which was related to PGE_2 and PGF_{2a} production (Botha et al., 1986). Various cancers have shown an elevation in the levels of PGE_2. However, apart from PGE_2 different other prostaglandins are involved in other cancers, like PGD_2 in colon cancer risk in ulcerative colitis (Vong et al., 2010), (TX) A_2 in colorectal cancer pathophysiology (Li et al., 2015; Dovizo et al., 2012), multiple myeloma (Liu et al., 2016) and lung cancer cell proliferation (Li et al., 2009).

COX-1 and COX-2 are similar in various aspects, like their structure and properties. These similarities also include the same product (PGH_2) that is yielded by both the isomers. However, despite such similarities, they also differ in various aspects like regulating expression, synthases, etc., which leads to various different tasks. Cyclooxygenase-1 is expressed in many tissues. Here the prostanoids that are derived from COX-1 have functions that are homeostatic in nature. The activity of COX-1 keeps up the prostanoid creation at a basal rate and permits a quick rise when there is a requirement of excess of free AA by cell membrane remodeling while cyclooxygenase-2 is the reason for the increased creation of prostanoids due to the inflammatory stimuli as well as growth factors during the event of inflammation and other pathological situations that also includes cancer (Ricciotti et al., 2011; Smith et al., 2000).

Various studies have reported the involvement of these enzymes (specifically COX-2) and PG products in inflammation that is related to cancer, including esophageal (Zhang, et al., 2013), gastrointestinal (Cheng et al., 2013; Cathcart et al., 2012), pancreatic cancers (Knab et al., 2014), breast (Glover et al., 2011) and cervical cancers (Parida et al., 2014), renal

(Kaminska et al., 2014), prostate (Shao et al., 2012), and bladder cancers (Gakis et al., 2014), skin cancers (Elmets et al., 2014; Rundhaug et al., 2011) head and neck cancers (Mends et al., 2009), hematological tumors (Ramon et al., 2013), and mesothelioma (Nuvoli et al., 2013). The COX-2 expression also leads to the characterization of tumor cells (Greenhough et al., 2009; Harris et al., 2007). Tumor diseases like colorectal cancer are because of transcriptional and post-transcriptional alterations (Dixon et al., 2013). The involvement of COX-1 in cancer has received less attention, unlike COX-2. Because cyclooxygenase-1 has a role in homeostatic functions, it was thought that it would not be involved in carcinogenesis. But there were occasional incidences of increase in the level of COX-1 expressions in various neoplastic disorders (Rouzer et al., 2009), The genetic disruption of COX-1 has been shown to be as efficient as COX-2 disruption in the reduction of intestinal (Chaulada et al., 2000) and skin tumorigenesis (Tiano et al., 2009) in mouse models, indicating that both COX-1 and COX-2 isoforms could cooperate in the carcinogenetic procedure.

16.4   ROLE OF COX-1 IN VARIOUS NEOPLASTIC DISORDERS

16.4.1   RENAL CELL CARCINOMA (RCC)

With the exception of the study of overexpression in an RCC rat model by Cyclooxygenase-1 mRNA (Okamoto et al., 2003), the expression of COX-1 was nearly unexplored. Interestingly, two latest immunohistochemical studies have demonstrated the relation amongst bad prognosis in RCC and Cyclooxygenase-1 overexpression (Yu et al., 2013) and the validity of the combined action of COX-1 and VEGF (Vascular Endothelial Growth Factor) in the histopathological prognosis of RCC (Osman et al., 2015).

16.4.2   SKIN CANCER

There is accumulated proof that COX-2 can be engaged in the pathophysiology of non-melanoma skin cancer, whereas the expression of Cyclooxygenase-1 in healthy tissue remains unchanged. However, both the cyclooxygenase isoforms are practically involved in the pathogenesis of basal cell carcinoma as per some preclinical genetic studies (Tang et al., 2010; Müller-Decker, 2011).

16.4.3   HEAD AND NECK CANCER

RT-PCR (reverse transcription-polymerase chain reaction), Western blotting, and Immunohistochemistry showed cyclooxygenase-1 overexpression in neoplastic cells and no standard mucosal expression to compare the concentrations of cyclooxygenase-1 expression between patients with head and neck cancer and ordinary mucosa (Erovic et al., 2008).

16.4.4   ESOPHAGEAL CANCER

In main human tumor samples, the growth factors angiogenic (VEGF-A) and lymphangiogenic (VEGF-C) as well as both cyclooxygenase isoforms suggested prospective COX-1 involvement in disease pathophysiology (Von et al., 2005). A study induced esophageal adenocarcinoma which was conducted on the PGE_2 pathway in a rat model along with gastroduodenal reflux caused by esophagojejunostomy (Piazeulo et al., 2012) suggested that there may be a correlation amongst both the cyclooxygenase isoforms. The study also reported that inflammatory lesions and tumor growth were reduced by the use of indomethacin (a dual COX inhibitor), while the COX-2 selective (MF-tricyclic) inhibitor was ineffective (Esquivias et al., 2012).

16.4.5   COLORECTAL CANCER

An examination of the expression profiles of Cyclooxygenase-1 and Cyclooxygenase-2 mRNA in tumor tissue compared to ordinary colorectal cancer patients in phase III (Dukes' C, Church et al., 2004) was done. The constitutive role of COX-1 was not subjected to variable expression as a change in the expression due to regulation of COX-1 was recorded in normal and malignant tissues, in accordance with the tumorigenic role of COX-1. In addition, the analysis of COX-1, COX-2, and mPGES expression levels of COX-1$^{-/-}$ and COX-2$^{-/-}$Apc Δ716 (Adenomatous Polyposis Coli) double-knockout mice showed that from the start of intestinal polyp development, the COX-1 was required and that the addition of COX-2 along with mPGES was needed in order to fasten the growth of polyps (Takeda et al., 2003). On this basis, a mechanistic collaboration was suggested in the subsequent polyp development between Cyclooxygenase-1 in the early phase of carcinogenesis and cyclooxygenase-2 in later. Early in the period of intestinal carcinogenesis, a signaling COX-1-PGE$_2$ was suggested to happen before COX-2 induction, related to the suppression of PG-Catabolizing (15-PGDH) (Smartt et al., 2012). According to some new studies, cyclooxygenase-1 is necessary for the maintenance, in addition to the conversion of preneoplastic cells induced by tumor promoters, to anchorage-independent growth capacity of colon cells (the main characteristics of malignant phenotype) (Li et al., 2014).

16.4.6   BREAST CANCER

In the clinically identifiable breast carcinoma samples, both isoforms (COX-1 and COX-2) are expressed, and COX-1 is mainly localized in stromal cells (Hwang et al., 1998; Fahlen et al., 2017). In comparison to normal tissue, the up-regulation of cyclooxygenase-1 gene expression was also proved by an assessment of whole breast carcinoma's genome expression (Haaknsen et al., 2011).

16.4.7   CERVICAL CANCER

More than 10 years ago, up-regulation of COX-1 in cervical carcinoma and COX-1 autocrine/paracrine COX-2 and PGE$_2$ receptor regulation and angiogenic factors were established *in vitro* (Sales et al., 2002). Interestingly lately, it has been shown that seminal plasma can encourage cervical tumor cell development *in vitro* and *in vivo* by activating both COX isoforms (Sutherland et al., 2012) and angiogenic chemokine inflammatory pathways (Sales et al., 2012).

16.4.8   ENDOMETRIAL CANCER

Possible participation of COX-1 in the early developmental phase of endometrial cancer was proposed, which was based on the enhanced expression of COX-1 mRNA in G$_1$ and G$_2$ grade endometrial cancer patients (Sugimoto et al., 2007). In addition, a potential function for COX-1 has been suggested in endometrial carcinogenesis (Dery et al., 2011).

16.4.9   OVARIAN CANCER

About 20 years back, cyclooxygenase-1 was initially recognized as a marker of ovarian cancer (Lee et al., 1995). Several studies in various models of mouse, hen, and humans of ovarian cancer (Gupta et al., 2003; Daikoku et al., 2005, 2006; Hales et al., 2008; Urick et al., 2006; Eilati et al., 2012) have reported COX-1 overexpression. COX-1 is suggested to be the principal enzyme for regulating PGE_2 production in ovarian cancer cells (Kino et al., 2005). The combined COX isoforms (COX-1, COX-2) mitigate invasion of gonadotropin induced tumor cells (Lau et al., 2010). Therefore, COX-1 and COX-2 are chief inflammatory markers characterizing fast increasing and very aggressive ovarian carcinomas (type II) (Ali et al., 2011).

16.4.10   HEMATOLOGICAL TUMORS

Acute myeloid (AML) and lymphoid leukemia (ALL) have been well reported in human cancer and acute lymphoid patients for the transcription of both the COX-1 and COX-2 isoforms, although COX-1 is expressed and active. The PGE_2 that is derived from COX-1 encourages the spontaneous development *in vitro* studies of AML leukemic blasts (Truffinet et al., 2007). In the different Cyclooxygenase-related biproducts, PGE_2 appears to have a role for *in vitro* growth of leukemic blast cells (Fiancette et al., 2011), expressing an important benefit from selective Cyclooxygenase-1 antagonism. Cyclooxygenase-1, but not cyclooxygenase-2, is also represented and is active enzymatically in main blasts in patients with (APL) acute promyelocytic leukemia (PML), a distinct AML subtype identified by the PML gene in chromosome 15 and the RAR-alpha (retinoic acid receptor-alpha) gene in chromosome 17.

16.5   COX-1 SELECTIVE INHIBITORS: ANTICARCINOGENIC ACTIVITY

The antagonism of some COX-2 inhibitors has been researched widely, and there are many extremely selective COX-2 inhibitors available (Tortorella et al., 2016). On the other hand, comparatively few COX-1-selective inhibitors were described (Vitale et al., 2016) and for anticancer activity, only some of them were investigated.

Name	SC-560	Mofezolac	FR122047
Structure			
Chemical Name	5-(4-chlorophenyl)-1-(4-methoxyphenyl)-3-(trifluoromethyl)pyrazole	(3,4-bis(4-methoxyphenyl)-5-isoxazolyl)acetic acid	1-((4,5-bis(4-methoxyphenyl)-2-thiazoyl)carbonyl)-4-methylpiperazine

16.5.1   SC-560 (5-(4-CHLOROPHENYL)-1-(4-METHOXYPHENYL)-3-(TRIFLUOROMETHYL)PYRAZOLE)

It is used to evaluate the role of COX-1-derived prostaglandins in inflammation and pain as a pharmacological instrument (Smith et al., 1998). SC-560 has been examined in several pathological circumstances and has been studied in various experimental *in vitro* and *in vivo* designs on colorectal and ovarian cancers, and also on other tumors.

16.5.1.1   ROLE IN THERAPY OF OVARIAN CANCER

The first study on the pharmacological behavior of SC-560 in ovarian cancer modeling showed elevated cyclooxygenase-1 levels in the ovarian tumor with extensive angiogenesis. The study was based on a histopathological pattern (Gupta et al., 2003). The antiproliferative effects of indomethacin and celecoxib were observed in in-vitro, SC-560 (selective and cyclooxygenase-2 non-COX isoforms, respectively) when 50–100 times more dose was administered in in-vivo structures of the same cancer cells known for the expression and activity of COX isoforms (Smith et al., 1998). In comparison, only SC-560 inhibited the VEGF secretion induced with AA at small doses, a dose-dependent effect that was reversed by PGE_2. Daikoku then demonstrated *in vivo* inhibitory growth of tumor effectiveness of SC-560 in ovarian cancer which was genetically engineered, and that were familiar to various genetic alterations associated with the disease, as

COX-1 overexpression (Daikoku et al., 2005, 2006). With respect to COX-1 downstream objectives, the (Peroxisome Proliferator-Activated Receptor Gamma-Extracellular signal Regulated Kinase) PPARδ-ERK signaling participation in human and murine ovarian cancer was experimentally evidenced (Daikoku et al., 2007). Li W in SKOV-3 xenograft model widely examined SC-560 for its in-vivo activity (Li et al., 2009–2012, 2015, 2014). The main expression of SKOV-3 cells in this model is the COX-1 isoform, determined by immunohistochemical cell specimens (Li et al., 2010), and the inhibitor-specific COX-1 dose attained a slight to moderate decrease in tumor development throughSC-560. Cisplatin (Li et al., 2014) or taxol (Li et al., 2012, 2014, 2015) were generally better than single drugs at different pharmacological endpoints, that includes apoptosis, angiogenesis, and proliferation in association with SC-560. There was elevated effectiveness of SKOV-3 system when a combination of SC-560 with the nonselective COX-inhibitor, Ibuprofen (Li et al., 2009) was administered. This elevation was also observed when SC-560 was given in combination with selective celebrcoxib inhibitor, Celecoxib (Li et al., 2011). This suggested a possible compensation in xenograft biology between the two isoforms that could be achieved if both COX-1 and COX-2 are inhibited. The *in vivo* impacts of SC-560 on the SKOV-3 system may be correlated from a mechanical point of perspective with treatment-independent PGE_2 reduced production and related angiogenesis inhibition. There is no definite proof that prostaglandin development in SKOV-3 cells is exclusive or predominantly dependent on COX-1. Moreover, COX-2 (Brenneis et al., 2006) may also be inhibited by *in vitro* SC-560 systems, and COX-independent impacts may add to the activity of antitumor agents. Some of the concerns are partially due to the cell line (SKOV-3) itself; in some instances, the COX-1 expression (Gupta et al., 2003) is reported to be negative. The contrast findings vary from the cell line source, from a technical issue to an antibody-cross-reactivity (Saed et al., 2008) to different experimental circumstances (i.e., *in-vitro* versus *in-vivo*). This is certainly not uncommon in cyclooxygenase literature. It is interesting to note that SC-560 also increases the sensitivity of pacli-taxel to the MDR_1/P-glycoprotein up-regulation of taxane-resistant OVC lines. A comparable impact was generated by the NS398 selective COX-2 inhibitor, which was not changed by the addition of PGE_2 (Lee et al., 2013). SC-560 also indicates the real option that it could be a potential lead for the treatment of ovarian cancer (Huang et al., 2014). Besides co-extrapolation with CMAP, the characterization of gene expression profiling produced an enormous repository of information on gene expression, explaining the newly identified feature. This provides data on the gene expression altered in several cell lines treated with > 1000 bioactive compounds (Lee et al., 2007).

16.5.1.2 ROLE IN THERAPY OF COLORECTAL CANCER

Grosch studied the impact of SC-560 on survival, development of cells and apoptosis of COX-1, and COX-2 modulated cancers, *in vitro* and *in vivo* in contrast to celecoxib against cells of colorectal cancer (Grosch et al., 2001). Irrelevant to the COX status, *in vitro* cell survival was impacted by both SC-560 and celecoxib, while apoptosis was induced by celecoxib alone. *In vivo*, both the compounds were active in the direction of xenograft HCT-15 (COX-2 deficient) but had no vital impact on tumors with HT-29 (COX-2 expressing), suggesting a general mechanism of action based on COX. Wu WK (Wu et al., 2009) also investigated the effects of SC-560 on colon cancer cells HT-29, showing that G1-S was accompanied with the transitional arrest and 3-kinase phosphoinositide (PI3K)-induced autophagy. HCT-116 colon cancer cells completely lacking COX expression and activity (Sheng et al., 1997), proliferation, inhibition, and cell cycle progression arrest *in vitro* caused by SC-560 have been researched. Lee showed that cell cycle regulator protein p21CIP1 had an impact on the growth inhibitory effect of HCT116 neurons (Lee et al., 2006). In addition, Sakoguchi-Okada N showed that the inhibition of surviving expression and Wnt/beta-catenin signaling pathway were associated with the growth and apoptotic effect of SC-560 (as well as other nonselective and COX-2-selective inhibitors on HCT-116 cells) (Sakoguchi et al., 2007). To find potential COX-related action mechanisms of NSAIDs, HCT-116 cells modified with the treatment-induced gene expression by using subtractive hybridization suppression were implicated for the tumour proliferation status (Jain et al., 2004). Interestingly, SC-560, which suggested possible contrasting impacts on the antitumor activity of NAG-1 (formally known as GDF15) and Thymosin-4 (TMSB5X), was caused by two cancer-based genes. In fact, NAG-1 codes for a TGF super-family of pleiotropic cytokines in a variety of cell kinds and included in a cell stress response program. A tumor-growth suppressive or improving induction impact of NAG-1 can be depending on its (acute or continuous) induction pattern and pathophysiology (Moon et al., 2017). Thymosin-4 induction could, too, potentially jeopardize SC-560 anti-carcinogenicity, involving thymosin-4 mechanistically in the metastasis (Wang et al., 2004;

Piao et al., 2004) and in the adverse prognosis of CRC (Gemoll et al., 2015). The dose required For effective inhibition of Human Lung cancer cell line such as H460, H358 and A549 are higher as compared to the ones needed for inhibiting the COX. SC-560 has shown to suppress the growth, inhibit reactive oxygen species production and cell proliferation in multiple myeloma at dose 10 times greater than those required for inhibiting the enzyme (Lee et al., 2006; Ding et al., 2006) In cancer cell lines HA22T/VGH and HuH-6, SC-560 therapy led to acute apoptosis and developmental inhibition. Combination therapy of coxib CAY10404 and SC-560 is linked to activation of the ERK1/2 signalling pathway.

16.5.2 MOFEZOLAC (5-(4-CHLOROPHENYL)-1-(4-METHOXYPHENYL)-3-(TRIFLUOROMETHYL)PYRAZOLE)

In Japan, Mofezolac was developed and marketed as a strong pain killer (Goto et al., 1998) among the few selective COX-1 inhibitors examined as prospective analgesics and antiplatelet agents, and its anticancer activity has almost solely been studied in experimental patterns on colorectal cancer. *In vitro* therapy of a COX-1-expressive RGMI cell line (non-transformed cells derived from rat gastric mucosa) by mofezolac induces a weak apoptotic impact, significantly autonomous of prostaglandin synthesis, with regard to indomethacin or sodium diclofenac (Kusuhara et al., 1998), and comparable conduct has also been observed in gastric adenocarcinoma cells of AGS, treated at levels comparable to those found at gastric mucosa after oral administration (Kusuhara et al., 1999). Mofezolac therapy decreases the growth of aberrant crypt foci (putative preneoplastic lesions) caused by azoxymethane (AOM) with respect to *in-vitro* colorectal cancer models, suppressing the amount of Apc knockout polyps. Mofezolac's effectiveness was comparable for both murine models to that of nimesulide, suggesting a tumorigenic function for both isoforms of cyclooxygenase (Kitamura et al., 2002). Accordingly, polyp development was suppressed better with combination therapy of COX-1-and COX-2-selective inhibitors rather than one single therapy in Apc knockout mice (Kitamura et al., 2004). In order to substantially reduce the occurrence, multiplicity, and volumes of AOM-inducing colon carcinomas (Niho et al., 2006), mofezolac inhibits preneoplastic lesions, thus confirming the pathophysiological function of COX-1 in AOM-induced intestinal carcinomas. With regards to mofezolac it is also interesting to note that beef tallow promoted cancer of the colon in the rats can be suppressed, thus indicating a potential advantage to high-fat populations (Miao et al., 2011).

16.5.3 FR122047 (1-((4,5-BIS(4-METHOXYPHENYL)-2-THIAZOYL) CARBONYL)-4-METHYL PIPERAZINE)

The COX-1-selective inhibitor, FR122047 was initially designed as a anti-platelet agent without ulcerative effects (Tanaka et al., 1994), and has been investigated as an analgesic (Ochi et al., 2000), or has been utilized as an instrument to investigate the participation of COX-1, and the function of the prostanoids produced in COX-1 and COX-2 processes in multiple types of inflammatory substances (Ochi et al., 2002, 2003). The antitumor activity by the FR122047 in MCF-7 breast cancer cells was examined *in vitro* (Jeong et al., 2010). FR122047 therapy inhibits MCF-7 cell's in-vitro cell development and leads to apoptotic cell death, which is mechanistically autonomous both from the development of ROS and PGE_2 associated therapy production. Further research has been carried out in the same group of (Jeong et al., 2011) MCF-7 cell death mechanisms caused by FR122047, demonstrating that the therapy FR122047 causes caspase-mediated apoptosis, while parallely stimulating the defensive autophagic reaction of the MCF-7 neurons. It is noteworthy that caspase-9 inhibits the cytoprotective self-reinforced process and therefore increases MCF-7's susceptibility to induced cell death by cell FR-122047.

Overall, COX-1 selective inhibitors are like other NSAIDs, and the COX-dependent mechanisms have been recorded in some instances, others being COX-independent. The *in vitro* effects of the tumor cycle characteristic for COX expression and activity are generally studied in preliminary testing of the anticancer components of COX inhibitors. The dose required for effective inhibition of Human Lung cancer cell line such as H460, H358 and A549 are higher as compared to the ones needed for inhibiting the COX. SC-560 has shown to suppress the growth, inhibit reactive oxygen species production and cell proliferation in multiple myeloma at dose 10 times greater than those required for inhibiting the enzyme (Lee et al., 2006; Ding et al., 2006) In cancer cell lines HA22T/VGH and HuH-6, SC-560 therapy led to acute apoptosis and developmental inhibition. Combination therapy of coxib CAY10404 and SC-560 is linked to activation of the ERK1/2 signalling pathway. The biological endpoint is usually connected with the cell cycle G_1 phase arrest and cell death, impairing cell development and proliferation. These impacts generally occur at levels of compounds which are much higher than the prevalent cytotoxic drug (Boccarelli et al., 2011), and more significant than the COX-inhibitor levels which are clinically significant. In fact, the real efficient COX inhibitor concentration in *in-vitro* systems could be less than what was stated because of a subtractive interaction with culture medium's serum proteins (Lin et al., 1987). Therefore, COX-1 inhibitors and traditional NSAIDs possess weak antiproliferative impacts in connection with enzyme inhibition while considering the caution against protein interaction. This likely represents the weak effect of *in vitro* development and proliferation conditions of COX-derived PGs. These molecules are not functioning as primary indicators of homeostasis alteration, but as amplification signal at tissue levels in the various inflammatory pathological circumstances in which PG activity has been examined (Ricciotti et al., 2011). The *in vitro* proliferation of tumor cells is unlikely, as demonstrated by an absence of effectiveness of COX inhibitors in resting tumor cells (Duan et al., 2006).

KEYWORDS

- **acute lymphoid leukemia**
- **cyclooxygenase**
- **G protein-coupled receptor**
- **lipopolysaccharide**
- **prostaglandin**
- **renal cell carcinoma**
- **reverse transcription polymerase chain reaction**
- **vascular endothelial growth factors**

REFERENCES

Ali-Fehmi, R., Semaan, A., Sethi, S., Arabi, H., Bandyopadhyay, S., Hussein, Y. R., Diamond, M. P., et al., (2011). Molecular typing of epithelial ovarian carcinomas using inflammatory markers. *Cancer*, *117*(2), 301–309.

Balkwill, F., & Mantovani, A., (2001). Inflammation and cancer: Back to Virchow? *Lancet*, *357*(9255), 539–545.

Ben-Neriah, Y., & Karin, M., (2011). Inflammation meets cancer, with NF-_B as the matchmaker. *Nat. Immunol.*, *12*(8), 715–723.

Boccarelli, A., Pannunzio, A., & Coluccia, M., (2011). The challenge of establishing reliable screening tests for selecting anticancer metal compounds. *Bioinorganic Medicinal Chemistry*, 175–196.

Botha, J. H., Robinson, K. M., Ramchurren, N., Reddi, K., & Norman, R. J., (1986). Human esophageal carcinoma cell lines: Prostaglandin production, biological properties, and behavior in nude mice. *J. Natl. Cancer Inst.*, *76*(6), 1053–1056.

Brenneis, C., Maier, T. J., Schmidt, R., Hofacker, A., Zulauf, L., Jakobsson, P. J., Scholich, K., & Geisslinger, G., (2006). Inhibition of prostaglandin E2 synthesis by SC-560 is independent of cyclooxygenase 1 inhibition. *FASEB J., 20*(9), 1352–1360.

Cathcart, M. C., O'Byrne, K. J., Reynolds, J. V., O'Sullivan, J., & Pidgeon, G. P., (2012). COX-derived prostanoid pathways in gastrointestinal cancer development and progression: Novel targets for prevention and intervention. *Biochim. Biophys. Acta., 1825*(1), 49–63.

Cheng, J., & Fan, X. M., (2013). Role of cyclooxygenase-2 in gastric cancer development and progression. *World J. Gastroenterol., 19*(42), 7361–7368.

Chulada, P. C., Thompson, M. B., Mahler, J. F., Doyle, C. M., Gaul, B. W., Lee, C., Tiano, H. F., et al., (2000). Genetic disruption of Ptgs-1, as well as Ptgs-2, reduces intestinal tumorigenesis in min mice. *Cancer Res., 60*(16), 4705–4708.

Church, R. D., Yu, J., Fleshman, J. W., Shannon, W. D., Govindan, R., & McLeod, H. L., (2004). RNA profiling of cyclooxygenases 1 and 2 in colorectal cancer. *Br. J. Cancer, 91*(6), 1015–1018.

Coussens, L. M., Zitvogel, L., & Palucka, A. K., (2013). Neutralizing tumor-promoting chronic inflammation: A magic bullet. *Science, 339*(6117), 286–291.

Daikoku, T., Tranguch, S., Chakrabarty, A., Wang, D., Khabele, D., Orsulic, S., Morrow, J. D., et al., (2007). Extracellular signal-regulated kinase is a target of cyclooxygenase-1-peroxisome proliferator-activated receptor-delta signaling in epithelial ovarian cancer. *Cancer Res., 67*(11), 5285–5292.

Daikoku, T., Tranguch, S., Trofimova, I. N., Dinulescu, D. M., Jacks, T., Nikitin, A. Y., Connolly, D. C., & Dey, S. K., (2006). Cyclooxygenase-1 is over expressed in multiple genetically engineered mouse models of epithelial ovarian cancer. *Cancer Res., 66*(5), 2527–2531.

Daikoku, T., Wang, D., Tranguch, S., Morrow, J. D., Orsulic, S., DuBois, R. N., & Dey, S. K., (2005). Cyclooxygenase-1 is a potential target for prevention and treatment of ovarian epithelial cancer. *Cancer Res., 65*(9), 3735–3744.

Dennis, E. A., & Norris, P. C., (2015). Eicosanoid stormin infection and inflammation. *Nat. Rev. Immunol., 15*(8), 511–523.

Ding, J., Tsuboi, K., Hoshikawa, H., Goto, R., Mori, N., Katsukawa, M., Hiraki, E., et al., (2006). Cyclooxygenase isozymes are expressed in human myeloma cells but not involved in anti-proliferative effect of cyclooxygenase inhibitors. *Mol. Carcinog., 45*(4), 250–259.

Dixon, D. A., Blanco, F. F., Bruno, A., & Patrignani, P., (2013). Mechanistic aspects of COX-2 expression in colorectal neoplasia. *Recent Results Cancer Res., 191*, 7–37.

Dovizio, M., Tacconelli, S., Ricciotti, E., Bruno, A., Maier, T. J., Anzellotti, P., Francesco, L. D., et al., (2012). Effects of celecoxib on prostanoid biosynthesis and circulating angiogenesis proteins in familial adenomatous polyposis. *J. Pharmacol. Exp. Ther., 341*(1), 242–250.

Duan, W., & Zhang, L., (2006). Cyclooxygenase inhibitors not inhibit resting lung cancer A549 cell proliferation. *Prostaglandins Leukot. Essent. Fat. Acids, 74*(5), 317–321.

Eilati, E., Pan, L., Bahr, J. M., & Hales, D. B., (2012). Age-dependent increase in prostaglandin pathway coincides with onset of ovarian cancer in laying hens. *Prostaglandins Leukot. Essent. Fat. Acids, 87*(6), 177–184.

Elmets, C. A., Ledet, J. J., & Athar, M., (2014). Cyclooxygenases: Mediators of UV-induced skin cancer and potential targets for prevention. *J. Investig. Dermatol., 134*(10), 2497–2502.

Erovic, B. M., Woegerbauer, M., Pammer, J., Selzer, E., Grasl, M. C., & Thurnher, D., (2008). Strong evidence for up-regulation of cyclooxygenase-1 in head and neck cancer. *Eur. J. Clin. Investig.*, *38*(1), 61–66.

Esquivias, P., Morandeira, A., Escartín, A., Cebrián, C., Santander, S., Esteva, F., García-González, M. A., et al., (2012). Indomethacin but not a selective cyclooxygenase-2 inhibitor inhibits esophageal adenocarcinogenesis in rats. *World J. Gastroenterol.*, *18*(35), 4866–4874.

Fahlén, M., Zhang, H., Löfgren, L., Masironi, B., Von, S. E., Von, S. B., & Sahlin, L., (2017). Expression of cyclooxygenase-1 and cyclooxygenase-2, syndecan-1 and connective tissue growth factor in benign and malignant breast tissue from premenopausal women. *Gynecol. Endocrinol.*, *33*(5), 353–358.

Fiancette, R., Vincent-Fabert, C., Guerin, E., Trimoreau, F., & Denizot, Y., (2011). Lipid mediators and human leukemic blasts. *J. Oncol.*, 389021.

Gakis, G., (2014). The role of inflammation in bladder cancer. *Adv. Exp. Med. Biol.*, *816*, 183–196.

Gemoll, T., Strohkamp, S., Schillo, K., Thorns, C., & Habermann, J. K., (2015). MALDI-imaging reveals thymosin beta-4 as an independent prognostic marker for colorectal cancer. *Oncotarget*, *6*(41), 43869–43880.

Glover, J. A., Hughes, C. M., Cantwell, M. M., & Murray, L. J., (2011). A systematic review to establish the frequency of cyclooxygenase-2 expression in normal breast epithelium, ductal carcinoma in situ, microinvasive carcinoma of the breast and invasive breast cancer. *Br. J. Cancer*, *105*(1), 13–17.

Goto, K., Ochi, H., Yasunaga, Y., Matsuyuki, H., Imayoshi, T., Kusuhara, H., & Okumoto, T., (1998). Analgesic effect of mofezolac, a non-steroidal anti-inflammatory drug, against phenylquinone-induced acute pain in mice. *Prostaglandins Other Lipid Mediat.*, *56*(4), 245–254.

Greenhough, A., Smartt, H. J., Moore, A. E., Roberts, H. R., Williams, A. C., Paraskeva, C., & Kaidi, A., (2009). The COX-2/PGE2 pathway: Key roles in the hallmarks of cancer and adaptation to the tumor microenvironment. *Carcinogenesis*, *30*(3), 377–386.

Grösch, S., Tegeder, I., Niederberger, E., Bräutigam, L., & Geisslinger, G., (2001). COX-2 independent induction of cell cycle arrest and apoptosis in colon cancer cells by the selective COX-2 inhibitor celecoxib. *FASEB J.*, *15*(14), 2742–2744.

Gudis, K., & Sakamoto, C., (2005). The role of cyclooxygenase in gastric mucosal protection. *Dig. Dis. Sci.*, *50*(1), S16–S23.

Gupta, R. A., Tejada, L. V., Tong, B. J., Das, S. K., Morrow, J. D., Dey, S. K., & DuBois, R. N., (2003). Cyclooxygenase-1 is overexpressed and promotes angiogenic growth factor production in ovarian cancer. *Cancer Res.*, *63*(5), 906–911.

Haakensen, V. D., Bjøro, T., Lüders, T., Riis, M., Bukholm, I. K., Kristensen, V. N., Troester, M. A., et al., (2011). Serum estradiol levels associated with specific gene expression patterns in normal breast tissue and in breast carcinomas. *BMC Cancer*, *11*, 332.

Hales, D. B., Zhuge, Y., Lagman, J. A., Ansenberger, K., Mahon, C., Barua, A., Luborsky, J. L., & Bahr, J. M., (2008). Cyclooxygenases expression and distribution in the normal ovary and their role in ovarian cancer in the domestic hen (*Gallus domesticus*). *Endocrine*, *33*(3), 235–244.

Hanahan, D., & Weinberg, R. A., (2011). Hallmarks of cancer: The next generation. *Cell*, *144*(5), 646–674.

Harris, R. E., (2007). Cyclooxygenase-2(cox-2) and the inflammogenesis of cancer. *Subcell. Biochem.*, *42*, 93–126.

Hirata, T., & Narumiya, S., (2011). Prostanoid receptors. *Chem. Rev.*, *111*(10), 6209–6230.

Huang, Y., Ju, B., Tian, J., Liu, F., Yu, H., Xiao, H., Liu, X., et al., (2014). Ovarian cancer stem cell-specific gene expression profiling and targeted drug prescreening. *Oncol. Rep.*, *31*(3), 1235–1248.

Hwang, D., Scollard, D., Byrne, J., & Levine, E., (1998). Expression of cyclooxygenase-1 and cyclooxygenase-2 in human breast cancer. *J. Natl. Cancer Inst.*, *90*(6), 455–460.

Jain, A. K., Moore, S. M., Yamaguchi, K., Eling, T. E., & Baek, S. J., (2004). Selective nonsteroidal anti-inflammatory drugs induce thymosin beta-4 and alter actin cytoskeletal organization in human colorectal cancer cells. *J. Pharmacol. Exp. Ther.*, *311*(3), 885–891.

Jeong, H. S., Choi, H. Y., Lee, E. R., Kim, J. H., Jeon, K., Lee, H. J., & Cho, S. G., (2011). Involvement of caspase-9 in autophagy-mediated cell survival pathway. *Biochim. Biophys. Acta*, *1813*(1), 80–90.

Jeong, H. S., Kim, J. H., Choi, H. Y., Lee, E. R., & Cho, S. G., (2010). Induction of cell growth arrest and apoptotic cell death in human breast cancer MCF-7 cells by the COX-1 inhibitor FR122047. *Oncol. Rep.*, *24*(2), 51–356.

Kaminska, K., Szczylik, C., Lian, F., & Czarnecka, A. M., (2014). The role of prostaglandin E2 in renal cell cancer development: Future implications for prognosis and therapy. *Future Oncol.*, *10*(14), 2177–2187.

Kino, Y., Kojima, F., Kiguchi, K., Igarashi, R., Ishizuka, B., & Kawai, S., (2005). Prostaglandin E2 production in ovarian cancer cell lines is regulated by cyclooxygenase-1, not cyclooxygenase-2. *Prostaglandins Leukot. Essent. Fat. Acids*, *73*(2), 103–111.

Kitamura, T., Itoh, M., Noda, T., Matsuura, M., & Wakabayashi, K., (2004). Combined effects of cyclooxygenase-1 and cyclooxygenase-2 selective inhibitors on intestinal tumorigenesis in adenomatous polyposis coli gene knockout mice. *Int. J. Cancer*, *109*(4), 576–580.

Kitamura, T., Kawamori, T., Uchiya, N., Itoh, M., Noda, T., Matsuura, M., Sugimura, T., & Wakabayashi, K., (2002). Inhibitory effects of mofezolac, a cyclooxygenase-1 selective inhibitor, on intestinal carcinogenesis. *Carcinogenesis*, *23*(9), 1463–1466.

Knab, L. M., Grippo, P. J., & Bentrem, D. J., (2014). Involvement of eicosanoids in the pathogenesis of pancreatic cancer: The roles of cyclooxygenase-2 and 5-lipoxygenase. *World J. Gastroenterol.*, *20*(31), 10729–10739.

Kulmacz, R. J., (2005). Regulation of cyclooxygenase catalysis by hydroperoxides. *Biochem. Biophys. Res. Commun.*, *338*(1), 25–33.

Kusuhara, H., Komatsu, H., Sumichika, H., & Sugahara, K., (1999). Reactive oxygen species are involved in the apoptosis induced by nonsteroidal anti-inflammatory drugs in cultured gastric cells. *Eur. J. Pharmacol.*, *383*(3), 331–337.

Kusuhara, H., Matsuyuki, H., Matsuura, M., Imayoshi, T., Okumoto, T., & Matsui, H., (1998). Induction of apoptotic DNA fragmentation by nonsteroidal anti-inflammatory drugs in cultured rat gastric mucosal cells. *Eur. J. Pharmacol.*, *360*(2/3), 273–280.

Lampiasi, N., Foderà, D., D'Alessandro, N., Cusimano, A., Azzolina, A., Tripodo, C., Florena, A. M., et al., (2006). The selective cyclooxygenase-1 inhibitor SC-560 suppresses cell proliferation and induces apoptosis in human hepatocellular carcinoma cells. *Int. J. Mol. Med.*, *17*(2), 245–252.

Langenbach, R., Loftin, C., Lee, C., & Tiano, H., (1999). Cyclooxygenase knockout mice: Models for elucidating isoform-specific functions. *Biochem. Pharmacol.*, *58*(8), 1237–1246.

Lau, M. T., Wong, A. S., & Leung, P. C., (2010). Gonadotropins induce tumor cell migration and invasion by increasing cyclooxygenases expression and prostaglandin E (2) production in human ovarian cancer cells. *Endocrinology, 151*(7), 2985–2993.

Lee, E., Choi, M. K., Han, I. O., & Lim, S. J., (2006). Role of p21CIP1 as a determinant of SC560 response in human HCT116 colon carcinoma cells. *Exp. Mol. Med., 38*(3), 325–331.

Lee, E., Choi, M. K., Youk, H. J., Kim, C. H., Han, I. O., Yoo, B. C., Lee, M. K., & Lim, S. J., (2006). 5-(4-chlorophenyl)-1-(4-methoxyphenyl)-3-trifluoromethylpyrazole acts in a reactive oxygen species-dependent manner to suppress human lung cancer growth. *J. Cancer Res. Clin. Oncol., 132*(4), 223–233.

Lee, G., & Ng, H. T., (1995). Clinical evaluations of a new ovarian cancer marker, COX-1. *Int. J. Gynaecol. Obstet., 49*, S27–S32.

Lee, J. K., Havaleshko, D. M., Cho, H., Weinstein, J. N., Kaldjian, E. P., Karpovich, J., Grimshaw, A., & Theodorescu, D., (2007). A strategy for predicting the chemosensitivity of human cancer and its application to drug discovery. *Proc. Natl. Acad. Sci. USA., 104*(32), 13086–13091.

Lee, J. P., Hahn, H. S., Hwang, S. J., Choi, J. Y., Park, J. S., Lee, I. H., & Kim, T. J., (2013). Selective cyclooxygenase inhibitors increase paclitaxel sensitivity in taxane-resistant ovarian cancer by suppressing P-glycoprotein expression. *J. Gynecol. Oncol., 24*(3), 273–279.

Li, H., Liu, K., Lisa, A. B., Zhao, Y., Wang, L., Sheng, Y., Oi, N., Limburg, P. J., Bode, A. M., & Dong, Z., (2015). Circulating prostaglandin biosynthesis in colorectal cancer and potential clinical significance. *EBio. Medicine, 2*(2), 165–171.

Li, H., Zhu, F., Chen, H., Cheng, K. W., Zykova, T., Oi, N., Lubet, R. A., Bode, A. M., Wang, M., & Dong, Z., (2014). 6-C-(E-phenylethenyl)-naringenin suppresses colorectal cancer growth by inhibiting cyclooxygenase-1. *Cancer Res., 74*(1), 243–252.

Li, W., Cai, J. H., Zhang, J., Tang, Y. X., & Wan, L., (2012). Effects of cyclooxygenase inhibitors in combination with taxol on expression of cyclin D1 and Ki-67 in a xenograft model of ovarian carcinoma. *Int. J. Mol. Sci., 13*(8), 9741–9753.

Li, W., Ji, Z. L., Zhuo, G. C., Xu, R. J., Wang, J., & Jiang, H. R., (2010). Effects of a selective cyclooxygenase-1 inhibitor in SKOV-3 ovarian carcinoma xenograft-bearing mice. *Med. Oncol., 27*(1), 98–104.

Li, W., Liu, M. L., Cai, J. H., Tang, Y. X., Zhai, L. Y., & Zhang, J., (2012). Effect of the combination of a cyclooxygenase-1 selective inhibitor and taxol on proliferation, apoptosis, and angiogenesis of ovarian cancer *in vivo*. *Oncol. Lett., 4*(1), 168–174.

Li, W., Tang, Y. X., Wan, L., Cai, J. H., & Zhang, J., (2015). Effects of combining Taxol and cyclooxygenase inhibitors on the angiogenesis and apoptosis in human ovarian cancer xenografts. *Oncol. Lett., 5*(3), 923–928.

Li, W., Wan, L., Zhai, L. Y., & Wang, J., (2014). Effects of SC-560 in combination with cisplatin or taxol on angiogenesis in human ovarian cancer xenografts. *Int. J. Mol. Sci., 15*(10), 19265–19280.

Li, W., Wang, J., Jiang, H. R., Xu, X. L., Zhang, J., Liu, M. L., & Zhai, L. Y., (2011). Combined effects of cyclooxygenase-1 and cyclooxygenase-2 selective inhibitors on ovarian carcinoma *in vivo*. *Int. J. Mol. Sci., 12*(1), 668–681.

Li, W., Xu, R. J., Lin, Z. Y., Zhuo, G. C., & Zhang, H. H., (2009). Effects of a cyclooxygenase-1-selective inhibitor in a mouse model of ovarian cancer, administered alone or in combination with ibuprofen, a nonselective cyclooxygenase inhibitor. *Med. Oncol., 26*(2), 170–177.

Li, X., & Tai, H. H., (2009). Activation of thromboxane A(2) receptors induces orphan nuclear receptor Nurr1 expression and stimulates cell proliferation in human lung cancer cells. *Carcinogenesis*, *30*(9), 1606–1613.

Lin, J. H., Cocchetto, D. M., & Duggan, D. E., (1987). Protein binding as a primary determinant of the clinical pharmacokinetic properties of non-steroidal anti-inflammatory drugs. *Clin. Pharmacokinet*, *12*(6), 402–432.

Liu, Q., Tao, B., Liu, G., Chen, G., Zhu, Q., Yu, Y., Yu, Y., & Xiong, H., (2016). Thromboxane A2 receptor inhibition suppresses multiple myeloma cell proliferation by inducing p38/c-Jun N-terminal Kinase (JNK) mitogen-activated protein kinase (MAPK)-mediated G2/M progression delay and cell apoptosis. *J. Biol. Chem.*, *291*(9), 4779–4792.

McAdam, B. F., Mardini, I. A., Habib, A., Burke, A., Lawson, J. A., Kapoor, S., & FitzGerald, G. A., (2000). Effect of regulated expression of human cyclooxygenase isoforms on eicosanoid and isoeicosanoid production in inflammation. *J. Clin. Invest.*, *105*(10), 1473–1482.

Mendes, R. A., Carvalho, J. F., & Waal, I. V., (2009). An overview on the expression of cyclooxygenase-2 in tumors of the head and neck. *Oral Oncol.*, *45*(10), e124–e128.

Miao, L., Shiraishi, R., Fujise, T., Kuroki, T., Kakimoto, T., Sakata, Y., Takashima, T., et al., (2011). Chemopreventive effect of mofezolac on beef tallow diet/azoxymethane-induced colon carcinogenesis in rats. *Hepato-gastroenterology*, *58*(105), 81–88.

Moon, Y., (2017). NSAID-activated gene 1 and its implications for mucosal integrity and intervention beyond NSAIDs. *Pharmacol. Res.*, *121*, 122–128.

Morita, I., (2002). Distinct functions of COX-1 and COX-2. *Prostaglandins Other Lipid Mediat.*, *68, 69*, 165–175.

Müller-Decker, K., (2011). Cyclooxygenase-dependent signaling is causally linked to non-melanoma skin carcinogenesis: Pharmacological, genetic, and clinical evidence. *Cancer Metastasis Rev.*, *30*(3/4), 343–361.

Niho, N., Kitamura, T., Takahashi, M., Mutoh, M., Sato, H., Matsuura, M., Sugimura, T., & Wakabayashi, K., (2006). Suppression of azoxymethane-induced colon cancer development in rats by a cyclooxygenase-1 selective inhibitor, mofezolac. *Cancer Sci.*, *97*(10), 1011–1014.

Nuvoli, B., & Galati, R., (2013). Cyclooxygenase-2, epidermal growth factor receptor, and aromatase signaling in inflammation and mesothelioma. *Mol. Cancer Ther.*, *12*(6), 844–852.

Ochi, T., & Goto, T., (2002). Differential effects of FR122047, a selective cyclo-oxygenase-1 inhibitor, in rat chronic models of arthritis. *Br. J. Pharmacol.*, *135*(5), 782–788.

Ochi, T., Motoyama, Y., & Goto, T., (2000). The analgesic effect profile of FR122047, a selective cyclooxygenase-1 inhibitor, in chemical nociceptive models. *Eur. J. Pharmacol.*, *391*(1/2), 49–54.

Ochi, T., Ohkubo, Y., & Mutoh, S., (2003). Role of cyclooxygenase-2, but not cyclooxygenase-1, on type II collagen-induced arthritis in DBA/1J mice. *Biochem. Pharmacol.*, *66*(6), 1055–1060.

Okamoto, T., Hara, A., & Hino, O., (2003). Down-regulation of cyclooxygenase-2 expression but up-regulation of cyclooxygenase-1 in renal carcinomas of the Eker (TSC2 gene mutant) rat model. *Cancer Sci.*, *94*(1), 22–25.

Osman, W. M., & Youssef, N. S., (2015). Combined use of COX-1 and VEGF immunohistochemistry refines the histopathologic prognosis of renal cell carcinoma. *Int. J. Clin. Exp. Pathol.*, *8*(7), 8165–8177.

Parida, S., & Mandal, M., (2014). Inflammation induced by human papillomavirus in cervical cancer and its implication in prevention. *Eur. J. Cancer Prev.*, *23*(5), 432–448.

Piao, Z., Hong, C. S., Jung, M. R., Choi, C., & Park, Y. K., (2014). Thymosin β4 induces invasion and migration of human colorectal cancer cells through the ILK/AKT/ β-catenin signaling pathway. *Biochem. Biophys. Res. Commun.*, *452*(3), 858–864.

Piazuelo, E., Santander, S., Cebrián, C., Jiménez, P., Pastor, C., García-González, M. A., Esteva, F., et al., (2012). Characterization of the prostaglandin E2 pathway in a rat model of esophageal adenocarcinoma. *Curr. Cancer Drug Targets*, *12*(2), 132–143.

Ramon, S., Woeller, C. F., & Phipps, R. P., (2013). The influence of Cox-2 and bioactive lipids on hematological cancers. *Curr. Angiogenes.*, *2*(2), 135–142.

Ricciotti, E., & FitzGerald, G. A., (2011). Prostaglandins and inflammation. *Arterioscler. Thromb. Vasc. Biol.*, *31*(5), 986–1000.

Rouzer, C. A. L. J., (2003). Marnett. Mechanism of free radical oxygenation of polyunsaturated fatty acids by cyclooxygenases. *Chem. Rev.*, *103*(6), 2239–2304.

Rouzer, C. A., & Marnett, L. J., (2009). Cyclooxygenases: Structural and functional insights. *J. Lipid Res.*, *50*, S29–S34.

Rundhaug, J. E., Simper, M. S., Surh, I., & Fischer, S. M., (2011). The role of the EP receptors for prostaglandin E2 in skin and skin cancer. *Cancer Metastasis Rev.*, *30*(3/4), 465–480.

Saed, G. M., (2008). Immunohistochemical staining of cyclooxygenases with monoclonal antibodies. *Methods Mol. Biol., 477*, 219–228.

Sales, K. J., Katz, A. A., Howard, B., Soeters, R. P., Millar, R. P., & Jabbour, H. N., (2002). Cyclooxygenase 1 is up-regulated in cervical carcinomas: Autocrine/paracrine regulation of cyclooxygenase-2, prostaglandin E receptors, and angiogenic factors by cyclooxygenase-1. *Cancer Res.*, *62*(2), 424–432.

Sales, K. J., Sutherland, J. R., Jabbour, H. N., & Katz, A. A., (2012). Seminal plasma induces angiogenic chemokine expression in cervical cancer cells and regulates vascular function. *Biochim. Biophys. Acta*, *1823*(10), 1789–1795.

Shao, N., Feng, N., Wang, Y., Mi, Y., Li, T., & Hua, L. X., (2012). Systematic review and meta-analysis of COX-2 expression and polymorphisms in prostate cancer. *Mol. Biol. Rep.*, *39*(12), 10997–11004.

Sheng, H., Shao, J., Kirkland, S. C., Isakson, P., Coffey, R. J., Morrow, J., Beauchamp, R. D., & DuBois, R. N., (1997). Inhibition of human colon cancer cell growth by selective inhibition of cyclooxygenase-2. *J. Clin. Investig.*, *99*(9), 2254–2259.

Smartt, H. J., Greenhough, A., Ordóñez-Morán, P., Talero, E., Cherry, C. A., Wallam, C. A., Parry, L., et al., (2012). β-catenin represses expression of the tumor suppressor 15-prostaglandin dehydrogenase in the normal intestinal epithelium and colorectal tumor cells. *Gut.*, *61*(9), 1306–13014.

Smith, C. J., Zhang, Y., Koboldt, C. M., Muhammad, J., Zweifel, B. S., Shaffer, A., Talley, J. J., et al., (1998). Pharmacological analysis of cyclooxygenase-1 in inflammation. *Proc. Natl. Acad. Sci. USA*, *95*(22), 13313–13318.

Smith, W. L., & Langenbach, R., (2001). Why there are two cyclooxygenase isozymes. *J. Clin. Invest.*, *107*(2), 1491–1495.

Smith, W. L., DeWitt, D. L., & Garavito, R. M., (2000). Cyclooxygenases: Structural, cellular, and molecular biology. *Annu. Rev. Biochem., 69*, 145–182.

Sugimoto, T., Koizumi, T., Sudo, T., Yamaguchi, S., Kojima, A., Kumagai, S., & Nishimura, R., (2007). Correlative expression of cyclooxygenase-*1*(Cox-1) and human epidermal growth factor receptor type-*2*(Her-2) in endometrial cancer. *Kobe J. Med. Sci.*, *53*(5), 177–187.

Sutherland, J. R., Sales, K. J., Jabbour, H. N., & Katz, A. A., (2012). Seminal plasma enhances cervical adenocarcinoma cell proliferation and tumor growth *in vivo*. *PLoS One*, *7*(3), e33848.

Takeda, H., Sonoshita, M., Oshima, H., Sugihara, K., Chulada, P. C., Langenbach, R., Oshima, M., & Taketo, M. M., (2003). Cooperation of cyclooxygenase 1 and cyclooxygenase 2 in intestinal polyposis. *Cancer Res., 63*(16), 4872–4877.

Tanaka, A., Sakai, H., Motoyama, Y., Ishikawa, T., & Takasugi, H., (1994). Antiplatelet agents based on cyclooxygenase inhibition without ulcerogenesis. Evaluation and synthesis of 4,5-bis(4-methoxyphenyl)-2-substituted thiazoles. *J. Med. Chem., 37*(8), 1189–1199.

Tang, J. Y., Aszterbaum, M., Athar, M., Barsanti, F., Cappola, C., Estevez, N., Hebert, J., et al., (2010). Basal cell carcinoma chemoprevention with nonsteroidal anti-inflammatory drugs in genetically predisposed PTCH1+ humans and mice. *Cancer Prev. Res., 3*(1), 25–34.

Tiano, H. F., Loftin, C. D., Akunda, J., Lee, C. A., Spalding, J., Dunson, D. B., Rogan, E. G., et al., (2002). Deficiency of either cyclooxygenase (COX)-1 or COX-2 alters epidermal differentiation and reduces mouse skin tumorigenesis. *Cancer Res., 62*(12), 3395–3401.

Tortorella, M. D., Zhang, Y., & Talley, J., (2016). Desirable Properties for 3rd Generation Cyclooxygenase-2 Inhibitors. *Mini Rev. Med. Chem., 16*(16), 1284–1289.

Urick, M. E., & Johnson, P. A., (2006). Cyclooxygenase 1 and 2 mRNA and protein expression in the Gallus domesticus model of ovarian cancer. *Gynecol. Oncol., 103*(2), 673–678.

Vitale, P., Panella, A., Scilimati, A., & Perrone, M. G., (2016). COX-1 inhibitors: Beyond structure toward therapy. *Med. Res. Rev., 36*(4), 641–671.

Von, R. B. H., Stein, H. J., Pühringer, F., Koch, I., Langer, R., Piontek, G., Siewert, J. R., et al., (2005). Coexpression of cyclooxygenases (COX-1, COX-2) and vascular endothelial growth factors (VEGF-A, VEGF-C) in esophageal adenocarcinoma. *Cancer Res., 65*(12), 5038–5044.

Vong, L., Ferraz, J. G., Panaccione, R., Beck, P. L., & Wallace, J. L., (2010). A pro-resolution mediator, prostaglandin D (2), is specifically up-regulated in individuals in long-term remission from ulcerative colitis. *Proc. Natl. Acad. Sci. USA., 107*(26), 12023–12027.

Wallace, J. L., Bak, A., McKnight, W., Asfaha, S., Sharkey, K. A., & MacNaughton, W. K., (1998). Cyclooxygenase 1 contributes to inflammatory responses in rats and mice: Implications for gastrointestinal toxicity. *Gastroenterology, 115*(1), 101–109.

Wang, W. S., Chen, P. M., Hsiao, H. L., Wang, H. S., Liang, W. Y., & Su, Y., (2004). Overexpression of the thymosin beta-4 gene is associated with increased invasion of SW480 colon carcinoma cells and the distant metastasis of human colorectal carcinoma. *Oncogene, 23*(39), 6666–6671.

Wu, W. K., Sung, J. J., Wu, Y. C., Li, H. T., Yu, L., Li, Z. J., & Cho, C. H., (2009). Inhibition of cyclooxygenase-1 lowers proliferation and induces macro autophagy in colon cancer cells. *Biochem. Biophys. Res. Commun., 382*(1), 79–84.

Yu, Y., Fan, J., Hui, Y., Rouzer, C. A., Marnett, L. J., Klein-Szanto, A. J., FitzGerald, G. A., & Funk, C. D., (2007). Targeted cyclooxygenase gene (ptgs) exchange reveals discriminant isoform functionality. *J. Biol. Chem., 282*(2), 1498–1506.

Yu, Z. H., Zhang, Q., Wang, Y. D., Chen, J., Jiang, Z. M., Shi, M., Guo, X., et al., (2013). Overexpression of cyclooxygenase-1 correlates with poor prognosis in renal cell carcinoma. *Asian Pac. J. Cancer Prev., 14*(6), 3729–3734.

Zhang, M., Zhou, S., Zhang, L., Ye, W., Wen, Q., & Wang, J., (2013). Role of cancer-related inflammation in esophageal cancer. *Crit. Rev. Eukaryot. Gene Expr., 23*(1), 27–35.

Zidar, N., Odar, K., Glavač, D., Jerše, M., Zupanc, T., & Štajer, D., (2009). Cyclooxygenase in normal human tissues-is COX-1 really a constitutive isoform, and COX-2 an inducible isoform? *J. Cell. Mol. Med., 13*(9b), 3753–3763.

CHAPTER 17

Microfluidic Devices in Capturing Circulating Metastatic Cancer Cell Clusters

SANDEEP ARORA, AJMER SINGH GREWAL, NEELAM SHARMA, and SUKHBIR SINGH

Chitkara College of Pharmacy, Chitkara University, Punjab, India

ABSTRACT

Metastasis is the leading reason behind tumor-associated mortality, and the spreading of tumor cells through the cardiovascular system is a critical stage in the metastatic progression. Circulating tumor cell clusters (CTC clusters) are effective initiators of metastasis and serve as potential biomarkers useful clinically for patients having cancer. Therefore, early detection and analysis of CTC clusters are significant for the early diagnosis, prognosis, and effective therapy of cancer, permitting satisfactory clinical results in the cancer patients. Accurate, precise, and consistent methods for isolation and detection of CTC clusters are required to achieve this clinical data. Over the past 20 years, microfluidic-based techniques had revealed great potential for isolation and detection of CTC clusters from the blood.

17.1 INTRODUCTION

So far, cancer is one of the prominent reasons for mortality in humans. Statistics indicated that 90% of deaths of cancer patients are associated with cancer metastasis, which is a complex process involving several steps: tumor cells first dislodge from a primary tumor, then invade the blood vessels, travel through the bloodstream, extravasate into a distant site, and finally form a new tumor as shown in Figure 17.1 (Joosse et al., 2015;

Cao et al., 2017; Zou and Cui, 2018). Detection of cancer predominantly comprises of conventional instrumentation and non-invasive methods. Generally, cancer diagnosis using conventional instrumentation methods is more complex, costly, and unsafe for the health of cancer patients. The non-invasive techniques represent to adjudging the phase of cancer progression or evaluating the consequence of cancer therapy by investigating the alterations of certain components in human urine and peripheral blood. Thus, the non-invasive detection techniques are more appropriate, precise, and harmless to the cancer patients, and have turned out to be the mainstream of cancer diagnosis in the prospect (Hyun and Jung, 2014; Chiu et al., 2018).

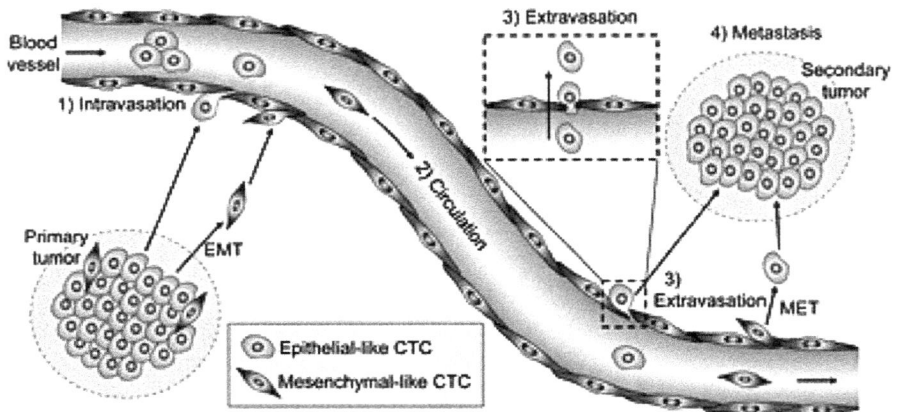

FIGURE 17.1   Stages of tumor metastasis and role of circulating tumor cell clusters in cancer metastasis (Reproduced from Cho et al., (2018) with permission from The Royal Society of Chemistry). (1) Tumor cells from primary cancer tissue invade blood vessels in the vicinity; (2) The invasive tumor cells circulate through the bloodstream; (3) CTC clusters adhere to blood vessel walls and extravasate to distant sites, resulting in metastasis; (4) Some of the metastatic tumor cells may go into a dormant state, while others develop into secondary tumors.

17.2   BIOLOGY OF CTC CLUSTERS

In metastasis, some tumor cells at the margins of the primary tumor attain mesenchymal-like phenotypes through the epithelial-to-mesenchymal transition (EMT), which offers motility to tumor cells (Nieto et al., 2016). These mobile tumor cells are able to enter nearby blood vessels and circulate throughout the body, and are therefore called circulating tumor cell (CTC) clusters. Due to coagulation with normal blood cells and genetic modification, fewer than 0.1% of CTC clusters escape from apoptosis and anoikis in the bloodstream (Méhes et al., 2001). According to the 'seed and soil' and 'mechanistic' theories (Fokas et al., 2007; Steeg, 2006), two hypotheses for the metastatic mechanism, CTC clusters that survive during circulation adhere to blood vessel walls and extravasate to distant sites to form secondary tumors. Some metastatic tumor cells go into a dormant state, while others colonize the new site. This depends on the metastatic microenvironment, in which the metastatic cells may have different expression patterns to the primary tumor cells (Cho et al., 2018).

17.3   CLINICAL IMPORTANCE OF CTC CLUSTERS

Effective cancer biomarkers can aid diagnosis, prognosis, and treatment, thereby improving clinical outcomes in cancer patients. Current techniques for monitoring cancer are limited to the assessment of cancer biomarkers in the serum and radiological imaging of tumor tissues. However, owing to the low sensitivity and specificity of these methods, precise techniques for monitoring cancer are still required. In current clinical evaluation, molecular characterization of cancer is typically based on the analysis of tumor cells that are biopsied from the primary tumor. The conventional biopsy is an invasive procedure, and it is sometimes difficult to access tumor sites, particularly if they are located inside the brain or lungs. In addition, repeated invasive biopsy, including bone marrow aspiration, may have a negative impact on patient compliance (Joosse et al., 2015). CTC clusters are promising independent biomarkers for the diagnosis, prognosis, and therapeutic efficacy of cancer (Cabel et al., 2017). In particular, early detection and characterization of CTC clusters are important to determine cancer diagnosis and appropriate treatment. Furthermore, the CTC isolation procedure is minimally invasive and cost-effective. Therefore, isolating and characterizing CTC clusters can be performed sequentially, providing real-time clinical information (Alix-Panabières and Pantel, 2013). Isolation of CTC is difficult owing to their extreme rarity in blood: typically, only 1 or 2 CTC per billion normal blood cells are present in patients with cancer (Hajba and Guttman, 2014). Although CTC isolation techniques have advanced over the course of more than 30 years, precise CTC isolation still remains technically challenging, especially during the early stages of cancer, when CTC clusters are present at extremely low frequencies. Many clinical studies have shown that EMT transition and clonal evolution lead to heterogeneity of surface markers on CTC clusters, and marker expression levels can change dramatically during therapy (Yu et al., 2013; Jordan et al., 2016). Consequently, CTC clusters exhibit highly variable levels of the epithelial marker epithelial cell adhesion molecule (EpCAM), which is the most widely used surface marker for CTC isolation. In addition, many CTC clusters in the bloodstream are masked by normal blood cells or coagulation factors, such as platelets. Thus, the heterogeneous surface markers and normal cells adhering to CTC clusters increase the difficulty of isolation strategies based on immune-affinity methods. Despite these difficulties, further progress in CTC isolation technologies will lead to deeper insight into the characteristics of cancer (Cho et al., 2018).

17.4   ROLE OF MICROFLUIDICS IN CTC CAPTURING

Microfluidic-based devices have had a chief influence on the research area of CTC. Such efforts have been facilitated by the automation of labor-intensive experimental processes involved in isolating and characterizing CTC clusters. As a consequence, the microfluidic field has been attaining pace especially in the supervision of the rare cells (Den Toonder, 2011). Various types of materials ranging from traditional silicon and glass to elastomers have been utilized for manufacturing these devices. The consumption of poly-dimethylsiloxane (PDMS), an elastomer, has made quick prototyping an easy and preferred technique, resulting in extensive applications of microfluidic-based devices for studying CTC clusters (Dong et al., 2013). Their smaller dimensions permit accurate and precise handling of fluid flow in the devices, transforming to superior control over the cells and smaller volumes furthermore require reduced reagents. Subsequent to the early success of utilizing CTC techniques in forecasting patient endurance, many microfluidic-based CTC isolation techniques have been advanced so far using immuno-affinity or physical separation procedures, as they present a better and compact technique with proficient utilization of the resources. Microfluidics for CTC isolation gained popularity with the reporting of the CTC-chip. Over the years, a great number of similar and inventive microfluidic platforms have advanced, each exploiting specific characteristics of the CTCs to isolate them from the blood cells. The different characteristics of CTCs could be biological (including target antigens), or physical (including size, density, and deformity) (Sun et al., 2011; Cho et al., 2018).

17.5   MICROFLUIDICS BASED TECHNIQUES FOR CAPTURING CTC CLUSTERS

17.5.1   LABEL-DEPENDENT TECHNIQUES

Label-dependent methods for positive CTC cluster isolation using epithelial-specific surface markers and negative CTC cluster isolation using leukocyte-specific surface markers are highly specific, allowing for very pure CTC clusters to be obtained from blood. Various types of label-dependent microfluidic-based techniques are classified in Table 17.1.

17.5.1.1   IMMUNOCAPTURE

Immunocapture, the most traditional among label-dependent methods for CTC isolation, is based on binding CTC clusters using cancer-specific antibodies or aptamers (Farokhzad et al., 2004). Positive immunocapture is the most common approach, and employs EpCAM-specific antibodies (Haber and Velculescu, 2014). In some cases, antibodies directed against alternative markers (e.g., prostate-specific membrane antigen [PSMA]), or combinations of antibodies (EpCAM, HER2, and EGFR) are used to isolate CTC clusters (Weissenstein et al., 2012; Lee et al., 2013). Alternatively, negative isolation methodologies focus on enriching CTCs by depleting white blood cells (WBCs) using anti-CD45 antibodies (Paterlini-Brechot and Benali, 2007). The immunocapture methods can be categorized as micropost array, chaotic mixing, meandering microchannel, nanostructure, or nanomaterial based on the structure and/or materials of the microchannel.

17.5.1.2   IMMUNOMAGNETOPHORESIS

Immunomagnetophoresis was one of the first methods to be developed for CTC isolation, and remains one of the most commonly used. In immuno-magnetophoresis, magnetic nano/microparticles bind to CTCs using tumor-specific antibodies or aptamers. Owing to its accuracy and ease of use, this isolation method has become widely adopted over the past decade (Miltenyi et al., 1990).

TABLE 17.1 Classification of Label-Dependent Microfluidics Based Techniques for Capture of CTC Clusters

Technique	Principle	Isolation Marker	Recovery (%)	References
Immuno-capture	Micropost array	EpCAM	82.7	Nagrath et al. (2007)
	Chaotic mixing	EpCAM	91.8	Stott et al. (2010)
	Meandering microchannel	PMSA	90.0	Dharmasiri et al. (2009)
	Nanomaterial mediation	EpCAM	80.0–96.4	Yoon et al. (2013)
	Nanostructures	EpCAM	> 95.0	Wang et al. (2011)
Immuno-magneto-phoresis	Direct capture and screening	EpCAM	90.0	Hoshino et al. (2011)
	Self-assembled magnetic beads	EpCAM	69.5	Autebert et al. (2015)
	Velocity control	EpCAM	> 90.0	Mohamadi et al. (2015)
	Micromixer	CD45	70.0	Luo et al. (2015)
	Current-induced lateral magnetophoresis	EpCAM	94.7	Plouffe et al., 2012
	Magnet-induced lateral magnetophoresis	EpCAM	> 90	Cho et al., 2017
Immuno-fluorescence	Immunostaining and detection	EpCAM and cytokeratin	94.0	Zhao et al. (2013)
Deterministic cell rolling	Cell-surface interaction	P-selectin	76.7	Choi et al. (2012)

17.5.1.3 IMMUNOFLUORESCENCE

Since conventional fluorescence-activated cell sorters (FACS) are limited by their large size and the requirement for trained personnel, microfluidic-based FACS devices have been developed within the past two decades (Zhao et al., 2013; Fu et al., 1999). Microfluidic-based FACS devices consist of a component for the detection of CTCs labeled by tumor-specific fluorescence-conjugated antibodies, as well as a sorting component for the isolation of detected CTCs using an integrated actuator. Once CTC clusters are identified by the immuno-fluorescence detector, the detected CTCs are isolated by the sorting actuator, which may be based on piezoelectric, hydrodynamic gating valve or optical switch modalities (Cho et al., 2010; Chen et al., 2010; Wang et al., 2005).

17.5.1.4   DETERMINISTIC CELL ROLLING

Several studies have taken an interesting approach to CTC isolation based on cellular adhesion with ligands and lateral passive cell rolling, which is called deterministic cell rolling (Choi et al., 2012). Deterministic cell rolling is based on ligand interactions between cells and the microchannel wall; ligand-interactive cells are laterally isolated by slanted ridges on the micro-channel floor, which alter the flow path of cells. However, this method is limited by low throughput due to incomplete cell rolling and the inability to use whole blood because of cell-surface blocking by blood substances (Choi et al., 2014; Karnik et al., 2008).

17.5.2   LABEL-INDEPENDENT TECHNIQUES

The key limitation of label-dependent methods is that they are often unable to capture CTCs with little or no expression of tumor-specific surface markers (Gossett et al., 2010). Conversely, size-based CTC isolation methods take advantage of the fact that CTCs are usually larger than normal blood cells and can, therefore, isolate CTC clusters independently of their surface marker phenotypes (Vona et al., 2000). Various types of label-independent microfluidic-based techniques for the capture of CTC clusters are classified in Table 17.2.

17.5.2.1   MECHANICAL FILTERING

Mechanical filtration is a representative label-free, size-based isolation method for CTCs. The main advantages of mechanical filtration methods are that they are simpler and have higher throughput than label-dependent methods. Furthermore, recent advanced microfabrication technologies can generate highly uniform and precise microstructures in filters, such as pores, pillars, and dams, which can increase cell isolation performance. Mechanical filters can be categorized into four types: microsieve, pillar, weir, and cross-flow (Ji et al., 2008).

TABLE 17.2 Classification of Label-Independent Microfluidics Based Techniques for Capture of CTC Clusters

Technique	Principle	Recovery (%)	References
Mechanical filtering	Microsieve	> 90.0	Hosokawa et al., 2010
	Microsieve (3D bilayer)	86.5	Zheng et al., 2011
	Piller capture array	> 80.0	Tan et al., 2010
	Weir	42.8	Xu et al., 2015
	Cross-flow	90.0	Park et al., 2016
Hydrodynamics	DLD	86.0	Loutherback et al., 2012
	DFF	85.0	Warkiani et al., 2016
	Two-stage DFF	97.2	Kim et al., 2014
	Microfluidic vortex	> 83.0	Sollier et al., 2014
Dielectrophoresis	DEP and FFF	75.0	Gascoyne et al., 2009
Acoustophoresis	Two-stage bulk acoustic wave	90.3	Augustsson et al., 2012
	Tilted-angle surface acoustic wave	84.3	Li et al., 2015
	Two-stage bulk acoustic wave and DEP trapping array	76.2	Antfolk et al., 2017

17.5.2.2   HYDRODYNAMICS

The hydrodynamic method is a size-based isolation approach based on the cell-size-dependent hydrodynamic inertial force during interactions between cells and microscale obstacles in continuous flow. Unlike the mechanical filtering method, this approach makes it easy to integrate subsequent microfluidic steps for the further manipulation of isolated CTCs and downstream analysis. Furthermore, the high flow velocity required to exert sufficient hydrodynamic inertial forces on cells enables high throughput (>10 mL h^{-1}).

17.5.2.3   ELECTROKINETICS

Dielectrophoresis (DEP) is an electrokinetic phenomenon that creates a force on cells when they are exposed to a non-uniform electric field. The magnitude of the DEP force depends on the size and dielectric properties of cells, and tumor cells have the size and dielectric properties that are distinct from normal blood cells. This makes the DEP method an efficient approach for isolating CTCs from the blood. In the early stages of DEP-based cell isolation, a discontinuous CTC isolation method using an interdigitated DEP electrode array was reported (Becker et al., 1995; Gascoyne et al., 1997).

17.5.2.4   ACOUSTOPHORESIS

Acoustophoresis (Laurell et al., 2007) is a cell manipulation method that has many advantages, such as being contact-free, label-free, simple, fast, biocompatible, and easy to integrate with other microfluidic technologies. When cells are exposed to a standing acoustic wave within a microchannel, they are forced toward the minimal acoustic pressure nodes. Because cells experience different magnitudes of the acoustic radiation force depending on their size, density, and compressibility, acoustophoresis has been used to manipulate blood cell subpopulations, viable, and nonviable cells and cancer cells (Dykes et al., 2011; Yang and Soh, 2012; Iranmanesh et al., 2015).

17.5.3   MULTI-STEP CTC ISOLATION METHODS

Although some microfluidic technologies for isolating CTCs based on a single principle have acceptable performance, each principle has inherent drawbacks. Multiple complementary isolation principles can, therefore, be merged and used together (Yan et al., 2017). Most multi-step isolation methods can be divided into pre-enrichment and isolation steps. The pre-enrichment part is usually based on a label-free method that allows for continuous CTC enrichment. As explained in Table 17.3, hydrodynamic approaches, such as DLD, DFF, PFF, mixing, and ensemble-decision aliquot ranking (eDAR), have been used for the pre-enrichment of CTC clusters; all of these methods are label-free. Subsequent isolation can be achieved based on label-dependent or label-independent methods, and isolated CTC clusters can be retrieved in either a continuous or discontinuous manner.

Immuno-magnetophoresis, cross-flow, and DEP have been employed for continuous CTC harvest. For discontinuous CTC capture, immunomagnetophoresis, immunocapture, and microsieve have been used. While immunomagnetophoresis can be applied for either continuous or discontinuous CTC harvest owing to the flexibility of usage for magnetic beads within microchannels, the immunocapture and microsieve methods can be used only for discontinuous CTC capture. Although some multi-step isolation methods achieve high performance, their fabrication process is typically complicated owing to the usage of multiple isolation principles. This is why most multi-step isolation platforms have been developed in a hybrid format instead of as on-chip devices (Liu et al., 2013). Furthermore, the cascaded isolation approach involves a complicated isolation procedure that may decrease the viability of isolated CTCs.

TABLE 17.3 Classification of Microfluidics Based Multi-Step Isolation Techniques for CTC Clusters

Type of Isolation	Pre-Enrichment	Principle	Isolation Marker	Recovery (%)	References
Continuous	DLD	Immuno-magneto-phoresis	EpCAM, CD16, CD45, CD66b	98.6	Ozkumur et al. (2013)
	DFF		EpCAM	93.28	Jack et al. (2016)
	PFF	Cross-flow	–	97.0	Lin et al. (2013)
	MOFF	DEP	–	75.2	Moon et al. (2011)
Discontinuous	Multi-mixing DLD	Immuno-magneto-phoresis	CD45	81.8	Lee et al. (2017)
	Hydrodynamic switching (eDAR)	Immuno-capture	EpCAM	90.6	Liu et al. (2013)
	Negative	Microsieve	EpCAM	90.0	Zhao et al. (2013)
	Immuno-magneto-phoresis	–	CD45	95.0	Gourikutty et al. (2016)

17.6 COMMERCIAL TOOLS FOR ISOLATION OF CTC CLUSTERS

Since the early 2000s, technologies for isolating CTC clusters have been consistently developed, some of which are now commercially available as automated platforms. The benefits of these commercialized technologies, such as their high performance, reproducibility, and ease to use, have been exploited in many cancer-related studies. The commercialized CTC isolation technologies can be classified into microfluidic or macroscale types, as well as label-dependent or label-independent types. Although they exhibit only a moderate level of performance, macroscale technologies have conventionally been used for isolating CTC clusters due to their simplicity, availability, and well-established procedures. However, with increasing emphasis being placed on the performance of CTC isolation, such as the recovery rate, purity, throughput, and viability, advanced microfluidic technologies have been developed and commercialized due to their advantages of outstanding performance, high reproducibility, integrative capacity, low price, and ease of automation. This section provides a brief explanation of commercialized technologies for CTC isolation, along with their characteristics and performance, as summarized in Table 17.4 (Ferreira et al., 2016; Cho et al., 2018).

TABLE 17.4 Summary of Various Commercial Tools for Isolation of CTC Clusters

Principle	Product Name	Company	Recovery (%)
Label-Dependent Tools			
Immuno-magnetophoresis (positive)	IsoFlux	Fluxion Biosciences	73.0
	Liquid Biopsy	Cynvenio Biosystems	78.0
	CellSearch	Menarini-Silicon Biosystems	> 85.0
	Adna Test	QIAGEN	100
	MagSweeper	Stanford University	62.0
	MACS CD326 (EpCAM) MicroBeads	Miltenyi Biotec	75.0
	Dynabeads Epithelial Enrich	ThermoFisher Scientific	64.0–70.0
	EasySep EpCAM	STEMCELL Technologies	25.0

TABLE 17.4 *(Continued)*

Principle	Product Name	Company	Recovery (%)
Immuno-magnetophoresis (negative)	MACS CD45 MicroBeads	Miltenyi Biotec	70.0–88.0
	Dynabeads CD45	ThermoFisher Scientific	87.4
	EasySep CD45 Depletion Kit	STEMCELL Technologies	58.0
	CanPatrol	SurExam BioTech	80.0–88.0
Immunocapture (meandering microchannel)	BioFluidica CTC Detection System	Biofluidica	83.1
Immunocapture (micropost array)	OncoCEE	Biocept	> 70.0
Immunocapture (*in vivo*)	CellCollector	GILUPI	41.0
Immunofluorescence	CytoTrack	CytoTrack	55.0
	CTCScope	ACD	71.0
Functional reaction (CAM assay)	Vita-Assay	Vitatex	50.0
Functional reaction (protein secretion)	EPISPOT	CHU, Montpellier, and UKE, Hamburg	37.0–100
Label-Independent Tools			
Mechanical filtration (weir)	Parsortix	ANGLE	42.0
Mechanical filtration (sieve)	Celsee PREP	Celsee Diagnostics	81.0
	ISET	Rarecells	88.0
	ScreenCell	Screencell	91.2
	CellSieve	CreatvMicroTech	98.0
	SmartBiopsy	CytoGen	86.7
DFF	ClearCell FX System	Clearbridge BioMedics	80.0
Microfluidic vortex	Vortex	Vortex Biosciences	51.0
Dielectrophoresis	ApoStream	ApoCell	69.9
Density gradient	OncoQuick	Greiner Bio-One	55.2
	AccuCyte	RareCyte	90.0

Source: Reproduced from: Cho et al. (2018) with permission from The Royal Society of Chemistry.

17.7   CONCLUSION

In summary, major developments in separation, isolation, and detection techniques of CTCs based on microfluidics were reviewed. These techniques consist of three classes: label-free, a label based, and multi-step isolation. Label-free techniques are, in general, grounded on the physical properties comprising of size, deformability, density, dielectric parameters, and viscosity. Size-based techniques usually suffer from the size overlap between CTC clusters and leukocytes, which has deprived isolation pureness. The clogging difficulties furthermore limit the flow rate and throughput. Label-based techniques are principally grounded on the affinity binding between CTC clusters and ligands. Most of these procedures necessitate pre-enrichment stages to make the sensitivity reach a satisfactory level. The pre-enrichment stages, such as immune-magnetic bead enrichment, will make the procedure of the diagnosis further complicated and upsurge the cost of time and expenditure. The authors are of the belief that the advancement of these inventive microfluidic-based CTC detection techniques will transform the strategy of tumor diagnosis and monitoring of cancer therapy in the forthcoming years.

KEYWORDS

- **capturing**
- **circulating tumor cells**
- **dielectrophoresis**
- **endometrial cancer**
- **isolation**
- **microfluidics**

REFERENCES

Alix-Panabières, C., & Pantel, K., (2013). Circulating tumor cells: Liquid biopsy of cancer. *Clin. Chem., 59*(1), 110–118.

Antfolk, M., Kim, S. H., Koizumi, S., Fujii, T., & Laurell, T., (2017). Label-free single-cell separation and imaging of cancer cells using an integrated microfluidic system. *Sci. Rep., 7*, 46507.

Augustsson, P., Magnusson, C., Nordin, M., Lilja, H., & Laurell, T., (2012). Microfluidic, label-free enrichment of prostate cancer cells in blood based on acoustophoresis. *Anal. Chem., 84*, 7954–7962.

Autebert, J., Coudert, B., Champ, J., Saias, L., Guneri, E. T., Lebofsky, R., Bidard, F. C., et al., (2015). High purity micro fluidic sorting and analysis of circulating tumor cells: Towards routine mutation detection. *Lab Chip, 15*, 2090–2101.

Becker, F. F., Wang, X. B., Huang, Y., Pethig, R., Vykoukal, J., & Gascoyne, P. R. C., (1995). Separation of human breast cancer cells from blood by differential dielectric affinity. *Proc. Natl. Acad. Sci. U.S.A., 92*, 860–864.

Cabel, L., Proudhon, C., Gortais, H., Loirat, D., Coussy, F., Pierga, J. Y., & Bidard, F. C., (2017). Circulating tumor cells: Clinical validity and utility. *Int. J. Clin. Oncol., 22*(3), 421–430.

Cao, J., Zhao, X. P., Younis, M. R., Li, Z. Q., Xia, X. H., & Wang, C., (2017). Ultrasensitive capture, detection, and release of circulating tumor cells using a nanochannel-ion channel hybrid coupled with electrochemical detection technique. *Anal. Chem., 89*, 10957–10964.

Chen, P., Feng, X., Hu, R., Sun, J., Du, W., & Liu, B. F., (2010). Hydrodynamic gating valve for microfluidic fluorescence-activated cell sorting. *Anal. Chim. Acta, 663*, 1–6.

Chiu, T. K., Chao, A. C., Chou, W. P., Liao, C. J., Wang, H. M., Chang, J. H., Chen, P. H., & Wude, M. H., (2018). Optically-induced-dielectrophoresis (ODEP)-based cell manipulation in a microfluidic system for high-purity isolation of integral circulating tumor cell (CTC) clusters based on their size characteristics. *Sens. Actuators B Chem., 258*, 1161–1173.

Cho, H., Kim, J., Jeon, C. W., & Han, K. H., (2017). A disposable microfluidic device with a reusable magnetophoretic functional substrate for isolation of circulating tumor cells. *Lab Chip, 17*, 4113–4123.

Cho, H., Kim, J., Song, H., Sohn, K. Y., Jeon, M., & Han, K. H., (2018). Microfluidic technologies for circulating tumor cell isolation. *Analyst, 143*(13), 2936–2970.

Cho, S. H., Chen, C. H., Tsai, F. S., Godin, J. M., & Lo, Y. H., (2010). Human mammalian cell sorting using a highly integrated micro-fabricated fluorescence-activated cell sorter (μFACS). *Lab Chip, 10*, 1567–1573.

Choi, S., Karp, J. M., & Karnik, R., (2012). Cell sorting by deterministic cell rolling. *Lab Chip, 12*, 1427–1430.

Choi, S., Levy, O., Coelho, M. B., Cabral, J. M., Karp, J. M., & Karnik, R., (2014). A cell rolling cytometer reveals the correlation between mesenchymal stem cell dynamic adhesion and differentiation state. *Lab Chip, 14*, 161–166.

Den, T. J., (2011). Circulating tumor cells: The grand challenge. *Lab Chip, 11*(3), 375–377.

Dharmasiri, U., Balamurugan, S., Adams, A. A., Okagbare, P. I., Obubuafo, A., & Soper, S. A., (2009). Highly efficient capture and enumeration of low abundance prostate cancer cells using prostate-specific membrane antigen aptamers immobilized to a polymeric micro fluidic device. *Electrophoresis, 30*, 3289–3300.

Dong, Y., Skelley, A. M., Merdek, K. D., Sprott, K. M., Jiang, C., Pierceall, W. E., Lin, J., et al., (2013). Microfluidics and circulating tumor cells. *J. Mol. Diagn., 15*(2), 149–157.

Dykes, J., Lenshof, A., Astrand-Grundstrom, I. B., Laurell, T., & Scheding, S., (2011). Efficient removal of platelets from peripheral blood progenitor cell products using a novel micro-chip based acoustophoretic platform. *PLoS One, 6*, e23074.

Farokhzad, O. C., Jon, S., Khademhosseini, A., Tran, T. N., Lavan, D. A., & Langer, R., (2004). Nanoparticle-aptamer bioconjugates: A new approach for targeting prostate cancer cells. *Cancer Res., 64*, 7668–7672.

Ferreira, M. M., Ramani, V. C., & Jeffrey, S. S., (2016). Circulating tumor cell technologies. *Mol. Oncol., 10*, 374–394.

Fokas, E., Engenhart-Cabillic, R., Daniilidis, K., Rose, F., & An, H. X., (2007). Metastasis: The seed and soil theory gains identity. *Cancer Metastasis Rev., 26*(3/4), 705–715.

Fu, Y., Spence, C., Scherer, A., Arnold, F. H., & Quake, S. R., (1999). A microfabricated fluorescence-activated cell sorter. *Nat. Biotechnol., 17*, 1109–1111.

Gascoyne, P. R., Noshari, J., Anderson, T. J., & Becker, F. F., (2009). Isolation of rare cells from cell mixtures by dielectrophoresis. *Electrophoresis, 30*, 1388–1398.

Gascoyne, P. R., Wang, X. B., Huang, Y., & Becker, F. F., (1997). Dielectrophoretic separation of cancer cells from blood. *IEEE Trans. Ind. Appl., 33*, 670–678.

Gossett, D. R., Weaver, W. M., Mach, A. J., Hur, S. C., Tse, H. T., Lee, W., Amini, H., & Di Carlo, D., (2010). Label-free cell separation and sorting in micro fluidic systems. *Anal. Bioanal. Chem., 397*, 3249–3267.

Gourikutty, S. B. N., Chang, C. P., & Poenar, D. P., (2016). An integrated on-chip platform for negative enrichment of tumor cells. *J. Chromatogr. B: Anal. Technol. Biomed. Life Sci., 1028*, 153–164.

Haber, D. A., & Velculescu, V. E., (2014). Blood-based analyses of cancer: Circulating tumor cells and circulating tumor DNA. *Cancer Discov., 4*, 650–661.

Hajba, L., & Guttman, A., (2014). Circulating tumor-cell detection and capture using micro fluidic devices. *Trends Anal. Chem., 59*, 9–16.

Hoshino, K., Huang, Y. Y., Lane, N., Huebschman, M., Uhr, J. W., Frenkel, E. P., & Zhang, X., (2011). Microchip-based immunomagnetic detection of circulating tumor cells. *Lab Chip, 11*, 3449–3457.

Hosokawa, M., Hayata, T., Fukuda, Y., Arakaki, A., Yoshino, T., Tanaka, T., & Matsunaga, T., (2010). Size-selective micro cavity array for rapid and efficient detection of circulating tumor cells. *Anal. Chem., 82*, 6629–6635.

Hyun, K. A., & Jung, H., (2014). Advances and critical concerns with the microfluidic enrichments of circulating tumor cells. *Lab Chip, 14*(1), 45–56.

Iranmanesh, Ramachandraiah, H., Russom, A., & Wiklund, M., (2015). On-chip ultrasonic sample preparation for cell based assays. *RSC Adv., 5*, 74304.

Jack, R. M., Grafton, M. M., Rodrigues, D., Giraldez, M. D., Griffith, C., Cieslak, R., Zeinali, M., et al., (2016). Ultra-specific isolation of circulating tumor cells enables rare-cell RNA profiling. *Adv. Sci., 3*, 1600063.

Ji, H. M., Samper, V., Chen, Y., Heng, C. K., Lim, T. M., & Yobas, L., (2008). Silicon-based microfilters for whole blood cell separation. *Biomed. Micro Devices, 10*, 251–257.

Joosse, S. A., Gorges, T. M., & Pantel, K., (2015). Biology, detection, and clinical implications of circulating tumor cells. *EMBO Mol. Med., 7*(1), 1–11.

Jordan, N. V., Bardia, A., Wittner, B. S., Benes, C., Ligorio, M., Zheng, Y., Yu, M., et al., (2016). HER2 expression identifies dynamic functional states within circulating breast cancer cells. *Nature, 537*(7618), 102–106.

Karnik, R., Hong, S., Zhang, H., Mei, Y., Anderson, D. G., Karp, J. M., & Langer, R., (2008). Nanomechanical control of cell rolling in two dimensions through surface patterning of receptors. *Nano Lett., 8*, 1153–1158.

Kim, T. H., Yoon, H. J., Stella, P., & Nagrath, S., (2014). Cascaded spiral microfluidic device for deterministic and high purity continuous separation of circulating tumor cells. *Biomicrofluidics, 8*, 064117.

Laurell, T., Petersson, F., & Nilsson, A., (2007). Chip integrated strategies for acoustic separation and manipulation of cells and particles. *Chem. Soc. Rev., 36*, 492–506.

Lee, H. J., Cho, H. Y., Oh, J. H., Namkoong, K., Lee, J. G., Park, J. M., Lee, S. S., et al., (2013). Simultaneous capture and in situ analysis of circulating tumor cells using multiple hybrid nanoparticles. *Biosens. Bioelectron., 47*, 508–514.

Lee, T. Y., Hyun, K. A., Kim, S. I., & Jung, H. I., (2017). An integrated microfluidic chip for one-step isolation of circulating tumor cells. *Sens. Actuators B Chem., 238*, 1144–1150.

Li, P., Mao, Z., Peng, Z., Zhou, L., Chen, Y., Huang, P. H., Truica, C. I., et al., (2015). Acoustic separation of circulating tumor cells. *Proc. Natl. Acad. Sci. U. S. A., 112*, 4970–4975.

Lin, B. K., McFaul, S. M., Jin, C., Black, P. C., & Ma, H., (2013). Highly selective biomechanical separation of cancer cells from leukocytes using micro fluidic ratchets and hydrodynamic concentrator. *Biomicrofluidics, 7*, 34114.

Liu, Z., Zhang, W., Huang, F., Feng, H., Shu, W., Xu, X., & Chen, Y., (2013). High throughput capture of circulating tumor cells using an integrated micro fluidic system. *Biosens. Bioelectron., 47*, 113–119.

Loutherback, K., D'Silva, J., Liu, L., Wu, A., Austin, R. H., & Sturm, J. C., (2012). Deterministic separation of cancer cells from blood at 10 mL/min. *AIP Adv., 2*, 42107.

Luo, W. Y., Tsai, S. C., Hsieh, K., & Lee, G. B., (2015). An integrated micro fluidic platform for negative selection and enrichment of cancer cells. *J. Micromech. Microeng., 25*, 084007.

Méhes, G., Witt, A., Kubista, E., & Ambros, P. F., (2001). Circulating breast cancer cells are frequently apoptotic. *Am. J. Pathol., 159*(1), 17–20.

Miltenyi, S., Muller, W., Weichel, W., & Radbruch, A., (1990). High gradient magnetic cell separation with MACS. *Cytometry, 11*, 231–238.

Mohamadi, R. M., Besant, J. D., Mepham, A., Green, B., Mahmoudian, L., Gibbs, T., Ivanov, I., et al., (2015). Nanoparticle-mediated binning and profiling of heterogeneous circulating tumor cell subpopulations. *Angew. Chem. Int. Ed. Engl., 54*, 139–143.

Moon, H. S., Kwon, K., Kim, S. I., Han, H., Sohn, J., Lee, S., & Jung, H. I., (2011). Isolating and concentrating rare cancerous cells in large sample volumes of blood by using dielectrophoresis and stepping electric fields. *Lab Chip, 11*, 1118–1125.

Nagrath, S., Sequist, L. V., Maheswaran, S., Bell, D. W., Irimia, D., Ulkus, L., Smith, M. R., et al., (2007). Isolation of rare circulating tumor cells in cancer patients by microchip technology. *Nature, 450*, 1235–1239.

Nieto, M. A., Huang, R. Y., Jackson, R. A., & Thiery, J. P., (2016). EMT: 2016. *Cell, 166*(1), 21–45.

Ozkumur, E., Shah, A. M., Ciciliano, J. C., Emmink, B. L., Miyamoto, D. T., Brachtel, E., Yu, M., et al., (2013). Inertial focusing for tumor antigen-dependent and-independent sorting of rare circulating tumor cells. *Sci. Transl. Med., 5*, 179–147.

Park, E. S., Jin, C., Guo, Q., Ang, R. R., Duffy, S. P., Matthews, K., Azad, A., et al., (2016). Continuous flow deformability-based separation of circulating tumor cells using micro fluidic ratchets. *Small, 12*, 1909–1919.

Paterlini-Brechot, P., & Benali, N. L., (2007). Circulating tumor cells (CTC) detection: Clinical impact and future directions. *Cancer Lett., 253*, 180–204.

Plouffe, B. D., Mahalanabis, M., Lewis, L. H., Klapperich, C. M., & Murthy, S. K., (2012). Clinically relevant microfluidic magnetophoretic isolation of rare-cell populations for diagnostic and therapeutic monitoring applications. *Anal. Chem., 84*, 1336–1344.

Sollier, E., Go, D. E., Che, J., Gossett, D. R., O'Byrne, S., Weaver, W. M., Kummer, N., et al., (2014). Size-selective collection of circulating tumor cells using Vortex technology. *Lab Chip, 14*, 63–77.

Stott, S. L., Hsu, C. H., Tsukrov, D. I., Yu, M., Miyamoto, D. T., Waltman, B. A., Rothenberg, S. M., et al., (2010). Isolation of circulating tumor cells using a microvortex-generating herringbone-chip. *Proc. Natl. Acad. Sci. U.S.A., 107*, 18392–18397.

Sun, Y. F., Yang, X. R., Zhou, J., Qiu, S. J., Fan, J., & Xu, Y., (2011). Circulating tumor cells: Advances in detection methods, biological issues, and clinical relevance. *J. Cancer Res. Clin. Oncol., 137*(8), 1151–1173.

Tan, S. J., Lakshmi, R. L., Chen, P., Lim, W. T., Yobas, L., & Lim, C. T., (2010). Versatile label free biochip for the detection of circulating tumor cells from peripheral blood in cancer patients. *Biosens. Bioelectron., 26*, 1701–1705.

Vona, G., Sabile, A., Louha, M., Sitruk, V., Romana, S., Schütze, K., Capron, F., et al., (2000). Isolation by size of epithelial tumor cells: A new method for the immunomorphological and molecular characterization of circulating tumor cells. *Am. J. Pathol., 156*, 57–63.

Wang, M. M., Tu, E., Raymond, D. E., Yang, J. M., Zhang, H., Hagen, N., Dees, B., et al., (2005). Butler, micro fluidic sorting of mammalian cells by optical force switching. *Nat. Biotechnol., 23*, 83–87.

Wang, S., Liu, K., Liu, J., Yu, Z. T., Xu, X., Zhao, L., Lee, T., et al., (2011). Highly efficient capture of circulating tumor cells by using nanostructured silicon substrates with integrated chaotic micro mixers. *Angew. Chem. Int. Ed. Engl., 50*, 3084–3088.

Warkiani, M. E., Khoo, B. L., Wu, L., Tay, A. K., Bhagat, A. A., Han, J., & Lim, C. T., (2016). Ultra-fast, label-free isolation of circulating tumor cells from blood using spiral microfluidics. *Nat. Protoc., 11*, 134–148.

Weissenstein, U., Schumann, A., Reif, M., Link, S., Toffol-Schmidt, U. D., & Heusser, P., (2012). Detection of circulating tumor cells in blood of metastatic breast cancer patients using a combination of cytokeratin and EpCAM antibodies. *BMC Cancer, 12*, 206.

Xu, L., Mao, X., Imrali, A., Syed, F., Mutsvangwa, K., Berney, D., Cathcart, P. J., et al., (2015). Optimization and evaluation of a novel size based circulating tumor cell isolation system. *PLoS One, 10*, e0138032.

Yan, S., Zhang, J., Yuan, D., & Li, W., (2017). Hybrid microfluidics combined with active and passive approaches for continuous cell separation. *Electrophoresis, 38*, 238–249.

Yang, A. H., & Soh, H. T., (2012). Acoustophoretic sorting of viable mammalian cells in a micro fluidic device. *Anal. Chem., 84*, 10756–10762.

Yoon, H. J., Kim, T. H., Zhang, Z., Azizi, E., Pham, T. M., Paoletti, C., Lin, J., et al., (2013). Sensitive capture of circulating tumor cells by functionalized graphene oxide nanosheets. *Nat. Nanotechnol., 8*, 735–741.

Yu, M., Bardia, A., Wittner, B. S., Stott, S. L., Smas, M. E., Ting, D. T., Isakoff, S. J., et al., (2013). Circulating breast tumor cells exhibit dynamic changes in epithelial and mesenchymal composition. *Science, 339*(6119), 580–584.

Zhao, M., Nelson, W. C., Wei, B., Schiro, P. G., Hakimi, B. M., Johnson, E. S., Anand, R. K., et al., (2013). New generation of ensemble-decision, aliquot ranking based on simplified microfluidic components for large-capacity trapping of circulating tumor cells. *Anal. Chem., 85*, 9671–9677.

Zhao, M., Schiro, P. G., Kuo, J. S., Koehler, K. M., Sabath, D. E., Popov, V., Feng, Q., & Chiu, D. T., (2013). An automated high-throughput counting method for screening circulating tumor cells in peripheral blood. *Anal. Chem., 85*, 2465–2471.

Metastatic Diseases

Zheng, S., Lin, H. K., Lu, B., Williams, A., Datar, R., Cote, R. J., & Tai, Y. C., (2011). 3D micro filter device for viable circulating tumor cell (CTC) enrichment from blood. *Biomed. Micro Devices, 13*, 203–213.
Zou, D., & Cui, D., (2018). Advances in isolation and detection of circulating tumor cells based on microfluidics. *Cancer Biol. Med., 15*(4), 335–353.

Index

For Product Safety Concerns and Information please contact our EU
representative GPSR@taylorandfrancis.com
Taylor & Francis Verlag GmbH, Kaufingerstraße 24, 80331 München, Germany